Anaesthesia: Review 12

Contents of *Anaesthesia: Review 11*

Edited by Leon Kaufman and Robert Ginsburg

ISBN 0443 050155

You can place your order by contacting your local medical bookseller or the Sales Promotion Department, Churchill Livingstone, Robert Stevenson House, 1–3 Baxter's Place, Leith Walk, Edinburgh EH1 3AF, UK Tel: (0131) 556 2424; Telex: 727511 LONGMN G; Fax (0131) 558 1278

Look out for *Anaesthesia Review* 13 in September 1996

Anaesthesia:
Review 12

Edited by

Leon Kaufman MD FRCA

Consulting Anaesthetist, University College Hospital, and St Mark's Hospital, London;
Honorary Senior Lecturer, Faculty of Clinical Sciences, University College, London, UK

Robert Ginsburg MB BS BSc FRCA

Consultant Anaesthetist, King's College Hospital, London, UK

CHURCHILL LIVINGSTONE
EDINBURGH LONDON MADRID MELBOURNE NEW YORK SAN FRANCISCO
AND TOKYO 1995

CHURCHILL LIVINGSTONE
Medical Division of Pearson Professional Ltd

Distributed in the United States of America by
Churchill Livingstone Inc., 650 Avenue of the Americas, New York,
N.Y. 10011, and by associated companies, branches and
representatives throughout the world.

First published 1995

ISBN 0 443 052425
ISSN 0263-1512

British Library Cataloguing in Publication Data
A catalogue record for this book is available from the British Library

Library of Congress Cataloging in Publication Data
is available

Produced by Longman Publishers Singapore Pte Ltd
Printed in Singapore

Contributors

T. M. Akthar BSc MB BS FFARCS(Ire)
Senior Registrar in Anaesthetics, Brook Hospital, London, UK

Tom Durcan MB BS FRCA
King's College Hospital, London, UK

Roger Fletcher MD FRCA
Department of Anaesthesia, Manchester Royal Infirmary, Manchester, UK
(formerly Department of Anaesthesia, University Hospital, Lund, Sweden)

David J. Gerrard FRCS
Research Fellow, Thrombosis Research Institute, King's College School of
Medicine and Dentistry, London, UK

John C Goldstone MD FRCA
Senior Lecturer, Academic Department of Anaesthesia, The Middlesex Hospital,
London, UK

Robert Ginsburg MB BS BSc FRCA
Consultant Anaesthetist, King's College Hospital, London, UK

Nicholas Harper MB BS FRCA
Basildon Hospital, Basildon, UK

Stephen P Hunt PhD
Senior Scientist, Division of Neurobiology, Laboratory of Molecular Biology,
MRC Centre, Cambridge, UK

J. Gareth Jones MD FRCP FRCA
Professor of Anaesthsia, University Department of Anaesthesia, University of
Cambridge Clinical School, Addenbrookes Hospital, Cambridge, UK

P. I. E. Jones FRCA
Consultant Anaesthetist, King's College Hospital, London, UK

Leon Kaufman MD FRCA
Consulting Anaesthetist, University College Hospital and St Mark's Hospital,
London; Honorary Senior Lecturer, Faculty of Clinical Sciences, University
College, London, UK

G. N. C. Kenny BSc MD FRCA
Senior Lecturer, University Department of Anaesthesia, Royal Infirmary, Glasgow, UK

Adrian R. Lloyd-Thomas MB FRCA
Consultant Paediatric Anaesthetist, Great Ormond Street Hospital for Children NHS Trust, London UK

A. T. Lovell BSc MB BS FRCA
Welcome Training Fellow, Academic Department of Anaesthesia, The Middlesex Hospital, London, UK

Rajesh Munglani MB BS DCH FRCA
Clinical Lecturer, University Department of Anaesthesia, University of Cambridge Clinical School, Addenbrookes Hospital, Cambridge, UK

Tim Nash MB BS FRCA DDBS RCOG
Consultant in Pain Management, The Walton Centre for Neurology and Neurosurgery, Liverpool, UK

Geraldine O'Sullivan FRCA
Consultant Anaesthetist, St Thomas' Hospital, London, UK

Graham J. Philpott MB BS FRCA
King's College Hospital, London, UK

C. S. Reilly MD FRCA
Head of Anaesthesia, Department of Surgical and Anaesthetic Sciences, Royal Hallamshire Hospital, Sheffield, UK

Lindsey T. A. Rylah MB BS MRCS MRCP FRCA
Consultant Anaesthetist, Basildon Hospital, Basildon, UK

John A. Skinner FRCS
Research Fellow, Thrombosis Research Institute, King's College School of Medicine and Dentistry, London, UK

N. P. Sutcliffe BSc MB ChB MRCP FRCA
Consultant Anaesthetist, Health Care International, Clydebank, UK

D. N. Tew BSc FRCA
Consultant in Anaesthesia and Intensive Care, Princess Margaret Hospital, Swindon, UK

Contents

Medicine relevant to anaesthesia

L. Kaufman

CARDIOVASCULAR

Assessment of perioperative cardiac risk

Goldman et al (1977) was one of the first physicians to analyse the cardiac risk factors in patients undergoing non-cardiac surgical operations. Since then there have been many other indices proposed (Detsky et al 1986, Clements et al 1991, Gold et al 1992, Charlson et al 1991, Seegobin et al 1991). Unfortunately anaesthetists have to rely on investigations performed by cardiologists who have access to modern equipment as a basis for their own assessment.

There are still many articles in the literature on this subject, suggesting that assessment of cardiac risk is unsatisfactory and even unpredictable. Dipyridamole thallium scintigraphy has been advocated by Boucher et al (1985), but Baron et al (1994) found that definite clinical evidence of coronary artery disease and age (greater than 65) were more important in predicting outcome of abdominoaortic surgery than invasive angiography.

Adams et al (1994) found that cardiac troponin I was a more sensitive and specific market of pericardial myocardial infarction than MB creatine kinase. Cardiac troponin I is a protein which is not found in skeletal muscle and hence does not result in increased levels in patients with acute or chronic skeletal muscle disorders. It has a high specificity for cardiac injury. Goldman (1994) has reviewed perioperative cardiac risk in view of these findings, noting that 50–75% of patients undergo expensive non-invasive cardiac tests, and it was felt that these should be restricted to patients who have some evidence of obvious cardiac disease. In these circumstances, if repeat testing is still positive the medical management is intensified and patients are referred for coronary arteriography and coronary bypass surgery. Goldman (1994) does not advocate the routine measurement of cardiac troponin I in all patients undergoing major non-cardiac surgery, but the test should be limited to those who are clearly at risk (see also review by Edwards & Reilly 1994). For advances in nuclear cardiology (see Zaret & Wackers 1993a, 1993b).

Myocardial infarction

Heavy physical exercise can promote the onset of acute myocardial infarction, especially in those who are unaccustomed to heavy physical exertion (Mittleman et al 1993), while regular physical exercise decreases the incidence of myocardial infarction (Willich et al 1993).

It has been suspected that brief periods of myocardial ischaemia might be cumulative, leading to infarction, but in fact the opposite appears to be the case. A brief period of coronary ischaemia, of as little as 3 min, followed by a period of 1 min reperfusion reduces the risk of myocardial necrosis (Marber et al 1994). Not to be forgotten on its own is right ventricular infarction, which accounts for nearly half of all inferior myocardial infarctions (Kinch & Ryan 1994).

Myocardial infarction may be reflected in increased levels of angiotensin-converting enzyme (ACE), which can lead to coronary vasoconstriction and growth of the smooth muscle in blood vessels or the development of atheroma (Espiner 1993). Following coronary angioplasty for acute myocardial infarction there is an increased level of free radicals (Grech et al 1993) and also serotonin (5-HT), which can lead to vasoconstriction distal to the area that has been dilated (Golino et al 1994). For details of coronary angioplasty see Landau et al (1994). Kellow (1994) has reviewed the renin–angiotensin system and ACE inhibitors in relationship to anaesthesia and the main problems appear to be hypotension and bradycardia. No further advice is offered regarding the use of spinal epidural anaesthesia and ideally the vasopressor of choice would be angiotensin II.

Another factor which may result in coronary insufficiency is that some patients appear to be dependent on nitric oxide (endothelium-derived relaxing factor, EDRF) to maintain coronary vasodilation and there may be some patients who have a deficiency of this vasodilator (Egashira et al 1993). Interestingly enough the vasodilator action of nitroglycerine and sodium nitroprusside is due to their conversion to nitric oxide. The hypotension in septic shock has been ascribed to excessive release of nitric oxide leading to vasodilatation, resistant to vasoconstrictors (Moncada & Higgs 1993). There are three isoforms of nitric oxide synthase, one of which is inducible (macrophage type). The inducible type is increased in response to cytokines or endotoxin as part of the inflammatory response and nitric oxide synthesis is increased in patients with septic shock. Selective inhibitors of the inducible isoform of nitric oxide synthase are being developed with the intention of treating the resistant vasodilatation (see Vallance & Collier 1994).

There is also the possibility that inhalation of nitric oxide may be of value in the treatment of pulmonary hypertension (Royston 1993).

The endothelins are a group of peptides which are released from endothelial cells causing cardiovascular and renal vasconstriction. They are extremely potent with a prolonged action and can also act directly on cardiac muscle. They also raise the level of atrial natriuretic peptide (ANP), which is a vasodilator.

Endothelin 1 prevents the release of renin, but stimulates the release of angiotensin II and aldosterone (Remuzzi & Benigni 1993).

Although elevation of the ST segment is a common abnormality in patients with myocardial infarction it is not a sensitive indicator for predicting the diagnosis of acute myocardial infarction (Adams et al 1993). Ten to twenty per cent of patients undergoing cardiac catheterization for angina-like chest pains have normal coronary angiograms (Editorial 1993a).

Guidelines for the early management of patients with myocardial infarction have been outlined by Weston et al (1994) and delay is one of the factors affecting outcome. Patients with obvious acute myocardial infarction should receive thrombolytic treatment within 90 min. Treatment involves the use of oxygen, aspirin, nitrates and adequate analgesia such as diamorphine, given with an antiemetic. Other drugs which might be required include adrenaline, atropine, lignocaine, frusemide and naloxone. Others have advocated the used of thrombolytic agents such as streptokinase, and reduction in mortality appears to be improved on treatment with thrombolysis together with aspirin (Anderson & Willerson 1993). For details on new plasminogen activators see Collen (1993) and for mechanism of action of aspirin see Patrono (1994).

Cardiomyopathy

Cardiac myopathies may be secondary to immune disorders, to infection, or may be inherited (Lange & Schreiner 1994, Kelly & Strauss 1994). β-Adrenergic blocking agents have been known to be of value in idiopathic dilated cardiomyopathy and the treatment of choice now appears to be with metoprolol, which improves symptoms and cardiac function and prevents clinical deterioration (Waagstein et al 1993).

Calcium channel blockers

Kenny (1994) has reviewed the dangers of overdose with calcium channel blockers and these result in vasodilatation, reduction in myocardial contractility and a depression of conduction at the sinoatrial and atrioventricular nodes. Patients become drowsy and confused and even comatose. There may be nausea and vomiting, hyperglycaemia due to reduction in the release of insulin and lactic acidosis due to poor tissue perfusion. Hypotension is a common feature. On electrocardiogram there may be sinus bradycardia, second- and third-degree heart block and even asystole. Treatment consists of gastric lavage, administration of activated charcoal, while hypotension may respond to intravenous fluids and intravenous calcium. Glucagon has been advocated as well as vasopressors such as isoprenaline, dopamine, dobutamine or noradrenaline. Bradycardia may respond to atropine or isoprenaline. A temporary pacemaker may be necessary. Pulmonary oedema may require treatment with diuretics or with mechanical ventilation.

Cardiac arrhythmias

The pathophysiology of ventricular tachycardia has been reviewed by Shenasa et al (1993), but the efficacy of treatment has only recently been evaluated by Mason et al (1993). They studied effects of imipramine, mexiletine, pirmenol, procainamide, propafenone, quinidine and sotalol and found that sotalol was more effective than all the other drugs in preventing recurrence of ventricular arrhythmias and reducing the mortality.

Cardiac surgery

There is still concern regarding neurological outcome following cardiac surgery. Newburger et al (1993) found that total circulatory arrest with deep hypothermia during open heart surgery in infants resulted in greater neurological disturbance than the use of low-flow cardiopulmonary bypass. In adults nuclear magnetic resonance (NMR) imaging of the brain revealed brain swelling in the immediate postoperative period (Harris et al 1993). Brain swelling may be due to microemboli, hypoperfusion or haemodilution. Coronary artery bypass surgery can still result in permanent neurophysiological deficiencies and there is a 2% incidence of stroke. Neurological damage includes confusion, memory loss, behavioural change as well as gross neurological deficits. Swain (1993) has reviewed the mechanisms of neurological damage. These may be due to emboli, alterations in blood flow, or drugs.

Baroreflex failure

The failure of the baroreflex has been reviewed by Manger (1993) in which there is lability of blood pressure, systolic and diastolic hypertension, tachycardia alternating with hypotension and bradycardia. Diagnosis may be confused with syncope, hyperthyroidism and phaeochromocytoma, but the condition appears to be related to damage to the glossopharyngeal and vagal nerves. The disorder is difficult to treat and although phenoxy-benzamine and methyldopa have been advocated to control the hypertension, clonidine apparently appears to be the most successful remedy. Robertson et al (1993), however, found that clonidine reduced the frequency of attacks but led to an increase in blood pressure and heart rate. Phentolamine, and nitroprusside, have also been advocated to control the hypertension.

Syncope

Fainting or neurocardiogenic shock has a much more favourable outcome than hypotension due to underlying cardiac disease. Syncope results from reduction in sympathetic activity. When a syncopal subject assumes the upright position there is increased parasympathetic activity and a reduction in plasma noradrenaline levels. Transient sinus cardiac arrest may ensue. In some instances there may be bradycardia, but with increased levels of adrenaline. Serotonia (5-HT) and an endogenous nitric oxide may also be implicated (Abboud 1993). Dickinson (1993) suggests that there may be 'collapse-firing' of venous baroreceptors. Sra et al (1993) found that artificial cardiac pacing was less effective than drug therapy in preventing syncope.

Patients with orthostatic hypotension associated with autonomic neuropathy and decreased red cell mass readily respond to erythropoietin, which increased the red cell volume (Hoeldtke & Streeten 1993).

Cardiac arrest

Cohen et al (1993) has assessed the value of active compression–decompression cardiac resuscitation in which passive relaxation in cardiopulmonary resuscitation (CPR) is converted into an active procedure by the use of a suction device which is hand-held (Ambu CardioPump). They found that active compression–decompression was more successful than standard resuscitation, with a survival rate at 24 h and neurological outcome better than standard CPR. Murphy et al (1994) have studied the views of elderly patients in relationship to CPR and found that most of them did not wish to be resuscitated when the consequences of survival had been explained to them. On the other hand Morgan et al (1994) found that some patients with carcinomatosis did wish to be resuscitated even though the medical attendants had issued 'do not resuscitate' orders. Hill et al (1994) found that few doctors in fact consulted patients to seek their views on resuscitation, and in their survey patients wished to discuss this with their doctors; in fact in the older age group their decision conflicted with that of the medical attendant. Doyal & Wilsher (1994) argued that competent elderly patients have a legal and moral right to decide whether to receive resuscitation or not.

There is discussion on whether relatives should be allowed to witness resuscitation and some feel this should not be discouraged (Whitlock 1994, Baskett 1994). Higgs (1994) felt that relatives' wishes should be accommodated in view of the fact that resuscitation is seen regularly on television, whereas Bloomfield (1994), who is a cardiologist, felt that it was less distressing for relatives if they were asked to leave the scene of resuscitation. Ambulance staff were often involved in resuscitation in the presence of relatives who found the experience terrifying.

The assessment of prognosis of patients who are still comatose following cardiac arrest has been outlined by Edgren et al (1994), who discuss the value of Glasgow and Glasgow-Pittsburgh coma scales. After 72 h it was shown that an absence of motor response to painful stimuli was prognostic of a poor outcome (see also Saltuari & Marosi 1994).

It is worth remembering that approximately 50% of patients who have been resuscitated have permanent neurological damage and the disability to be such that it might be considered to be worse than not surviving (Jaffe & Landau 1993).

The problems of the persistent vegetative state (PVS) have been discussed in detail by the Multi-Society Task Force on PVS (1994a, 1994b).

RESPIRATION

Asthma

Asthma may be induced by exercise, but inhalation of heparin appears to prevent this without affecting the release of histamine (Ahmed et al 1993). Colds and viral infections affecting the respiratory tract often increase symptoms and reduce peak flow (Nicholson et al 1993).

Partridge (1994) has outlined guidelines for self-management in asthmatic patients and it is interesting that many patients are unhappy with advice given on the use of a peak flow meter. These may not necessarily be strictly accurate, especially in children (Sly et al 1994). There is little information about long-term outcome of asthmatics, but Barnes (1993) has suggested that the early treatment with inhaled steroids results in better long-term management. A synthetic trifluoninated glucocorticoid, fluticasone propionate, has been advocated, but apparently it appears to be no better than conventional low-dose beclomethasone or budesonide (*Drug and Therapeutics Bulletin* 1994). Prolonged inhalation of β-agonists such as salbutamol lead to tolerance and increase the sensitivity of the bronchial tract to inhaled allergins (Cockcroft et al 1993, Britton 1993). Nitric oxide can be detected in the expiratory gases of normal subjects and it is produced in inflammatory and epithelial cells of the lower respiratory tract. The levels are significantly higher in asthmatic patients and these can be reduced by treatment with inhaled steriods. Measurement of exhaled nitric oxide may be a useful measure of efficacy of treatment (Kharitonov et al 1994).

Acute respiratory distress syndrome (ARDS)

Beale et al (1993) have reviewed ARDS and suggest that a better term is acute lung injury. There is still a mortality of 60% and the term ARDS should only apply to the more severe forms of respiratory failure. ARDS itself involves not only the lungs, but is a systemic disease involving tissue injury such as occurs in severe sepsis. Multiple organ failure involving the kidney and lungs has also been discussed by McClelland et al (1993) in which they attempt to develop a risk prediction system. Aerosolized prostacyclin (PGI_2) decreased the pulmonary hypertension, presumably by vasodilatation (Walmrath et al 1993). The place of extracorporeal gas exchange still remains to be determined (Sim & Evans 1993).

Steltzer et al (1994) have studied oxygen delivery and oxygen uptake in critically ill patients and found that increasing oxygen delivery and consumption did not result in an increase in survival rate, particularly in patients with ARDS and sepsis.

Dyspnoea

Patients with advanced cancer often suffer from dyspnoea. It is often a predictor of the life expectancy for carcinoma of the pancreas. Even without obvious causes of dyspnoea such as ascites and anaemia, dyspnoea appears to be associated with hypoxaemia, but the cause is unknown. Walsh (1993) advocated the use of small doses of chlorpromazine, while Bruera et al (1993)' found that inhalation of oxygen improved dyspnoea even at rest. It is sometimes difficult to determine whether dyspnoea is of cardiac or pulmonary origin and Davis et al (1994) found that plasma brain natriuretic peptide (BNP) was raised in patients with heart failure, but not in the dyspnoea associated with primarily lung disorders.

Sleep apnoeic syndrome

Continuous positive airway pressure (CPAP) is recommended for sleep apnoeic syndrome. Engleman et al (1994) found there was a low acceptance rate about using the equipment at night, the average time being only just over 3 h. It did in fact improve daytime cognitive function.

Mechanical ventilation

This has been reviewed in detail by Tobin (1994) and he draws attention to the fact that there are dangers of high-inspired oxygen tension and the possible hazards of the use of tidal volumes based on 10–15 ml/kg, which appears to produce damage to the basement membrane of the lung. Lung injury increases markedly when the plateau pressure is high and he advocates reducing the tidal volume to 5–7 ml/kg, with plateau pressure not higher than 35 cmH$_2$O. This may lead to an increased arterial carbon dioxide tension (Paco$_2$) and he advocates paying more attention to pH than Paco$_2$. The controversies regarding the use of positive end-expiratory pressure (PEEP) are discussed although it is claimed that it does not decrease the amount of extravascular lung water. Despite the advances in other modes of ventilation such as high-frequency ventilation or inverse-ratio ventilation it appears that there is no evidence to indicate they improve the patient's survival. The avoidance of complications is discussed and the criteria for discontinuing ventilatory support. If the arterial oxygen tension (PaO$_2$) is less than 60 mmHg when FiO$_2$ is 0.4 or more, weaning is unlikely to be successful. Another predictor is the ratio of respiratory frequency to tidal volume during 1 min of spontaneous respiration, and if this is less than 100 breaths/min per litre it indicates that weaning is likely to be successful.

Cough

Cough is a known side effect of angiotensin converting-enzyme inhibitors (ACEI) and in fact it may produce dyspnoea and bronchospasm. ACE is able to inactivate bradykinin and substance P and it may well be that inhibitors increase the plasma levels of these mediators. It is known that bradykinin can produce bronchoconstriction in asthmatic subjects (Lunde et al 1994).

REM sleep

Surgery and anaesthesia interfere with normal sleep patterns and Rosenberg et al (1994) found that REM sleep decreased on the first night after operation, but increased on the second and third nights and was associated with hypoxaemia.

KIDNEY

Diuretics

It has been reported that there are variations in response to loop diuretics, especially when administered by mouth. This applies particularly to frusemide, whose absorption is affected by food in that there is a delay in gastric emptying. The effect of delayed gastric emptying has no effect on bumetanide.

Frusemide causes a transient increase in plasma renin activity and also increases excretion of renal prostaglandins, which may affect its diuretic action. The efficacy of frusemide is altered by non-steroidal anti-inflammatory drugs (NSAIDs), which inhibit synthesis of prostaglandins. Paracetamol is a weak inhibitor of prostaglandin synthesis, but is still able to attenuate the rise in plasma renin activity and reduce the urine excretion of prostaglandins. It had little effect on diuresis (Martin & Prescott 1994).

Sudden cardiac arrest amongst hypertensives may result from the use of thiazide diuretics and this is dose-related and is due to hypokalaemia and hypomagnesaemia. Siscovick et al (1994) found that the mortality was reduced when a thiazide was combined with a potassium-sparing diuretic, when compared with thiazides alone or combined with potassium supplements.

DIABETES

Insulin-dependent diabetes mellitus (IDDM) is thought to be an autoimmune disease in which there is damage to the β cells of the pancreas. Studies in mice indicate there is a pre-diabetic phase when a critical mass of β cells has not been destroyed. Attempts have been made to stimulate the immune system and more recently specific β cell autoantigens such as glutamic acid decarboxylase have been targeted. The use of synthetic peptide (P277) given to pre-diabetic mice prevented the onset of the disease and reduced the frequency of hyperglycaemia. P277 decreased the damage to the islet cells by increasing the anti-idiotypic T-lymphocytes (Elias & Cohen 1994). Another approach has been to use Freund's complete adjuvant (CFA) and BCG vaccine. Shehadeh et al (1994) were able to show that BCG led to a clinical remission in patients for 3–6 months.

In patients with IDDM there is an incidence of microvascular and neurological complications but intensive insulin therapy delays the onset and progression, especially of retinopathy, nephropathy and neuropathy (Diabetes Control and Complications Trial Research Group 1993, see Lasker 1993). However, there was an increased incidence of severe hypoglycaemia. Others believe that the successful treatment depends on intermittent intravenous therapy (Aoki et al 1993).

Microalbuminuria is a sensitive indicator that renal and cardiovascular disease will develop and it has been shown in these patients that there is insulin resistance (Yip et al 1993, Barnett & Bain 1993).

The incidence of diabetic nephropathy has also been shown by Bojestig et al (1994) to decrease as a result of better control of blood sugar, a feature that has been confirmed by Amiel (1993a). The use of captopril delays the progression of diabetic nephropathy and this effect does not depend on its antihypertensive action (Editorial 1993b)

There have been reports of unawareness of hypoglycaemia, especially in patients on human insulin. However, in patients with insulinoma severe hypoglycaemia may be asymptomatic as it appears that prolonged low blood glucose concentration increases the ability of the brain cells to take up glucose (Amiel 1993b, Mitrakou et al 1993). The infusion of lactate appears to be protective to brain function during hypoglycaemia (Maran et al 1994).

Insulin resistance is a major risk factor also in the development of non-insulin-dependent diabetes mellitus (NIDDM) (Lillioja et al 1993). Insulin is also a potent vasodilator, but this is impaired in hypertensive and in obese subjects, possibly resulting in increased peripheral resistance associated with hypertension, a feature which occurs in diabetic patients (Feldman & Bierbrier 1993). The pathogenesis is discussed by Yki-Jarvinen (1994) and it appears that a positive family history is also of importance. The management of NIDDM is discussed by Williams (1994) and this includes diet, change in lifestyle, the use of sulphonylureas which stimulate insulin secretion and biguanides which reduce absorption of glucose and also inhibit glucose production in the liver. Acarbose and miglitol inhibit α-glucosidases in the intestine, impairing digestion of polysaccharides and hence glucose absorption. The use of insulin in NIDDM is often restricted to incidents such as infection or myocardial infarction, during pregnancy and in the perioperative period.

Perioperative management

Raucoules-Aime et al (1994) have recommended that intravenous bolus of 10 units of insulin every 2 h effectively controls blood sugar at operation and can be used when an insulin infusion pump is not available. However, Hall (1994) expressed concern about the widespread adoption of this regime.

CENTRAL NERVOUS SYSTEM

The clinical syndromes involving myotonia have been reviewed by Russell & Hirsch (1994). They also discuss the hazards of various anaesthetic agents, but often forgotten is that patients with dystrophia myotonica die not during anaesthesia or of possible drug interactions. These patients may die because of failure to appreciate that the muscles involved in respiration are wasted and this includes the accessory muscles of respiration, namely the sternomastoids and pectoral muscles. There is also wasting of the laryngeal muscles and intubation can be readily performed without a muscle relaxant. There is a high postoperative mortality associated with administration of respiratory depressant drugs. The myopathy also affects the cardiac muscle, resulting in sudden death (Kaufman 1962).

Epilepsy

Many of the antiepileptic agents interfere with the destruction of γ-aminobutyric acid (GABA), e.g. vigabatrin. Benzodiazepines increase the action of GABA at the receptor site. A new antiepileptic agent, gabapentin, has no effect on $GABA_A$ or $GABA_B$ receptors and has no action on GABA metabolism. It appears to bind in a specific manner to a protein in certain regions of the brain. It does not induce liver enzymes and its main disadvantage is that the half-life is only 5–7 h. No significant drug interactions have been reported and its main indication is for patients with refractory partial seizures. As yet it is not advocated as the sole drug for treatment but as add-on therapy to reduce the side effects of other antiepileptic drugs (Chadwick 1994).

Migraine

Welch (1993) has reviewed the management of migraine. Acute migraine can be managed symptomatically with analgesic drugs such as aspirin, paracetamol, propoxyphene and codeine, although pethidine may be used for patients who do not respond to antimigraine drugs, or in whom these drugs are contraindicated, such as pregnancy, peripheral artery or coronary artery disease. For mild to moderate severe attacks NSAIDs are of value and they often reduce the severity of the attack, but not its duration. Ergotamine is effective in 50% of cases, while dihydroergotamine given intravenously was effective in 90% of attacks, but because of their vasoconstrictor properties these drugs should be avoided in patients with vascular disease. Sumatriptan, a recently introduced 5-HT agonist, is effective when given subcutaneously, but there are side effects such as flushing, tingling, neck stiffness and occasionally tightness or pain in the chest. Sumatriptan is a highly selective agonist of the D subtype of 5-HT$_1$ receptors. Ergotamine and dihydroergotamine are less selective at this receptor site. Other agents used in the treatment of migraine include dopamine antagonists such as metoclopramide, chlorpromazine and prochlorperazine, but side-effects particularly in young people include dystonia and tardive dyskinesia.

Parkinsonism

Parkinsonism is caused by the reduction of dopamine acting as a neurotransmitter. There are two dopamine receptors, D1 and D2, and it appears that dopamine D2A receptors are involved when dopamine agonists are administered. Therapy in the management of Parkinson's disease has been reviewed by Calne (1993) and this may include symptomatic treatment which involves anticholinergic agents that correct the disparity between dopamine and acetyleholine. They control tremor, but have little effect on rigidity or dyskinesia. Amantadine, on the other hand, improves rigidity and dyskinesia. However, the main drug in use is L-dopa, which unfortunately has many side effects, but these may be reduced by the administration of a decarboxylase inhibitor. Dopamine itself does not cross the blood–brain barrier. Other synthetic dopamine agonists being evaluated include cabergoline, ropinirole and nitecapone, which is an inhibitor of COMT.

Synthetic dopamine agonists include bromocriptine and pergolide, while selegiline, an inhibitor of monoamine oxidase B (MAO-B) is often beneficial. MAOs are now divided into type A and type B. MAO-A preferentially degrades the neurotransmitters 5-HT, adrenaline and noradrenaline as well as dopamine, but MAO-B is only involved in destruction of dopamine. Thus MAO-B inhibitors may be of value in the treatment of Parkinson's disease. Lazabemide is a newly-introduced reversible and selective inhibitor of MAO-B (Guentert et al 1994). Claims have also been made for the surgical transplantation of fetal tissue.

Depression

Tricyclic antidepressants are widely used in the management of depression, but are not devoid of side effects. Buckley et al (1994) found that overdose with dothiepin was associated with cardiac arrhythmias and convulsions. The use of monoamine oxidase inhibitors (MAOIs) are limited because of the interaction with analgesics such as pethidine and hypertensive crisis associated with vasopressors. As already mentioned, two types of MAO are recognized, an A and a B (the A being associated with depression). The A form deaminates 5-HT and noradrenaline, while the B type acts on phenylethylamine and benzylamine. Meclobemide is highly selective in inhibiting MAO type A and has no effect on type B. It does not appear to have any effect on the sympathetic or adrenal gland and is inactive at muscarinic dopaminergic, serotoninergic, adrenergic, opioid or benzodiazepine receptors. There are few adverse reactions and there are no drug interactions with tricyclic antidepressants. The metabolism of the drug is prolonged in the presence of cimetidine, and it is advisable to avoid the use of pethidine. The drug is given after meals as there may be problems with absorption of tyramine in the intestine (Freeman 1993).

The treatment of schizophrenia involves the use of antipsychotic drugs that have some affinity for dopamine at the D_2 receptor site, which unfortunately results in abnormal movements. It has been found that blockade of the 5-HT receptor (S_2) reduces this side effect. This has led to the development of risperidone, a benzisoxazole derivative, which is a potent S_2 and D_2 antagonist. It does produce slight postural hypotension and increases prolactin, which affects menstruation. Drug interactions might be anticipated with dopamine agonists if there is concomitant Parkinsonism (Livingston 1994).

Tetanus

Sun et al (1994) reviewed cases of tetanus that occurred in Hong Kong, mostly in heroin addicts who took the drug intravenously and either the drug or the needles were contaminated with a tetanus organism. The commonest presenting symptom was pain or stiffness of the neck, followed by trismus and dysphagia, and within 24 h muscle spasm developed. Pulmonary and gastrointestinal complications were common as well as autonomic dysfunction characterized by tachycardia, profuse sweating, labile blood pressure, hyperpyrexia and cardiac arrhythmias. Treatment was with labetalol and propranolol. Intrathecal tetanus immunoglobin reduced the mortality and management also included tracheostomy and artificial ventilation.

CARCINOID

Veall et al (1994) have reviewed the anaesthetic management of patients undergoing laparotomy for carcinoid syndrome. The symptoms occur when the patients have hepatic secondaries and these include flushing, diarrhoea and bronchospasm. There may also be pulmonary and tricuspid valve fibrosis as carcinoid tumours secrete not only 5-HT but also histamine, bradykinin, tachykinin and prostaglandins. A recent development in the treatment has been the introduction of an analogue of somatostatin, octreotide. Preoperative assessment should be directed to the control of bronchospasm and to note any complications such as tricuspid regurgitation or pulmonary stenosis. Diarrhoea may lead to severe water and electrolyte loss and indicates there is an alteration in motor function of the small intestine and colon (Von der Ohe et al 1993). Veall et al (1994) favour the use of etmidate or propofol for induction of anaesthesia and a nondepolarizing muscle relaxant such as atracurium or vecuronium. Anaesthesia was maintained with isoflurane and fentanyl. Most of the problems at operation were cardiovascular and bronchospasm was conspicuously absent. Postoperative pain relief was with fentanyl (patient-controlled) or extradural analgesia with bupivacaine and fentanyl.

NEUROLEPTIC MALIGNANT SYNDROME

The neuroleptic malignant syndrome is recognized by the presence of fever, rigidity, autonomic instability and altered consciousness. Bristow & Kohen (1993) suggest that many of the cases are not genuine in that raised levels of creatine kinase are not specific to the disorder; the enzyme may be raised following intramuscular injections, hyperactivity and catatonia. In some instances the temperature is due to a febrile disorder.

MALIGNANT HYPERTHERMIA

The physiology of hyperthermia is outlined by Simon (1993). Hyperthermia may be a physiological response to exercise, occurs in heat stroke when there is impaired dissipation of heat and in dehydration where a decrease in blood volume leads to peripheral vasoconstriction and decreased sweating.

Malignant hyperthermia in anaesthesia is often precipitated by halogenated inhalational agents and suzamethonium. The neuroleptic malignant syndrome occurs in 0.2% of patients who receive neuroleptic drugs, of which haloperidol is predominant.

Hyperthermia occurs in thyrotoxicosis and in hyperparathyroidism and phaeochromocytoma. Drugs likely to result in hyperthermia include anticholinergic agents such as atropine but cocaine, amphetamines, alcohol and salicylates may also be involved. There is an increase in oxygen consumption, increase in heart rate and the patients with pre-existing disorders may develop cardiac ischaemia, arrhythmias, hypertension and even congestive cardiac failure. Metabolic abnormalities associated with hyperthermia include hypoxaemia, respiratory alkalosis, metabolic acidosis, hypokalaemia and hyperkalaemia, hypernatraemia and hypoglycaemia. Temperatures as high as 42°C can be tolerated, mortality being related to the severity of the pre-existing disease rather than the increased temperature. Heat stroke and malignant hyperthermia have a high mortality.

Until recently in vitro tests of muscle contracture in response to halothane and caffeine have been accepted criteria for susceptibility of patients to malignant hyperpyrexia. A recent search on DNA has suggested that there may be a genetic test based on DNA, but Hopkins et al (1994) strongly advised against the use of this test as a sole arbiter of diagnosis.

SMOKING

There has been debate recently regarding cardiovascular surgery for patients who persistently smoke. Powell & Greenhalgh (1994) reaffirm that no smoker should be denied urgent surgery, despite the fact that results of cardiac bypass surgery are less successful. Results of surgery are likely to be less successful in smokers who not only have severe arterial disease but also asthma which is accenuated by smoking. Many patients, presenting for operation, who are said to have asthma are being treated with bronchodilators, but refuse to discontinue smoking. The human cost of tobacco use has been discussed by Bartecchi et al (1994) and MacKenzie et al (1994). In the USA smoking-related diseases account for 20% of deaths and a quarter of all deaths in ages between 35–64. Smoking affects the cardiovascular system by increasing platelet aggregation, vasomotor activity which leads to a prothrombotic state and to coronary vasospasm. Not only does it result in carcinoma of the lung, but also carcinoma of the mouth, pharynx, larynx, oesophagus, stomach, pancreas, cervix, kidney, ureter and bladder. In the USA cigarette smoking is the commonest cause of pulmonary illness and death. Smokers may exhibit a decline in FEV_1 (forced expiratory volume in 1 s) at the rate of more than 60 ml per year (see Crapo 1994). In women lung cancer has surpassed the death rate from breast cancer. Women who take contraceptives and smoke are more likely to die of cardiovascular disease than those who do not.

In the USA it is estimated that there are 2000 deaths a year from non-smoking adults, attributable to passive smoking. Breakdown products of nicotine such as cotinine can be measured in the urine and measurement of this marker coincides with acute exacerbation of asthma when non-smokers are exposed to cigarette smoke (Boyle 1993, Chilmonczyk et al 1993).

SICKLE CELL DISEASE

Platte et al (1994) found that 50% of patients with sickle cell anaemia survive beyond the fifth decade. The highest mortality was amongst patients who had symptoms such as acute episode of pain, acute chest syndrome or stroke.

Acute painful episodes is a feature of sickle cell disease and Griffin et al (1994) found that a short course of high-dose methylprednisolone was effective in decreasing the duration of severe pain in children, but unfortunately when therapy ceased there was an increase in the attacks of pain. Another approach in patients with end-stage β-thalassaemia has been to alter the fetal haemoglobin genes by the use of the nucleoside analogue azacitidine (Lowrey & Nienhuis 1993).

REFERENCES

Abboud F M 1993 Neurocardiogenic syncope. N Engl J Med 328: 1117–1118
Adams J, Trent R, Rawles J 1993 Earliest electrocardiographic evidence of myocardial infarction: implications for thrombolytic treatment. Br Med J 307: 409–413
Adams J E, Sicard G A, Allen B T et al 1994 Diagnosis of perioperative myocardial infarction with measurement of cardiac troponin I. N Engl J Med 330: 670–674
Ahmed T, Garrigo J, Danta I 1993 Preventing bronchoconstriction in exercise-induced asthma with inhaled heparin. N Engl J Med 329: 90–95
Amiel S A 1993a Diabetic control and complications: better control means fewer microvascular complications. Br Med J 307: 881–882
Amiel S A 1993b Reversal of unawareness of hypoglycemia. N Engl J Med 329: 876–877
Anderson H V, Willerson J T 1993 Thrombolysis in acute myocardial infarction. N Engl J Med 329: 703–709
Aoki T T, Benbarka M M, Okimura M C et al 1993 Long-term intermittent intravenous insulin therapy and type 1 diabetes mellitus. Lancet 342: 515–518
Barnes P J 1993 Asthma: what is there left to find out? Firstly, why and how do people become asthmatic? Br Med J 307: 814–815
Barnett A H, Bain S C 1993 Microalbuminuria and insulin resistance in diabetes mellitus. Lancet 342: 880–881
Baron J-F, Mundler O, Bertrand M et al 1994 Dipyridamole-thallium scintigraphy and gated radionuclide angiography to assess cardiac risk before abdominal aortic surgery. N Engl J Med 330: 663–669
Bartecchi C E, MacKenzie T D, Schrier R W 1994 The human costs of tobacco use. N Engl J Med 330: 907–912
Baskett P J F 1994 Should relatives be allowed to watch resuscitation? Doctors need to be trained to work in public. Br Med J 308: 1689
Beale R, Grover E R, Smithies M, Bihari D 1993 Acute respiratory distress syndrome (ARDS): no more than a severe acute lung injury? Br Med J 307: 1335–1339
Bloomfield P 1994 Should relatives be allowed to watch resuscitation? Good information and time with the body are more important. Br Med J 308: 1688–1689
Bojestig M, Arnqvist H J, Hermansson G et al 1994 Declining incidence of nephropathy in insulin-dependent diabetes mellitus. N Engl J Med 330: 15–18
Boucher C A, Brewster D C, Darling R C et al 1985 Determination of cardiac risk by dipyridamole-thallium imaging before peripheral vascular surgery. N Engl J Med 312: 389–394
Boyle P 1993 The hazards of passive – and active – smoking. N Engl J Med 328: 1708–1709
Bristow M F, Kohen D 1993 How 'malignant' is the neuroleptic malignant syndrome? Br Med J 307: 1223–1224
Britton J 1993 Tolerance to beta-agonists in asthma therapy. Lancet 342: 818–819

Bruera E, de Stoutz N, Velasco-Leiva A, Schoeller T, Hanson J 1993 Effects of oxygen on dyspnoea in hypoxaemic terminal-cancer patients. Lancet 342: 13–14

Buckley N A, Dawson A H, Whyte I M, Henry D A 1994 Greater toxicity in overdose of dothiepin than of other tricyclic antidepressants. Lancet 343: 159–162

Calne D B 1993 Treatment of Parkinson's Disease. N Engl J Med 329: 1021–1027

Chadwick D 1994 Gabapentine. Lancet 343: 89–91

Charlson M E, MacKenzie R, Gold J P et al 1991 Risk for postoperative congestive heart failure. Gynecol Obstet 172: 95–104

Chilmonczyk B A, Salmun L M, Megathlin K N et al 1993 Association between exposure to environmental tobacco smoke and exacerbations of asthma in children. N Engl J Med 328: 1660–1665

Clements I P, Kaufman U P, Bailey K R et al 1991 Electrocardiographic prediction or myocardial area at risk. Mayo Clin Proc 66: 985–990

Cockcroft D W, McParland C P, Britto S A et al 1993 Regular inhaled salbutamol and airway responsiveness to allergen. Lancet 342: 833–837

Cohen T D, Goldner B G, Maccaro P C et al 1993 A comparison of active compression–decompression cardiopulmonary resuscitation with standard cardiopulmonary resuscitation for cardiac arrests occurring in the hospital. N Engl Med 329: 1918–1921

Collen D 1993 Towards improved thrombolytic therapy. Lancet 342: 34–36

Crapo R O 1994 Pulmonary-function testing. N Engl J Med 331: 25–30

Davis M, Espiner E, Richards G, Billings J et al 1994 Plasma brain natriuretic peptide in assessment of acute dyspnoea. Lancet 343: 440–444

Detsky A S, Abrams H B, McLaughlin J R et al 1986 Predicting cardiac complications in patients undergoing non-cardiac surgery. J Gen Intern Med 1: 211–219

Diabetes Control and Complications Trial Research Group 1993 The effect of intensive treatment of diabetes on the development and progression of long-term complications in insulin-dependent diabetes mellitus. N Engl J Med 329: 977–986

Dickinson C J 1993 Fainting precipitated by collapse-firing of venous baroreceptors. Lancet 342: 970–972

Doyal L, Wilsher D 1994 Withholding and withdrawing life sustaining treatment from elderly people: towards formal guidelines. Br Med J 308: 1689–1692

Drug and Therapeutics Bulletin 1994 Fluticasone propionate for asthma prophylaxis. 32 (No 4): 25–27

Edgren E, Hedstrand U, Kelsey S et al 1994 Assessment of neurological prognosis in comatose survivors of cardiac arrest. Lancet 343: 1055–1059

Editorial 1993a Chest pain with normal coronary angiograms. N Engl J Med 328: 1706–1708

Editorial 1993b Slowing the progression of diabetic nephropathy. N Engl J Med 329: 1496–1497

Edwards N D, Reilly C S 1994 Detection of perioperative myocardial ischaemia. Br J Anaesth 72: 104–115

Egashira K, Inou T, Hirooka Y et al 1993 Evidence of impaired endothelium-dependent coronary vasodilatation in patients with angina pectoris and normal coronary angiograms. N Engl J Med 328: 1659–1664

Engleman H M, Martin S E, Dery I J, Douglas N J 1994 Effect of continuous positive airway pressure treatment on daytime function in sleep apnoea/hypopnoea syndrome. Lancet 343: 572–575

Elias D, Cohen I R 1994 Peptide therapy for diabetes in NOD mice. Lancet 343: 704–706

Espiner E 1993 Myocardial infarction: kindred hearts and coronaries. Lancet 341: 995–996

Feldman R D, Bierbrier G S 1993 Insulin-mediated vasodilation: impairment with increased blood pressure and body mass. Lancet 342: 707–709

Freeman H 1993 Moclobemide. Lancet 342: 1528–1532

Gold B S, Young M E, Kinman J L et al 1992 The utility of preoperative electrocardiograms in the ambulatory surgical patient. Arch Intern Med 152: 301–305

Goldman L 1994 Assessment of perioperative cardiac risk. N Engl J Med 330: 707–711

Goldman L, Caldera D L, Nussbaum S R et al 1977 Multifactorial index of cardiac risk in noncardiac surgical procedures. N Engl J Med 297: 845–850

Golino P, Piscione F, Claude M D et al 1994 Local effect of serotonin released during coronary angioplasty. N Engl J Med 330: 523–528

Grech E D, Dodd N J F, Bellamy C M et al 1993 Free-radical generation during angioplasty reperfusion for acute myocardial infarction. Lancet 341: 990–992

Griffin T C, McIntire D, Buchanan G R 1994 High-dose intravenous methylprednisolone therapy for pain in children and adolescents with sickle cell disease. N Engl J Med 330: 733–737

Guentert T W, Golford N H G, Pfefen J P, Dingemanse J 1994 Mixed linear and non-linear disposition of lazabemide, a reversible and selective inhibitor of monoamine oxidase. Br J Clin Pharmacol 37: 545–552

Hall G M 1994 Insulin administration in diabetic patients: a return of the bolus? Br J Anaesth 72: 1–2

Harris D N F, Bailey S M, Smith P L C et al 1993 Brain swelling in first hour after coronary artery bypass surgery. Lancet 342: 586– 587

Higgs R 1994 Should relatives be allowed to watch resuscitation? Relatives' wishes should be accommodated. Br Med J 308: 1688

Hill M E, MacQuillan G, Forsyth M, Heath D A 1994 Cardiopulmonary resuscitation: who makes the decision? Br Med J 308: 1677

Hoeldtke R D, Streeten D H P 1993 Treatment of orthostatic hypotension with erythropoietin. N Engl J Med 329: 611–615

Hopkins P M, Halsall P J, Ellis F R 1994 Diagnosing malignant hyperthermia. Anaesthesia 49: 373–375

Jaffe A S, Landau W M 1993 Death after death: the presumption of informed consent for cardiopulmonary resuscitation – ethical paradox and clinical conundrum. Neurology 43: 2173–2178

Kaufman, L 1962 Disordered respiration in dystrophia myotonica. MD thesis, Edinburgh University

Kelly D P, Strauss A W 1994 Inherited cardiomyopathies. N Engl J Med 330: 913–919

Kellow N H 1994 The renin-angiotensin system and angiotensin converting enzyme (ACE) inhibitors. Anaesthesia 49: 613–622

Kenny J 1994 Treating overdose with calcium channel blockers. Br Med J 308: 992–993

Kharitonov S A, Yates D, Robbins R A et al 1994 Increased nitric oxide in exhaled air of asthmatic patients. Lancet 343: 133–135

Kinch J W, Ryan T J 1994 Right ventricular infarction. N Engl J Med 330: 1211–1217

Landau C, Lange R A, Hillis L D 1994 Percutaneous transluminal coronary angioplasty. N Eng J Med 330: 981–993

Lange L G, Schreiner G F 1994 Immune mechanisms of cardiac disease. N Engl J Med 330: 1129–1135

Lasker R D 1993 The diabetes control and complications trial. Implications for policy and practice. N Engl J Med 329: 1035–1036

Lillioja S, Mott D M, Spraul M et al 1993 Insulin resistance and insulin secretory dysfunction as precursors of non-insulin-dependent diabetes mellitus. N Engl J Med 329: 1988–1892

Livingston M G 1994 Risperidone. Lancet 343: 457–460

Lowrey C H, Nienhuis A W 1993 Brief report: treatment with azacitidine of patients with end-stage β-thalassemia. N Engl J Med 329: 845–848

Lunde H, Hedner T, Samuelsson O et al 1994 Dyspnoea, asthma and bronchospasm in relation to treatment with angiotensin converting enzyme inhibitors. Br Med J 308: 16–21

MacKenzie T D, Bartecchi C E, Schrier R W 1994 The human costs of tobacco use. N Engl J Med 330: 975–980

Manger W M 1993 Baroreflex failure: a diagnostic challenge. N Engl J Med 329: 1494–1495

Maran A, Cranston I, Lomas J et al 1994 Protection by lactate of cerebral function during hypoglycaemia. Lancet 343: 16–20

Marber M, Walker D, Yellon D 1994 Ischaemic preconditioning: new insight into myocardial protection. Br Med J 308: 1–2

Martin U, Prescott L F 1994 The interaction of paracetamol with frusemide. Br J Clin Pharmacol 37: 464–467

Mason J W for the Electrophysiologic Study versus Electrocardiographic Monitoring Investigators 1993 A comparison of seven antiarrhythmic drugs in patients with ventricular tachyarrhythmias. N Engl J Med 329; 452–458

McClelland P, Gilbertson A A, Percy D et al 1993 Severe combined acute renal and respiratory failure (SCARRF): the development of a risk prediction system. Br J Intensive Care (November): 407–414

Mitrakou A, Fanelli C, Veneman T et al 1993 Reversibility of awareness of hypoglycemia in patients with insulinomas. N Engl J Med 329: 834–839

Mittleman M A, Maclure M, Tofler G H et al 1993 Triggering of acute myocardial infarction by heavy physical exertion: protection against triggering by regular exertion. N Engl J Med 329: 1677–1683

Moncada S, Higgs A 1993 The L-arginine-nitric oxide pathway. N Engl J Med 329: 2002–2012

Morgan R, King D, Prajapati C, Rowe J 1994 Views of elderly patients and their relatives on cardiopulmonary resuscitation. Br Med J 308: 1677–1678

Multi-Society Task Force on PVS 1994a Medical aspects of the persistent vegetative state (first of two parts). N Engl J Med 330: 1499–1508

Multi-Society Task Force on PVS 1994b Medical aspects of the persistent vegetative state (second of two parts). N Engl J Med 330: 1572–1579

Murphy D J, Burrows D, Santilli S et al 1994 The influence of the probability of survival on patients' preferences regarding cardiopulmonary resuscitation. N Engl J Med 330: 545–549

Newburger J W, Jonas R A, Wernovsky G et al 1993 A comparison of the perioperative neurologic effects of hypothermic circulatory arrest versus low-flow cardiopulmonary bypass in infant heart surgery. N Engl J Med 329: 1057–1064

Nicholson K G, Kent J, Ireland D C 1993 Respiratory viruses and exacerbations of asthma in adults. Br Med J 307: 982–986

Partridge M 1994 Asthma: guided self management. Br Med J 308: 547–550

Patrono C 1994 Aspirin as an antiplatelet drug. N Engl J Med 330: 1287–1294

Platt O S, Brambilla D J, Rose W F et al 1994 Mortality in sickle cell disease. N Engl J Med 330: 1639–1644

Powell J T, Greenhalgh R M 1994 Arterial bypass surgery and smokers: no smoker should be denied urgent surgery to prevent amputation, stroke or death. Br Med J 308: 607–608

Raucoules-Aime M, Ichai C, Roussell L J et al 1994 Comparison of two methods of iv insulin administration in the diabetic patient during the perioperative period. Br J Anaesth 72: 5–10

Remuzzi G, Benigni A 1993 Endothelins in the control of cardiovascular and renal function. Lancet 342: 589–593

Robertson D, Hollister A S, Biaggioni I et al 1993 The diagnosis and treatment of baroreflex failure. N Engl J Med 329: 1449–1455

Rosenberg J, Wildschiodt G, Pederson M H et al 1994 Late postoperative nocturnal episodic hypoxaemia and associated sleep pattern. Br J Anaesth 72: 145–150

Royston D 1993 Inhalational agents for pulmonary hypertension. Lancet 342: 941–942

Russell S H, Hirsch N P 1994 Anaesthesia and myotonia. Br J Anaesth 72: 210–216

Saltuari L, Marosi M 1994 Coma after cardiac arrest: will he recover all right? Lancet 343: 1052

Seegobin R D, Goodland F C, Wilmshurst T H et al 1991 Postoperative myocardial damage in patients with coronary artery disease undergoing major non cardiac surgery. Can J Anaesth 38: 1005–1011

Shehadeh N, Calcinaro F, Bradley B J et al 1994 Effect of adjuvant therapy on development of diabetes in mouse and man. Lancet 343: 706–707

Shenasa M, Borggrefe M, Haverkamp W et al 1993 Ventricular tachycardia. Lancet 341: 1512–1519

Sim K M, Evans T W 1993 Supporting the injured lung: the benefits of extracorporeal gas exchange in adults remain unproved. Br Med J 307: 1293–1294

Simon H B 1993 Hyperthermia. N Engl J Med 329: 483–487

Siscovick D S, Raghunathan T E, Psaty B M, Koepsell T D et al 1994 Diuretic therapy for hypertension and the risk of primary cardiac arrest. N Engl J Med 330: 1852–1857

Sly P D, Cahill P. Willet K, Burton P 1994 Accuracy of mini peak flow meters in indicating changes in lung function in children with asthma. Br Med J 308: 572–574

Sra J S, Jazayeri M R, Avitall B et al 1993 Comparison of cardiac pacing with drug therapy in the treatment of neurocardiogenic (vasovagal) syncope with bradycardia or asystole. N Engl J Med 328: 1085–1090

Steltzer H, Hiesmayr M, Mayer N et al 1994 The relationship between oxygen delivery and uptake in the critically ill: is there a critical or optimal therapeutic value? A meta-analysis. Anaesthesia 49: 229–236

Sun K O, Chan Y W, Cheung R T F et al 1994 Management of tetanus: a review of 18 cases. J R Soc Med 87: 135–137

Swain J A 1993 Cardiac surgery and the brain. N Engl J Med 329: 1119–1120

Tobin M J 1994 Mechnical ventilation. N Engl J Med 330: 1056–1061

Vallance P, Collier J 1994 Biology and clinical relevance of nitric oxide. Br Med J 309: 453–457

Veall G R Q, Peacock J E, Bax N D S, Reilly C S 1994 Review of the anaesthetic management of 21 patients undergoing laparotomy for carcinoid syndrome. Br J Anaesth 72: 335–341

Von der Ohe M R, Camilleri M, Kvols K L, Thomforde G M 1993 Motor dysfunction of the small bowel and colon in patients with the carcinoid syndrome and diarrhea. N Engl J Med 329: 1073–1078

Waagstein F, Bristow M R, Swedberg K et al 1993 Beneficial effects of metoprolol in idiopathic dilated cardiomyopathy. Lancet 342: 1441–1446

Walmrath D, Schneider T, Pilch J et al 1993 Aerosolised prostacyclin in adult respiratory distress syndrome. Lancet 342: 961–962

Walse D 1993 Dyspnoea in advanced cancer. Lancet 342: 450–451

Welch K M A 1993 Drug therapy of migraine. N Engl J Med 329: 1476–1483

Weston C F M, Penny W J, Julian D G et al 1994 Guidelines for the early management of patients with myocardial infarction. Br Med J 308: 767–771

Whitlock M 1994 Should relatives be allowed to watch resuscitation? The doctor's perspective. Br Med J 308: 1687–1688

William G 1994 Management of non-insulin-dependent diabetes mellitus. Lancet 343: 95–100

Willich S N, Lewis M, Lowel H et al 1993 Physical exertion as a trigger of acute myocardial infarction. N Engl J Med 329: 1684–1690

Yip J, Mattock M B, Morocutti A et al 1993 Insulin resistance in insulin-dependent diabetic patients with microalbuminuria. Lancet 342: 883–887

Yki-Jarvinen H 1994 Pathogenesis of non-insulin-dependent diabetes mellitus. Lancet 343: 91–95

Zaret B L, Wackers F J 1993a Nuclear cardiology (first of two parts). N Engl J Med 329: 775–783

Zaret B L, Wackers F J 1993b Nuclear cardiology (second of two parts). N Engl J Med 329: 855–863

2

Ventilation strategies to improve oxygenation in patients with the adult respiratory distress syndrome

A. T. Lovell   J. C. Goldstone

Artificial ventilation is a widespread technique often used in patients whose primary organ dysfunction is non-respiratory. For these patients mechanical ventilation usually results in normal blood gases. For patients with severe acute lung injury, conventional volume-cycled ventilation is often inadequate, and maximum oxygenation requires optimizing mechanical support.

PATHOPHYSIOLOGY OF SEVERE ACUTE RESPIRATORY FAILURE

Adult respiratory distress syndrome (ARDS) is precipitated by direct damage to the lung, e.g. gastric aspiration, or secondary to distant disease, e.g. sepsis. Despite differing aetiologies, some common pathophysiological features emerge. Activation and degranulation of leucocytes stimulate release of a cascade of cytokines, resulting in endothelial disruption and damage following diverse initiating stimuli. Many attempts at interruption or modulation of cytokine pathways have not so far met with success, and treatment is directed towards support of the damaged lung whilst awaiting natural recovery (Kollef & Schuster 1995).

The early phase of acute lung injury is characterized by oedema and rising lung weight. This fact has been recognized by pathologists for many years, and widespread oedema not only confined to the dependent lung has now been demonstrated in vivo by computed tomography (CT) scanning (Gattinoni et al 1988, 1991). A two-compartment model of the severely injured lung has been developed, one of which is fluid laden, non-compliant and non-ventilated, whilst the other is remarkably normal. Mechanical ventilation attempts to recruit as many alveoli as possible whilst maintaining ventilated alveoli patent. Whilst mechanical ventilation attempts to maximize oxygenation within some alveoli it leads to further damage. Repeated opening and closing of airways add to the shearing effect and may lead to further lung injury, as well as avoiding over-distension of the more normal lung regions. Recognition that only a small part of the lung is playing a part in gas exchange has given rise to the concept of the *baby lung*.

STRATEGIES TO IMPROVE OXYGENATION

Postural changes

Although changing posture to the prone position is associated with an improvement in arterial oxygenation in most cases, this improvement is variable. If gas exchange improves, it is usually progressive and may take hours to become apparent. In some patients who initially respond, blood gas deterioration may occur again if the prone posture is maintained for a prolonged period. When these patients are returned to the supine position the improvements in gas exchange are unpredictably maintained. Further, when the patient is turned repeatedly the effects of the manoeuvre may produce progressively less improvement and occasionally gas exchange may deteriorate.

Gattinoni et al (1994) used fine-cut chest CT scans in patients with normal and acutely injured lungs to demonstrate the gas exchange defect in damaged lungs. They found an exponential decrease in the amount of gas per unit volume of lung tissue with dorsal progression through a supine normal lung. When the subject is turned to the prone position, the regional inflation distribution changes markedly, increasing dorsally and decreasing ventrally. However, unlike the supine position the gas distribution is far more homogeneous.

In patients with lung damage in the supine position there is a similar exponential decrease in the amount of aerated lung tissue as one travels dorsally. However, Pelosi et al (1994) showed that due to oedema and infiltration even at the most ventral surface, the lungs are only half as well aerated as usual. The ventilation that does occur in these severely damaged lungs occurs preferentially in the non-dependent areas of the lungs. Without positive end-expiratory pressure (PEEP) there is virtually complete alveolar collapse or consolidation in the posterior half of the lungs. PEEP produces a more uniform distribution of ventilation to include and recruit the dependent lung regions. When the patient is turned prone, the inflation gradient reverses and is again characteristically homogeneous. As in the supine position the dependent alveoli are collapsed.

Permissive hypercapnia

During mechanical ventilation in normal lungs normocapnia is usually easily achieved. Acute hypercapnia has many deleterious effects when the patient is breathing spontaneously, encouraging the belief that normocapnia is an important ventilatory goal (Table 2.1).

Achieving normocapnia in those with severe lung injury is at a cost. Critically ill patients are often hypermetabolic with a large physiological dead space, and therefore have a large ventilatory requirement. Tidal volumes of 10–15 ml/kg were frequently required and the high minute ventilation necessitates high peak and mean airway pressures.

Table 2.1   Effects of hypercapnia

Hypoxia
Reduction in tissue oxygen uptake
Hyperkalaemia
Vasodilatation
Increase in cerebral blood flow and volume
Increase in intracranial pressure
Stimulation of the sympathetic nervous system
    Hypertension
    Tachycardia

The avoidance of further lung injury by hypoventilation has begun to receive a higher priority than achieving normocapnia. Initially this approach was taken with severe asthma by Darioli & Perret (1984) and subsequently has been applied to ARDS by Hickling et al (1990). Dreyfuss et al (1988) have shown that high inspiratory volumes as much as high pressures create further lung damage. In man, Hickling (1990) studied the effect of permissive hypercapnia and showed a 60% improvement in outcome compared to predicted mortality. However, this study was retrospective and used a historical control group. In a randomized controlled trial of permissive hypercapnia in ARDS, Amato et al (1993) found improvement in oxygenation and lower airway pressures in the hypercapnic group but overall mortality was unchanged. This was, however, only a small study and until a large study is completed the potential for improvements in patients treated with permissive hypercapnia will remain uncertain.

Consequences of permissive hypercapnia.

During prolonged hypercapnia extracellular acidosis is common. The majority of the effects of acute hypercapnia are related to changes in the intracellular pH (pH_{in}). As carbon dioxide is freely diffusible acute hypercapnia initially results in similar changes to intracellular and extracellular pH. However, within 3 h pH_{in} has returned to 90% of normal because of intracellular buffering and cellular proton pumps. Extracellular pH correction, on the other hand, is extremely slow, relying upon renal compensation mechanisms, and should not therefore be used as an indicator of pH_{in}.

The circulatory effects of hypercapnia are dominated by the direct depression of the myocardium, although this may be balanced by the degree of sympathetic stimulation produced. Myocardial irritability can be increased and the consequent arrhythmias may limit the use of permissive hypercapnia. Effects on the peripheral circulation are almost entirely confined to direct vasodilatation which, combined with the potential myocardial depression, may lead to hypotension. Permissive hypercapnia is associated with a significant increase in pulmonary vascular resistance, and reductions in the alveolar–arterial PO_2 gradient and shunt fraction. These changes are regardless of the changes in cardiac output. It is thought that the improvement in oxygenation reflects either a generalized pulmonary vasoconstriction, or possibly enhanced vasoconstriction in hypoxic lung regions.

The metabolic effects of permissive hypercapnia are largely confined to hyperkalaemia and problems with oxygen uptake by haemoglobin. Ultimately renal compensation mechanisms will return the extracellular pH to near normal, but this is a very gradual process. Additionally hypercapnia alters the pharmacokinetics and pharmacodynamics of some drugs, notably aminoglycosides. Although many of the consequences of hypercapnia are minor, in particular cases they may limit the desirability of this technique.

Recruitment therapy

Traditional techniques for managing severe lung injury were based on large-volume hyperventilation in order to effectively clear carbon dioxide and reopen collapsed airways. Since the development of the concept of the *baby lung* and with the increasing use of permissive hypercapnia the use of much smaller tidal volumes, often in the range of 5–8 ml/kg, has become the norm and other strategies aimed at recruitment of the collapsed and fluid-filled airways have been developed. The two most widely used are the addition of PEEP and inverse ratio ventilation (IRV).

Positive end-expiratory pressure

The most direct way of recruiting non-ventilated alveoli is with the addition of PEEP, titrated to maintain an adequate tissue oxygen delivery with an acceptable inspired oxygen concentration. Optimal values for PEEP and tidal volumes can be determined from static pressure–volume curves; Ranieri et al (1991) showed that patients who have reached the plateau of the curve may benefit from a smaller tidal volume and are unlikely to benefit from further increments of PEEP. If it is not possible to measure the static pressure–volume relationship then the effect of increased PEEP on airway pressure can be observed. An increment in airway pressure of less than the increase in PEEP implies that recruitment must be occurring, whereas an increment greater than the increase in PEEP suggests that the lung has moved beyond its maximum compliance and that the PEEP should be reduced (Fig. 2.1).

Numerous studies have established that lung water is not reduced by PEEP, and may on occasion be increased. The actions of PEEP that explain the improvement in oxygenation are re-expansion of collapsed alveoli, redistribution of fluid to the more compliant perivascular space and layering of fluid within the alveoli. When the recruited airways are continuously splinted open, alveolar wall shear stresses are much reduced and alveoli are no longer collapsing during every expiration, reducing the degree of volume-related lung injury. That PEEP can successfully recruit lung volume has been very clearly demonstrated using chest CT scans by Gattinoni and his colleagues (Gattinoni et al 1988).

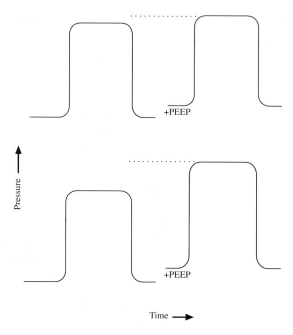

Fig. 2.1 Effects on airway pressure of adding PEEP. Upper panel shows the effect of adding PEEP whilst alveoli are recruitable. Note the rise in peak pressure is less than the PEEP increment. Lower panel shows the effect of adding PEEP when no further alveoli are recruitable and over-distension is occurring. Note the rise in peak pressure is greater than or equal to the PEEP increment.

For a long time it was thought that the application of PEEP to patients with obstructive lung disease was contraindicated since it would cause yet further hyperinflation. More recently it has been realized that these patients can have significant levels of intrinsic PEEP ($PEEP_i$) and in these circumstances the application of PEEP to levels less than $PEEP_i$ will in fact unload the inspiratory muscles and not be associated with further dynamic hyperinflation (Tobin & Lodato 1989).

Inverse ratio ventilation

Most recent interest in recruitment therapy has moved towards IRV. This technique was first described in neonates by Reynolds (1971). He found that by prolonging the duration of inspiration it was possible to improve oxygenation. Since then numerous studies in adults have confirmed the utility of IRV and today Inspiratory: Expiratory (I : E) ratios as high as 4 : 1 are employed, although the principles underlying this mode of ventilation do not necessarily require the actual inversion of the I : E ratio. The rationale behind the use of an extended inspiratory time is to manipulate the pattern of applied pressure to achieve lung recruitment without causing over-inflation of the relatively normal alveoli.

During conventional ventilation mean alveolar pressure ($P_{\bar{A}}$) corresponds directly to alveolar recruitment, intrapulmonary shunt reduction and arterial oxygenation. $P_{\bar{A}}$ cannot be directly measured but rises with increases in minute ventilation, PEEP or changes in inspiratory flow characteristics. Increases in mean airway pressure ($P_{\bar{aw}}$) will increase $P_{\bar{A}}$ to a variable degree. However, not all methods of increasing $P_{\bar{aw}}$ are equivalent. Gas exchange improves and intrapulmonary shunt decreases even if $P_{\bar{aw}}$ is kept constant but PEEP is applied.

In theory prolongation of the inspiratory time will increase $P_{\bar{aw}}$ without increasing peak pressure despite a constant tidal volume and PEEP level. This is only true so long as the encroachment on expiration is not at the expense of generating dynamic hyperinflation and $PEEP_i$. Extending the inspiratory time to generate $PEEP_i$ has, however, been used as a method of preventing the collapse of unstable alveoli. The generation of $PEEP_i$, however, will either increase the peak pressure or if pressure-limited ventilation is used then the tidal volume must fall. If $PEEP_i$ is generated it will act in concert with any external PEEP in preventing alveolar collapse.

Extending the inspiratory time may improve gas exchange independent of effects on $P_{\bar{aw}}$. In severely injured lungs poorly inflated alveoli have longer than normal time constants and require a longer inspiratory time to inflate fully. Additionally non-aerated alveoli may require a more sustained inflation pressure in order to open. Lastly, prolonged inspiration will facilitate gas mixing.

IRV can be generated either by using a pressure-controlled ventilator (PC-IRV) or a volume-controlled ventilator with an inspiratory hold facility (VC-IRV). VC-IRV has the advantage of ensuring a delivered tidal volume, gives good control over the inspiratory flow characteristics, is readily available on most intensive therapy unit (ITU) ventilators and allows a gradual transition to IRV from conventional ventilation. However, it is extremely uncomfortable for the patient and usually requires deep sedation. There is no control of peak pressure when volume cycling is used and so dangerously high peak pressures can be generated, especially by coughing against the ventilator or repeatedly triggering extra breaths. For this reason muscle relaxants are often used during VC-IRV.

PC-IRV in many ways represents a safer although less familiar strategy for the application of IRV. With PC-IRV there is precise control over the peak pressure. Changes in frequency or respiratory impedance will change the delivered tidal volume, which necessitates continuous monitoring of expired minute volume. However, coughing against the ventilator will not lead to dangerously high airway pressures. PC-IRV is generally much better tolerated than VC-IRV and as a result often requires lower levels of sedation.

With any technique that is associated with dynamic hyperinflation and a potential for the generation of $PEEP_i$ there is a risk of ventilator-induced lung damage. The use of large tidal volumes (15–20 ml/kg) with this technique has been associated with a 23% pneumothorax rate. With studies using smaller tidal volumes the pneumothorax rate is far lower. Inevitably if $PEEP_i$ is generated then cardiac output may be impaired and oxygen delivery may need to be ensured via measurement of cardiac output.

The overall effect of IRV in patients is rather unpredictable and therapy must be carefully individualized. The potential benefits are considerable. Poelaert et al (1991) reported a 35% decrease in peak pressure at the same time as a 17% increase in cardiac output on switching to PC-IRV from conventional ventilation. However, no randomized outcome studies have been published to date. The widespread use of IRV must be cautious with full assessment of the potential risks and benefits. As a result guidelines as to which patients should receive IRV are somewhat contradictory (Marcy 1994, Marcy & Marini 1991, East et al 1992). Usually IRV is only used once it is impossible to achieve acceptable oxygenation with acceptable conventional ventilatory parameters. Attempts to prolong the inspiratory time in these patients should be made gradually since these patients are already unstable and rapid institution of this ventilatory strategy can precipitate a crisis. Many people prefer to use VC-IRV for gradual introduction of IRV, later switching to PC-IRV once the change in ventilatory parameters is complete. It must be stressed that many of the benefits of IRV can be achieved by changing the I : E ratio to 1 : 1 rather than formally reversing the I : E ratio.

High-frequency ventilation

Conventional attempts at mechanical ventilation attempt to duplicate the normal bulk flow of gas, with tidal volumes and frequencies in or near the physiological range. As lung function deteriorates conventional strategies frequently fail to provide adequate carbon dioxide clearance or oxygen delivery without considerable potential for barotrauma or cardiovascular depression. High-frequency ventilation (HFV) comprises three ventilatory techniques depending on the ventilatory frequency used. HFV is characterized by the use of small tidal volumes – in some circumstances less than the anatomical dead space. As a consequence of the smaller tidal volumes the peak airway pressures are lower than with conventional ventilation, although the frequency × tidal volume product is far greater. The arguments in favour of the use of HFV generally hinge around the reduction in pressure swings which may reduce the incidence of barotrauma, and the improvement in ventilation and perfusion matching consequent on the different gas delivery technique. Jet ventilators work on the principle that an injector creates a high velocity *jet* of gas that is directed into the lung. These jets are small, typically 1–3 mm in diameter, and can be positioned either proximally or distally within the airway. As a rule the more distally placed the lower the functional dead space, but inevitably the greater the risk that movement will direct the jet into a single lung. Jet ventilators can entrain gas, giving rise to augmentation of the tidal volume. As with conventional ventilation exhalation is dependent on passive lung recoil (Table 2.2).

Table 2.2 Factors affecting the tidal volume

Jet driving pressure
Injector size
Inspiratory time
Frequency
Size of endotracheal tube
Presence of entrainment gas
Presence of auto PEEP

Volume and flow measurements during HFV are difficult especially at higher frequencies. Proximal airway pressure monitoring must be several centimetres distal to the jet orifice in order to provide a reasonable representation of peak and mean airway pressures. As frequencies rise, especially near resonant frequencies, alveolar pressures can greatly exceed measured proximal pressures due to the induction of standing waves and gas trapping.

Under conventional ventilation, with bulk flow gas transport, alveolar ventilation depends upon frequency (f) and tidal (V_T) and dead space (V_D) volumes, $V_A = f(V_T - V_D)$. Clearly with jet ventilation, as V_T approaches or becomes less than V_D this relationship breaks down and gas transport has to occur by different methods (Table 2.3).

Table 2.3 Methods of gas transport during jet ventilation

Bulk flow of gas
Pendelluft
Coaxial flow
Taylor dispersion
Molecular diffusion

Although the relative importance of these mechanisms is still unclear, bulk flow still accounts for appreciable gas transport especially near to the major airways. Pendelluft movement of gas may be particularly pronounced in lungs with marked heterogeneity. It is likely that the contributions of the different mechanisms will change according to differences in lung pathology and ventilator settings. Predicting gas exchange as a result of ventilator settings is difficult under non bulk flow conditions, and generally $V_A \propto f V_T^2$.

The alveolar to capillary gas transport, as in conventional ventilation, depends upon matching $\dot{V}_A/\dot{Q}$ ratios. Thus the mean alveolar pressure and functional residual capacity play a considerable role. Because of the induction of standing waves or gas trapping mean airway pressure may significantly underestimate mean alveolar pressure. The easiest method to manipulate $P_{\overline{aw}}$ is the application of PEEP or increasing inspiratory time. Increasing inspiratory time will increase V_T and therefore V_A unless gas trapping occurs, in which case V_T will fall.

Studies by Carlton et al (1983) and MacIntyre et al (1986) with jet ventilation in adults have so far shown that reasonable gas exchange is possible with lower peak pressures but without improvement in outcome. The major problems related to the use of jet ventilation are due to inadequate humidification, physical damage due to jet impingement and gas trapping. Recently studies have started to be performed using ultra-high-frequency jet ventilators, the preliminary results of which suggest that it may be possible to gain a marked improvement in outcome. Other groups are looking at combining pressure-limited ventilation at low frequencies with jet ventilation in the hope of keeping the benefits of jet ventilation without its drawbacks.

Nitric oxide

Until the recognition by Moncada (Palmer et al 1987) in 1987 that nitric oxide (NO) was in fact endothelial-derived relaxing factor (EDRF) most anaesthetists considered that NO was a potentially very dangerous pollutant. Moncada et al (1991) have recently demonstrated that NO is a key biological molecule. In the body NO is synthesized from the terminal guanidino nitrogen of L-arginine and diffuses to the adjacent vascular endothelium, where it exerts its vasodilator effects via a cGMP-mediated pathway. Its biological half-life is about 3 s, being inactivated by extremely avid binding to haemoglobin, to which it binds 1500 times more strongly than carbon monoxide. NO undoubtedly plays a major role in hypoxic pulmonary vasoconstriction (HPV), hypoxia to a $PO_2 < 4$ kPa inhibiting the formation of NO and thereby leading to vasoconstriction. Because of the fact that NO is inactivated by contact with haemoglobin inhaled NO has the unique opportunity to produce pulmonary vasodilatation without having effects on the systemic circulation – an effect that cannot be achieved with the current intravenous vasodilators. NO functions in the pulmonary circulation even when there has been considerable damage to the endothelium by free radical attack, and this renders it even more useful.

The usual dose range is 20–80 p.p.m. although effects are sometimes seen at doses as low as 0.25 p.p.m. The effects of administration of NO are often dramatic (Frostell et al 1993, Hurford & Zapol 1994). There is a concentration dependent reduction in pulmonary hypertension due to a reduction in pulmonary vascular resistance. In some patients there is a consequential rise in right ventricular ejection fraction, indicating how valuable this reduction in right ventricular afterload can be. The changes in pulmonary artery pressures occur without any systemic changes. The pulmonary vasodilatation occurs within 3 min of commencing NO inhalation and disappears within 3 min of its withdrawal. Tachyphylaxis has not been seen even when NO has been used for up to 53 days. Importantly, Pison et al (1993) showed that the pulmonary vasodilatation caused by inhaling low levels of NO occurs in the region of the well-ventilated alveoli, giving rise to a marked reduction in intrapulmonary shunt and an improvement in PaO_2.

Inhaled NO is a potent bronchodilator. This may explain why occasionally there have been reports of bronchospasm following abrupt withdrawal of NO. The use of inhaled NO in ARDS has much to recommend it from a theoretical point of view since it should be distributed only to the ventilated and not the collapsed and fluid-filled alveoli. Rossaint et al (1993) have amply confirmed these theoretical advantages. The magnitude of the haemodynamic response to inhaled NO is dependent upon the degree of pulmonary hypertension present. This may be related to the fact that NO is usually produced in the lungs and it is possible that some patients with ARDS may have problems producing NO.

Safety of inhaled NO

The interest in the use of inhaled NO is tempered by concerns over its toxicity. NO is a common environmental pollutant and workplace exposure limits in the USA are currently set at 25 p.p.m. for an 8 h per day exposure. However, there are no long-term toxicology studies. The potential for NO toxicity is two-fold. When NO is avidly bound to haemoglobin the haemoglobin is converted to methaemoglobin. Usually methaemoglobin levels remain within the normal range during low-level NO therapy but this is not always the case. The rapid oxidation of NO to NO_2, which is then transformed into nitric and nitrous acids with the potential for severe lung injury, constitutes a far more worrying problem. Foubert et al (1993) have reported that the rate of this reaction is proportional to the oxygen concentration and the square of the NO concentration. As a result it is recommended that the concentration of NO and oxygen are kept as low as possible and the contact time within the ventilation system is kept as short as possible. In any case patients receiving NO therapy, inspired NO and NO_2 should be monitored and methaemoglobin levels assayed daily.

CONCLUSIONS

Over the last 10 years there have been enormous advances in our understanding of the management of severe lung injury. The concept of the *baby lung* has now been almost universally accepted and with this the consequent need for permissive hypercapnia. Together this has led to a complete rethinking of the ventilation strategy in severe lung injury. As a result tidal volumes of 5–8 ml/kg are now commonplace along with attempts to try to limit peak inflation pressures below 35–40 cmH$_2$O. In those patients unventilatable by conventional strategies, newer techniques such as inverse ratio ventilation may have a role, although at present this must still be considered somewhat experimental. For patients with pulmonary hypertension the addition of inhaled nitric oxide has much to recommend it, although long-term outcome studies are still awaited. The theoretical promise offered by jet ventilation has so far failed to be demonstrated despite several good clinical trials. Perhaps the most impressive finding regarding the ventilatory management of severe lung injury is that of Morris et al (1992) who showed that by careful attention to detail the mortality from conventional ventilatory techniques in severe lung injury can be vastly reduced.

REFERENCES

Amato M, Barbas C, Medeiros D et al 1993 Improved lung mechanics and oxygenation achieved through a new approach to mechanical ventilation in ARDS: the importance of reducing the 'mechanical stress' on the lung. Am Rev Respir Dis 147: A890

Carlton G C, Howland W S, Ray C et al 1983 High frequency jet ventilation: a prospective randomized evaluation. Chest 84: 551–559

Darioli R, Perret C 1984 Mechanical controlled hypoventilation in status asthmaticus. Am Rev Respir Dis 129: 385–387

Dreyfuss D, Soler P, Basset G et al 1988 High inflation pressure pulmonary edema: respective effects of high airway pressure, high tidal volume, and positive end-expiratory pressure. Am Rev Respir Dis 137: 1159–1164

East T, Böhm S, Wallace C et al 1992 A sucessful computerized protocol for clinical management of pressure control inverse ratio ventilation in ARDS patients. Chest 101: 697–710

Foubert L, Latimer R D, Oduro A 1993 Vasodilators (including angiotensin-converting enzyme inhibitors and coronary dilators). Curr Opin Anaesthesiol 6: 152–157

Frostell C G, Blomqvist H, Hedenstierna G et al 1993 Inhaled nitric oxide selectively reverses human hypoxic pulmonary vasoconstriction without causing systemic vasodilation. Anesthesiology 78: 427–435

Gattinoni L, Pesenti A, Bombino M et al 1988 Relationships between lung computed tomographic density, gas-exchange and PEEP in acute respiratory failure. Anesthesiology 69: 824–832

Gattinoni L, Pelosi P, Vitale G et al 1991 Body position changes redistribute lung computed tomographic density in patients with acute respiratory failure. Anesthesiology 74: 15–23

Gattinoni L, Pelosi P, Valenza F et al 1994 Patient positioning in acute respiratory failure. In: Tobin M J (ed) Principles and practice of mechanical ventilation. McGraw-Hill, New York, pp 1067–1076

Hickling K 1990 Ventilatory management of ARDS: can it affect the outcome? Intensive Care Med 16: 216–226

Hickling K, Henderson S, Jackson R 1990 Low mortality associated with low volume pressure limited ventilation with permissive hypercapnia in severe adult respiratory distress syndrome. Intensive Care Med 16: 372–377

Hurford W E, Zapol W M 1994 Nitric oxide inhalation in the intensive care unit. Curr Opinion Anaesthesiol 7: 153–160

Koller M H, Schuster D P 1995 The acute respiratory distress syndrome. N Engl J Med 332: 27–37

MacIntyre N R, Follett V, Deitz J L et al 1986 Jet ventilation at 100 bpm in adult respiratory failure. Am Rev Respir Dis 134: 897–901

Marcy T W 1994 Inverse ratio ventilation. In Tobin M J (ed) Principles and practice of mechanical ventilation. McGraw-Hill, New York, pp 319–331

Marcy T, Marini J 1991 Inverse ratio ventilation in ARDS: rationale and implementation. Chest 100: 494–504

Moncada S, Palmer R M J, Higgs E A 1991 Nitric oxide: physiology, pathophysiology and pharmacology. Pharmacol Rev 43: 109–142

Morris A, Wallace C, Clemer T et al 1992 Final report: computerized protocol controlled clinical trial of new therapy which includes $ECCO_2R$ for ARDS. Am Rev Respir Dis 145: A184

Palmer R M J, Ferrige A G, Moncada S 1987 Nitric oxide release accounts for the biological activity of endothelium-derived relaxation factor. Nature 327: 524–526

Pelosi P, D'Andrea L, Vitale G et al 1994 Vertical gradient of regional lung inflation in adult respiratory distress syndrome. Am J Respir Crit Care Med 149: 8–13

Pison U, Lopez F A , Heidelmeyer C F et al 1993 Inhaled nitric oxide reverses hypoxic pulmonary vasoconstriction without impairing gas exchange. J Appl Physiol 74: 1287–1292

Poelaert J I, Vogelaers D P, Colardyn F A 1991 Evaluation of the hemodynamic and respiratory effects of inverse ratio ventilation with a right ventricular ejection fraction catheter. Chest 99: 1444–1450.

Ranieri V M, Eissa N T, Corbeil C et al 1991 Effects of positive end-expiratory pressure on alveolar recruitment and gas exchange in patients with the adult respiratory distress syndrome. Am Rev Respir Dis 144: 544–551

Reynolds E 1971 Effects of alterations in mechanical ventilator settings on pulmonary gas exchange in hyaline membrane disease. Arch Dis Child 47: 152–159

Rossaint R, Falke K F, Lopez F et al 1993 Inhaled nitric oxide for the adult respiratory distress syndrome. N Engl J Med 328: 399–405

Tobin M T, Lodato R F 1989 Peep, auto PEEP and waterfalls. Chest 96: 449–451

3

Monitoring end-tidal carbon dioxide tension during anaesthesia

R. Fletcher

In this review of the use of end-tidal carbon dioxide monitoring in anaesthesia and intensive care, I will restrict myself to two main issues. The first is the use of capnography as a tool for monitoring metabolism and cardiopulmonary function. I will argue that in this latter role it has much in common with pulse oximetry, and is scarcely less valuable. Secondly, I will discuss the relationship between end-tidal and arterial carbon dioxide tension ($PE'CO_2$ and $PaCO_2$ respectively) and suggest some ways to improve non-invasive estimation of $PaCO_2$ from $PE'CO_2$ during mechanical ventilation.

CAPNOGRAPHY AS A GENERAL MONITORING TOOL DURING ANAESTHESIA

Figure 3.1 shows the chain of events involved in the transport of carbon dioxide, one of the end-products of metabolism, from its production in the cell to its elimination at the airway opening. The flux of carbon dioxide measured at the airway opening ($\dot{V}CO_2$), can be modified or interrupted at a number of points. Thus at the cellular level, stress, muscular activity (Fig. 3.2) and hyperthermia increase $\dot{V}CO_2$; anaesthesia, muscle relaxants and hypothermia reduce it. The first sign of malignant hyperthermia is an increase in cellular metabolism, leading to an increase in $\dot{V}CO_2$. Transport of venous blood from the tissues to the pulmonary capillary can be suddenly interrupted by surgical manipulation, cardiac arrest and arrhythmia, and other causes of reduced cardiac output. Hypovolaemia due to bleeding produces a more gradual reduction in $PE'CO_2$ (Fig. 3.3). Pulmonary embolism may prevent perfusion of all or part of the lung. Finally, cessation of or a reduction in ventilation, as in accidental disconnection, bronchial intubation, or a change in ventilatory volume due to changes in lung mechanics, will affect $\dot{V}CO_2$ and end-tidal $PE'CO_2$. During controlled ventilation, a reduction in $\dot{V}CO_2$ may be caused by a change in expired minute volume ($\dot{V}_E$) due to leakage from the tubing. With pressure-controlled ventilation, it may also be due to increased airway resistance or decreased compliance. If $PE'CO_2$ is suddenly and significantly reduced, but $\dot{V}_E$ is unchanged, pulmonary embolism should be strongly suspected (Fig. 3.4).

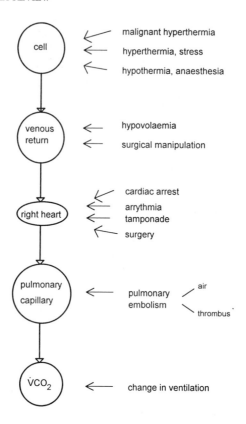

Fig. 3.1 Flow scheme to show the chain of events involved in the transport of carbon dioxide from the cell to the airway opening.

Oesophageal intubation is easily detected; absence of carbon dioxide after a couple of breaths is diagnostic. Rebreathing in closed systems, and even incorrect assembly of systems (Sames & Wilkinson 1994) can be detected with capnography.

Thus a sudden change in $PE'CO_2$ is as much a warning of a possible cardiopulmonary problem as is a sudden change in arterial blood oxygen saturation (SaO_2). In pulse oximetry, a change in SaO_2 does not tell the anaesthetist where the problem lies. It may be due to a change in inspired oxygen fraction, to reduced ventilation, or a right–left shunt due to atelectasis. Reduction in signal strength may also convey information, e.g. poor peripheral perfusion, and/or low cardiac output. The anaesthetist must consider each of these possibilities.

Similarly, with capnography, when $PE'CO_2$ changes, the anaesthetist must discover which step in the transport chain from mitochondrion to airway opening has been affected: cellular metabolism, pulmonary perfusion or ventilation. A change in the shape of the capnogram may assist diagnosis;

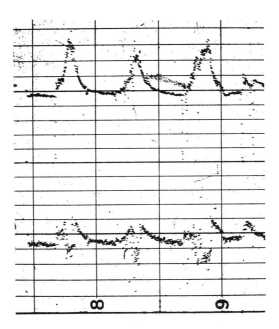

Fig. 3.2   Tracings obtained from a patient with tetanus. Upper tracing: minute carbon dioxide elimination, which shows cyclical increases approximately every 45 min. Lower tracing: PE′CO$_2$, which increases in parallel with $\dot{V}CO_2$. Some breaths are, however, interrupted by the patient triggering the ventilator, before expiration is complete, resulting in a lower PE′CO$_2$. Giving muscle relaxants would have prevented the enormous increases in muscle metabolism. (Courtesy of L. Nordström.)

e.g. cardiogenic oscillations in the case of pulmonary embolism, or a steeping of the slope of the 'alveolar plateau' in airways obstruction. It may be argued that hypoxia is the most important single catastrophe that can occur during anaesthesia, and therefore capnography is bound to be of less significance. The potential of capnography as a general cardiopulmonary function monitor has, however, been underestimated in most countries, the Netherlands being a notable exception (Smalhout & Kalenda 1975). More widespread use of capnography would have prevented many deaths caused by accidental oesophageal intubation.

It should also be noted that capnography gives breath-by-breath monitoring, whereas with pulse oximetry there is both biological and apparatus delay. During the operation of pulmonary banding, performed to reduce pulmonary perfusion in conditions such as ventricular septal defect, capnography gives an immediate indication of reduced pulmonary flow, whereas the pulse oximeter reacts considerably later. This delay can also be seen during surgery on the pulmonary vasculature in infants with Fallot's tetralogy (Fig. 3.5).

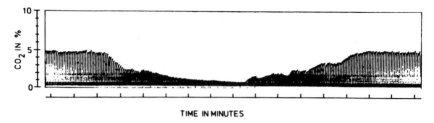

TIME IN MINUTES

Fig. 3.3 Reduction in PE′CO$_2$ due to hypovolaemia caused by bleeding. Reduced cardiac output and pulmonary artery pressure cause a large alveolar dead space and Pa′CO$_2$– PE′CO$_2$ difference. As the circulation is restored, PE′CO$_2$ rises again. (Courtesty of B. Jonson).

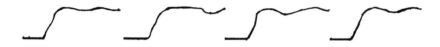

Fig. 3.4 Capnograms obtained from 14-year-old boy undergoing neurosurgery. PE′CO$_2$ had suddenly fallen from 4.5 kPa to 2.5 kPa and air could be heard in the heart. Note that, beause of cardiogenic oscillations, no two tracings have the same appearance – a diagnostic finding in pulmonary embolism.

CAN WE ESTIMATE PaCO$_2$ FROM PE′CO$_2$

All anaesthetists are familiar with the concept of a PaCO$_2$ to PE′CO$_2$ difference. Why are PaCO$_2$ and PE′CO$_2$ usually not equal? During anaesthesia with controlled or spontaneous ventilation, gas exchange is imperfect. This implies that alveolar PCO$_2$ and PaCO$_2$ are not in equilibrium, i.e. there is an alveolar dead space. The ideal ventilation/perfusion ratio is about 1; we have a cardiac output of about 5 litres, and the alveoli receive a ventilation of about 5 litres. Physiological or pathological conditions that create a spectrum of ventilation/perfusion ($\dot{V}/\dot{Q}$) ratios which differ from unity cause an alveolar dead space. How this affects gas exchange can be understood with the aid of simple lung models, such as were first used by Folkow & Pappenheimer (1955), Otis et al (1956) and Severinghaus & Stupfel (1957), in order to explain the relationship between $\dot{V}/\dot{Q}$ ratios and the lung's mechanical properties.

One group of individuals who demonstrate zero or very small PaCO$_2$– PE′CO$_2$ differences are infants and children (Fletcher et al 1986, Stokes et al 1986).

Model 1: children

Children have an almost perfect lung, here represented by a single compartment with an alveolar PCO$_2$ which is in equilibrium with PaCO$_2$ (Fig. 3.6). When expired carbon dioxide is plotted against expired volume (the

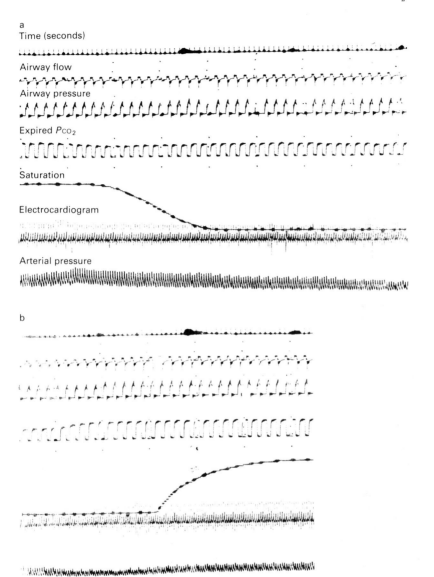

a
Time (seconds)

Airway flow

Airway pressure

Expired Pco$_2$

Saturation

Electrocardiogram

Arterial pressure

b

Fig. 3.5 These tracings were obtained during an operation for the creation of a Blalock–Taussig shunt in an infant with Fallot's tetralogy. The pulmonary vasculature proved to be unusually reactive; manipulation of the pulmonary artery caused an immediate increase in pulmonary vascular resistance and an increase in intracardiac right–left shunting. The figure shows that carbon dioxide elimination is reduced long before measured SaO$_2$. Similarly, carbon dioxide elimination recovers before the pulse oximeter has registered any improvement. Whereas the capnograph reacts to changes in pulmonary perfusion from breath to breath, there is biological and electronic delay before the pulse oximeter shows a change in SaO$_2$. The electronic delay is due to averaging; the biological delay is due to the time it takes for desaturated blood to reach the extremities. In the case of right-left shunting, there is further delay before the maximum change in SaO$_2$ is registered, as it takes time for the desaturated blood to circulate through the body and return to the left heart, further reducing SaO$_2$.

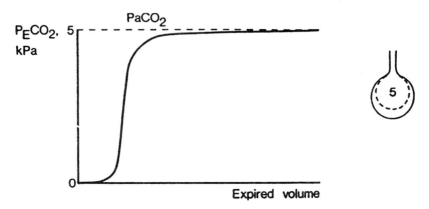

Fig. 3.6 Lung model 1: children. The lung is regarded as a single compartment – the vertical height of the lungs is too small to significantly affect the distribution of inspiratory gas or pulmonary flow. Arterial blood and alveolar gas are in equilibrium: zero $PaCO_2 - PE'CO_2$ difference. (From Fletcher 1980.)

carbon dioxide single breath test, $SBTCO_2$) or, less satisfactorily, against time (the capnogram) we find that phase III of the curve, the unfortunately named 'alveolar plateau', is almost horizontal. In other words, after the airway dead space gas has been washed out, expired gas PCO_2 is almost constant throughout the breath. $PaCO_2 - PE'CO_2$ is zero. In healthy children, a measurable $PaCO_2 - PE'CO_2$ may be seen during anaesthesia if atelectases have formed (Fig. 3.7), in which case it is caused partly by the 'apparent' dead space of right–left shunting (Fletcher & Larsson 1986; see model 4 below). Also interventions such as retracting the lung during thoracotomy (Fig. 3.8) may considerably affect carbon dioxide elimination.*

Model 2: adults

Even in healthy adults, the vertical height of the lung affects gas exchange and $PaCO_2 - PE'CO_2$ in two ways, through its effects on lung mechanics and pulmonary perfusion.

Gravity causes variation in alveolar size. At end-expiration the alveoli and airways in basal or dependent regions are 'squashed' (hence the reason for airway closure in older subjects), while in the uppermost 'non-dependent' regions the alveoli and airways are relatively expanded. Since dependent and non-dependent alveoli have different sizes at end-expiration, it follows that they function on different parts of their pressure–volume curves. This

---

* What slope there is to phase III in healthy children depends partly upon the continued generation of carbon dioxide into a shrinking alveolar compartment, and partly upon 'stratified inhomogeneity', i.e. variation in PCO_2 along the terminal respiratory unit (see model 2).

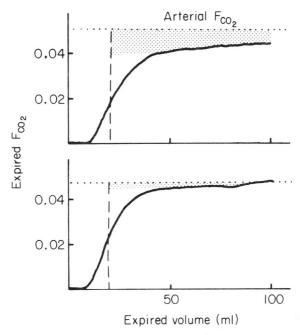

Fig. 3.7   Atelectasis. Carbon dioxide single-breath tests obtained from an 11-month-old child undergoing operation for coarctation of the aorta. The upper tracing shows an alveolar dead space caused by atelectasis, with a PaCO$_2$ – PE'CO$_2$ difference of 0.5 kPa. Functional residual capacity (FRC), measured by SF$_6$, at this time was 130 ml, PaO$_2$ was 13.4 kPa, with an FiO$_2$ of 0.5. The lower tracing was obtained after manual hyperinflation of the lungs, when FRC increased to 174 ml and PaO$_2$ increased to 36 kPa. Zero PaCO$_2$ – PE'CO$_2$ difference. (From Fletcher & Larsson 1986, reproduced with permission from the editor of *Anaesthesia*.)

affects their filling; although they are nominally 'in parallel', not only do they fill to different extents (i.e. their ventilation per unit volume varies), but also they fill and empty *asynchronously*. Variation in ventilation per unit volume amongst parallel compartments is an important cause of the $\dot{V}/\dot{Q}$ mismatch and PaCO$_2$ – PE'CO$_2$. The asynchronous emptying also causes expired PCO$_2$ to increase with increasing expired volume – see below.

Gravity also affects pulmonary perfusion. The lesser circulation is a low-pressure system, and thus while dependent regions are well perfused, non-dependent ones may be totally unperfused (West 1974). Thus gravity affects both ventilation and perfusion, which explains why even in *healthy* anaesthetized adults, some $\dot{V}/\dot{Q}$ mismatch is common, resulting in a measurable PaCO$_2$ – PE'CO$_2$ difference.

Airways disease. Thus $\dot{V}/\dot{Q}$ mismatch occurs to some extent in all adults, even in the awake state. During anaesthesia and in the presence of airways

---

* During controlled ventilation, variations in alveolar pressure may cause cyclical changes in pulmonary flow. However, this is probably a less important cause of $\dot{V}/\dot{Q}$ mismatch than gravity-dependent variation in ventilation and perfusion (Fletcher & Jonson 1984).

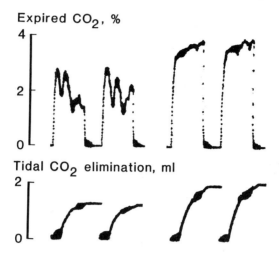

Expired CO$_2$, %

Tidal CO$_2$ elimination, ml

Fig. 3.8   Thoracotomy in a child. While the upper lung was retracted (first two tracings), the capnogram showed large variations in expired PCO$_2$. When the lung was released, the capnogram assumed a normal form and the volume of carbon dioxide eliminated increased. (Reproduced with permission from Fletcher R in: Hutton P, Prys-Roberts C eds. Anaesthesia and intensive care. Saunders, 1994.)

disease, e.g. asthma, bronchitis and emphysema, variations in ventilation per unit volume and the spread of $\dot{V}/\dot{Q}$ ratios are increased. Computer simulations of lung function show that it is the *variation* in airway resistance, rather than high resistance per se, that causes $\dot{V}/\dot{Q}$ spread. An increased inspiratory resistance obviously increases the work of breathing, but it is variation in resistance that causes some alveoli to fill preferentially and have low PCO$_2$s, and others to fill slowly and have high PCO$_2$s. This is always inefficient.

  Carbon dioxide elimination in airways disease. The factors that produce uneven ventilation and asynchronous emptying are also responsible for variations in ventilation/perfusion ratios and alveolar PCO$_2$ (West et al 1957a, 1957b). Thus well-ventilated, 'fast' alveoli, which empty early in expiration, have *by definition* the highest $\dot{V}/\dot{Q}$ ratios and therefore the lowest PCO$_2$ – the excreted carbon dioxide is diluted in the alveoli. Poorly ventilated alveoli empty late and have *by definition* the lowest $\dot{V}/\dot{Q}$ ratios and consequently the highest PCO$_2$ (alveolar PCO$_2$ approaches the venous level). This form of alveolar dead space has been described as having sequential causes. Figure 3.9 shows two 'parallel' compartments with different time constants, different $\dot{V}/\dot{Q}$ ratios and different PCO$_2$s. The 'alveolar plateau' slopes upwards. This reflects early emptying of low-PCO$_2$ alveoli and late emptying of high-PCO$_2$ alveoli, for the mechanism that delays filling also delays emptying (Otis et al 1956).

What causes the PaCO$_2$ – PE'CO$_2$ difference in airways disease?

The expirate is *ventilation weighted*; since most ventilation occurs by definition in high-$\dot{V}/\dot{Q}$, low-PCO$_2$ areas, the PCO$_2$ of the expirate tends to be

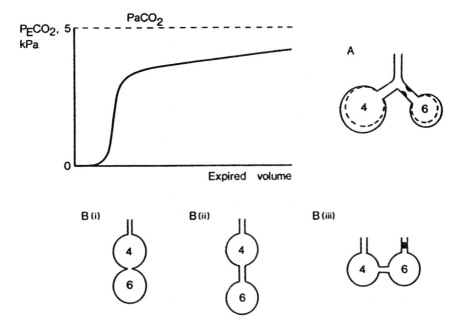

Fig. 3.9 Lung model 2: four mechanisms for 'sequential' alveolar dead space, the dead space commonly seen in adults. Model A illustrates uneven ventilation of asynchronously emptying **parallel** compartments with different pre-expiratory PCO$_2$s. Model B shows three possible **series** mechanisms (Cumming 1978) causing uneven ventilation secondary to defective mixing. Imperfect inert gas mixing (i) has been demonstrated even in the absence of gravity (Michels & West 1978). In centrilobular emphysema (ii) such 'series' mixing defects may be grossly exaggerateed. Thus the last part of the unit to empty has the highest PCO$_2$, which again contributes to the slope of phase III. Finally, West (1971) describes how a similar effect can be obtained due to collateral ventilation. When the respiratory bronchiole is obstructed (iii) morphologically **parallel** units can be ventilated in **series** via adjacent units. All three models thus show late emptying of high-PCO$_2$ alveoli, whether at the regional level or within the level of the terminal respiratory units. In each case the differences in pre-expiratory PCO$_2$ are secondary to uneven ventilation, although probably over-perfusion of the lung as in congenital heart disease with left–right shunting may contribute to model A. (From Fletcher 1980.)

low. The composition of the arterial blood is, however, *perfusion-weighted*. PaCO$_2$ must therefore reflect the high PCO$_2$ of well perfused but poorly ventilated alveoli. It is this difference in the weightings of the expirate and arterial blood that causes the PaCO$_2$ – PE$'$CO$_2$ difference.

Other mechanisms. Traditional thinking has centred on the concept of 'parallel, between units' mechanisms for dead space, i.e. compartments with different pre-expiratory PCO$_2$s, emptying asynchronously. Cumming (1978) suggests the presence of *series* dead space. He describes (G. Cumming, personal communication 1979) a *within-units* mixing defect – 'stratified inhomogeneity in the terminal respiratory unit' – in which the degree of mixing varies axially along the unit, the worst ventilated, lowest $\dot{V}/\dot{Q}$ (highest PCO$_2$) alveoli being found distally or peripherally (Fig. 3.9B). Additional evidence for this can be found in the data of Michels & West (1978) obtained during aircraft 'zero g' dives. With the effect of gravity on the lung abolished, the alveolar plateau for various inert gases still demonstrated a slight slope, even in healthy subjects. This is evidence of a within-units mixing defect (Cumming 1979).

Alveolar dead space in both healthy adults and those with lung disease can thus be explained by both parallel and series mechanisms; all lead to a sloping alveolar plateau.

Is the $PaCO_2 - PE'CO_2$ difference constant?

We thus expect to find a significant $PaCO_2 - PE'CO_2$ during anaesthesia with controlled or spontaneous ventilation in adults. The magnitude of this $PaCO_2 - PE'CO_2$ depends to a significant extent on the ventilatory pattern. One can deduce from Figure 3.9 that *increasing tidal volume* (V_T) *should reduce $PaCO_2 - PE'CO_2$*, and decreasing V_T should increase it. Table 3.1, based on Fletcher & Jonson (1984), shows the results of an investigation in which patients were ventilated at two different ventilator settings, which gave the same $PaCO_2$. $PaCO_2 - PE'CO_2$ was significantly less with low frequency, large tidal volume ventilation. Figure 3.10 shows the individual values in patients in the same study.

Also, those patients who demonstrated the greatest difference in $PaCO_2 - PE'CO_2$ between the two ventilator settings were those who had the steepest sloping 'alveolar plateaus'. The reason for this is that the patients with the steepest slopes are those that have the most uneven ventilation and thus greatest spread of $\dot{V}/\dot{Q}$ ratios. These subjects therefore benefit most from the change to low-frequency, large tidal volume ventilation. At small tidal volumes, the inspiratory gas goes chiefly to non-dependent, 'fast', high $\dot{V}/\dot{Q}$, low-PCO_2 compartments. When inspiratory time and tidal volume are increased, dependent, 'slow', low-$\dot{V}/\dot{Q}$, high-PCO_2 compartments receive proportionately more gas, and thus make a greater contribution to the expirate (Rehder et al 1977). Another effect of more even distribution of the inspirate at larger tidal volumes is that the slope of the alveolar plateau is reduced (Fletcher & Jonson 1984).

The rather linear, upward sloping phase III seen in most patients suggests that further increase in V_T would result in $PaCO_2 - PE'CO_2$ becom-

Table 3.1 Comparison of $PaCO_2$-$PE'CO_2$ at two different ventilator settings in 79 patients. Mean $Paco_2$ in both groups was 4.2 kPa

	Mean ventilatory rate (min⁻¹)	Mean tidal volume (litres)	Median $PaCO_2 - PE'CO_2$ (kPa)
Small tidal volumes	16	0.46	0.67
Large tidal volumes	9	0.75	0.41***

***$p < 0.001$ compared to other setting.

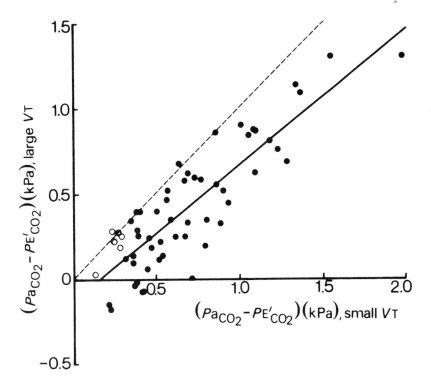

Fig. 3.10 PaCO$_2$– PE′CO$_2$ differences during small tidal volume, relatively high-frequency ventilation related to the same variable at large tidal volume, low-frequency ventilation. (Reproduced from Fletcher & Jonson 1984, with permission from the editor of the British Journal of Anaesthesia.)

ing zero; this may in fact occur at steady state at large tidal volumes. This does not imply a zero dead space, however, since $\dot{V}/\dot{Q}$ scatter (implicit in a sloping phase III) is *always associated with an alveolar dead space* (West 1969).

PaCO$_2$ – PE′CO$_2$ differences in the anaesthetic patient population: the effect of age and smoking.

Figure 3.11 shows the spread of values encountered in adults (and children) during anaesthesia with controlled ventilation. The older the patient, the more difficult it is to estimate PaCO$_2$ from PE′CO$_2$! However, the estimate may be improved by knowledge of the patient's smoking history (Fletcher 1987) and by performing a simple ventilatory manoeuvre (Fletcher 1993) – see below.

The relationship between age and PaCO$_2$ – PE′CO$_2$ is influenced by smoking habits (Figure 3.12). In non-smokers, and in those ex-smokers who had ceased smoking more than 6 months previously, we found no age dependent increase in either dead space fraction (Fletcher & Jonson 1981)

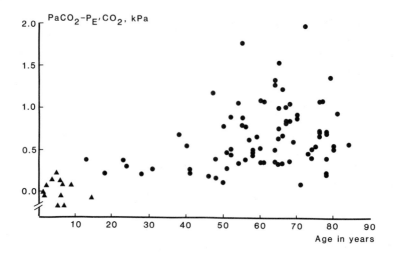

Fig. 3.11 $PaCO_2 - PE'CO_2$ differences during anaesthesia with controlled ventilation. The circles represent adult patients (from Fletcher & Jonson 1984). The triangles represent children with normal pulmonary circulation (from Fletcher et al 1986). Reproduced with permission from: Hutton P, Prys-Roberts C eds. Anaesthesia and intensive care. Saunders, 1994.

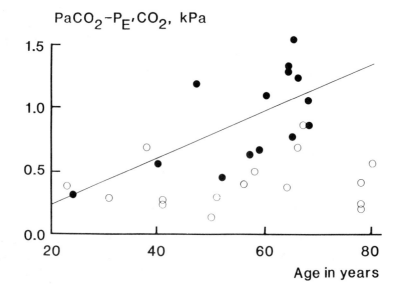

Fig. 3.12 Relationship between $PaCO_2 - PE'CO_2$, age and smoking habits in patients ventilated at a mean rate of 17 breaths per minute. Open circles = non-smokers and ex-smokers. Closed circles = smokers. The regression line refers only to the group of smokers ($r = 0.64$, $p = 0.02$); non- and ex-smokers showed no relationship between $PaCO_2 - PE'CO_2$ and age. (Reproduced from Fletcher 1987, with permission from the editor of Acta Anaesthesiologica Scandinavica.)

or in $PaCO_2 - PE'CO_2$. However, in smokers, $PaCO_2 - PE'CO_2$ increased significantly with age (Fletcher 1987). In a later study in which there were proportionately more ex-smokers, the same trend was found, although no longer statistically significant (Fletcher 1993). However, the more recent study demonstrated that smokers and ex-smokers over the age of 65 years nevertheless had a different response to changes in ventilator setting compared to non-smokers of any age. If whilst ventilating patients at a rate of 20 min^{-1} one suddenly halves the ventilatory rate, the response of the $PE'CO_2$ during the next few breaths can be instructive. In patients with good lung function $PE'CO_2$ is reduced; in those with poor function it can increase by $0.1-0.4$ kPa. The magnitude of the increase is positively correlated to the original $PaCO_2 - PE'CO_2$ at the higher frequency (Fletcher 1993).

Can the $PaCO_2 - PE'CO_2$ difference ever be negative at steady state? In principle, yes. It should be remembered that end-tidal sampled gas represents gas from the lowest-$\dot{V}/\dot{Q}$, highest-PCO_2 alveoli; $PaCO_2$ represents the temporal, perfusion-weighted mean of all alveolar PCO_2s. Thus negative $PaCO_2 - PE'CO_2$ differences may arise without implying active excretion of carbon dioxide against a concentration gradient. Negative $PaCO_2 - PE'CO_2$ differences have been reported during exercise (Jones et al 1979), probably because alveolar PCO_2 varies cyclically more when VCO_2, ventilation and cardiac output are increased. During anaesthesia with controlled ventilation we found that 9 of 79 patients ventilated at frequencies of 9–10 min^{-1} had small negative differences of -0.01 to -0.17 kPa (Fletcher & Jonson 1984). Some of these negative differences could of course be due to experimental error (see below).

UNUSUAL CAUSES OF INCREASED $PaCO_2-PE'CO_2$

Model 3: pulmonary embolism

In pulmonary embolism, perfused and unperfused compartments may have similar mechanical properties, but contribute differing PCO_2s to the expirate. In Figure 3.13, compartments A and B give PCO_2s of 5 and 0 kPa respectively, so that mixed alveolar gas has a PCO_2 of 2.5 kPa, while $PaCO_2$ is 5 kPa. In reality, even in regions whose pulmonary artery is totally occluded, some carbon dioxide is found in the alveoli. Bronchial artery perfusion causes some carbon dioxide elimination in 'unperfused' alveoli, and carbon dioxide-rich gas from the airway dead space is aspirated at the beginning of each inspiration. Furthermore, local homeostatic reflexes may reduce ventilation of the unperfused lung compartment.

In this model, unperfused alveoli empty synchronously with perfused alveoli. This is alveolar dead space of *non-sequential* causes, and is associated with a flat 'alveolar plateau'. In fact, the combination of a flat 'alveolar plateau' with a large alveolar dead space and large (e.g. 2–3 kPa) $PaCO_2 -$

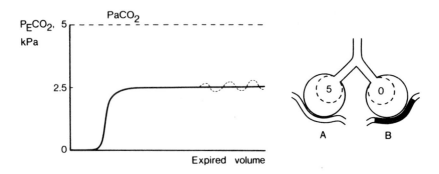

Fig. 3.13 Model 3: pulmonary embolism – alveolar dead space of non-sequential causes. Alveolus A is unperfused; its PCO_2 is therefore zero. Cardiogenic oscillations may be seen (dotted line). (From Fletcher 1980.)

$PE'CO_2$ difference is virtually diagnostic of pulmonary embolism (Eriksson et al 1985)(but see model 4).

Another pathognomonic sign of pulmonary embolism is the presence of cardiogenic oscillations (Fowler & Read 1961). These are due to the action of the heart, which by its cycle influences the filling and emptying of adjacent pulmonary segments. If some of these segments contain alveolar gas with low PCO_2, and others have a high PCO_2, then the PCO_2 of the expirate will vary in synchrony with the cardiac cycle. Figure 3.4 shows a capnogram obtained from a patient in whom air embolism occurred during neurosurgery (in spite of use of the supine position!).

Model 4: right–left shunting

In atelectasis and cyanotic heart disease, some venous blood reaches the left side of the heart without passing through the capillaries of ventilated alveoli. The right–left shunt thus formed affects not only arterial oxygenation but also carbon dioxide elimination; since the venous blood is rich in carbon dioxide, $PaCO_2$ must be higher than alveolar capillary PCO_2 and therefore higher than $PE'CO_2$. The single breath test appears as in Figure 3.14. It will be noticed that there is a close resemblance to the state of affairs in pulmonary embolism, in which a large alveolar dead space and large $PaCO_2 - PE'CO_2$ is observed; however, there are no cardiogenic oscillations.

Does the increased $PaCO_2 - PE'CO_2$ in cyanotic heart disease imply an alveolar dead space? The answer to this question rather depends on one's definition of dead space. If dead space implies the presence of compartments with high or infinite $\dot{V}/\dot{Q}$ ratios, then the derangement of gas exchange associated with cyanotic heart disease is not a dead space; in fact a right–left shunt represents an area of zero $\dot{V}/\dot{Q}$, since $\dot{V}$ for the shunted blood is zero. However, seen from the child's point of view, all the drawbacks of a dead space are present. Compared to a normal child, the 'blue

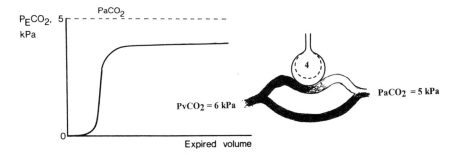

Fig. 3.14   Model 4: right–left intracardiac shunting. Venous blood, PCO$_2$ 6 kPa, is mixed with blood from the pulmonary veins, PCO$_2$ 4 kPa, to produce a PaCO$_2$ of 5 kPa (approximately.) Since pulmonary vein and alveolar gas are in equilibrium, PE´CO$_2$ is also 4 kPa. PaCO$_2$ – PE´CO$_2$ is thus about 1 kPa. Observe that, in orde to clear the blood of a given volume of carbon dioxide, the child mut have a greater ventilatory volume than a normal child. Intrapulmonary shunting produces the same picture. See also Table 3.2

baby' has to increase its work of breathing in order to eliminate a given $\dot{V}CO_2$. This increased ventilation is necessary because, in order to maintain a PaCO$_2$ of say 5 kPa, alveolar PCO$_2$ must be 'hyperventilated' down to say 4 kPa, implying a veno-alveolar PCO$_2$ difference of 2 kPa as against the normal 1 kPa. One way of circumventing the ambiguity is to use the terms *apparent* or *virtual* to describe the dead space associated with right–left shunting.

Table 3.2 compares some blood gas values at different stages in the central circulation in normal and cyanotic children. In this case the cyanotic child has a PaCO$_2$ – PE´CO$_2$ difference of 1 kPa with an arterial oxygen saturation of 75%; this is compatible with a haemoglobin level of about 180 g/litre.

Thus, in right–left shunting, arterial desaturation and an PaCO$_2$ – PE´CO$_2$ difference go hand in hand. Figure 3.15 shows the theoretical relationship; as a rule of thumb, each 10% reduction in SaO$_2$ is associated with an obligatory increase in the PaCO$_2$ – PE´CO$_2$ difference of about 0.4 kPa (Fletcher 1991). The relationship is influenced chiefly by haemoglobin (Hb) concentration, but even by PaCO$_2$ and respiratory quotient (RQ). The

Table 3.2   Gas exchange variables in a child with a 50% right–left intracardiac shunt.

		Right heart blood	Pulmonary capillary blood	End-tidal gas	Arterial blood	Arterial–end-tidal differences
Normal child	PCO$_2$ (kPa)	6	5	5	5	0
	O$_2$ saturation (%)	70	100		100	
Cyanotic child	PCO$_2$ (kPa)	6	4	4	5	1
50% RL shunt	O$_2$ saturation (%)	50	100		75	

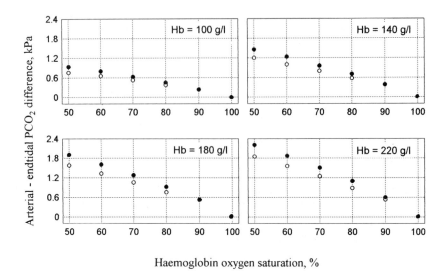

Fig. 3.15   Theoretical relationship between $PaCO_2 - PE'CO_2$, SaO_2, haemoglobin concentration and $PaCO_2$ in cyanotic children. The upper, infilled circles are for $PaCO_2 = 5$ kPa, the lower open circles are for $PaCO_2 = 4$ kPa. Hb concentration, $PaCO_2$ and respiratory quotient are the principal factors that modify the relationship between $PaCO_2 - PE'CO_2$ and SaO_2. RQ is assumed to be 0.8.

greater the Hb, the greater the effect of desaturation on $Paco_2 - PE'CO_2$. (If the arterial – pulmonary end-capillary oxygen difference is large because of a high Hb concentration, then the arterial – pulmonary end-capillary carbon dioxide difference must also be large, in order to preserve the RQ.)

$PaCO_2 - PE'CO_2$ during thoracic surgery

During thoracic surgery in the lateral position, the vertical height of the thorax is greater than in the supine position, and thus the effect of gravity on lung mechanics, i.e. uneven ventilation, and on perfusion, is increased. In accordance with West's concepts (West 1974), one would expect to find unperfused alveoli in the upper lung, especially when pulmonary arterial pressure is low. In fact, dead space and the arterial–end-tidal difference do decrease as pulmonary artery pressure increases (O. Werner personal communication 1992, Werner et al 1984a).

When the pleura is opened, the upper lung assumes a new pressure/volume characteristic. It fills and empties more easily and therefore receives a greater proportion of the tidal volume than in the intact thorax. In addition, its perfusion also increases, leading to increased upper lung carbon dioxide elimination (Werner et al 1984b). (Figure 3.8 shows the effect on carbon dioxide elimination of *retracting* the upper lung during thoracotomy in a child.) If PE′CO$_2$ is measured in both lungs simultaneously, i.e. using two capnographs, then upper lung PE′CO$_2$ is always less than lower lung PE′CO$_2$ (Werner et al 1984b). The difference between the two values is least when the pleura is open.

One-lung ventilation (OLV) can be expected to affect the PaCO$_2$ – PE′CO$_2$ difference. Following Werner's observation (personal communication 1992), one would expect perhaps that the alveolar dead space, and therefore PaCO$_2$ – PE′CO$_2$, would decrease when the switch is made from two-lung to one-lung ventilation, since the potential alveolar dead space of the over-ventilated, under-perfused upper lung is now eliminated. But in fact, PaCO$_2$ – PE′CO$_2$ during OLV is as great as during two-lung ventilation; it ranges from 0.2 to 2.5 kPa (Yam et al 1994). A probable reason for this is that OLV creates a large right–left shunt through the unventilated lung (Malmkvist et al 1989), and this can be expected to create a large PaCO$_2$ – PE′CO$_2$ difference – see lung model 4.

Why prefer the plot of expired PCO$_2$ against volume to expired PCO$_2$ against time?

Only by plotting PaCO$_2$ against volume can one use the information available in the expirate. During controlled ventilation, expiration takes the form of a 'die-way' exponential, and therefore most of the expirate leaves early. On the time plot, the main changes in expired PCO$_2$ are thus compressed into a small space. Later in the expiration, a flat 'alveolar plateau' may appear, but this contains very little information as the expiratory flow rate is low. To the untrained observer, even patients with marked expiratory obstruction can appear to have a normal tracing on the time plot! In addition, if one plots percentage carbon dioxide or FCO$_2$ against volume, the area under the curve becomes the volume of carbon dioxide in the breath, from which dead space ratios and V̇CO$_2$ can be calculated. The area under the curve of carbon dioxide plotted against time has no useful units.

A note on the measurement of PaCO$_2$ – PE′CO$_2$ differences

The measurement of PaCO$_2$ – PE′CO$_2$ differences requires analysis of both expired gas and blood gas PCO$_2$. Thus the capnograph and the blood gas analyser must be cross-calibrated, i.e. agree with each other when presented with gas and blood samples with the same PCO$_2$. Failure to cross-calibrate can lead to large errors in measured PaCO$_2$ – PE′CO$_2$ (Fletcher 1995).

To avoid such errors in a scientific study only one capnograph and one blood gas analyser should be used. When purchasing test gases with which to calibrate the capnograph, e.g. 4–5% carbon dioxide in equal parts nitrous oxide/oxygen, the manufacturer's claimed carbon dioxide content should be ignored. Instead one should assume that the blood gas analyser is correct – indeed, since blood gas analysers cannot be calibrated, one has no choice! One then determines the carbon dioxide content of the test gas via the blood gas analyser. Previously I have done this by tonometry, but some newer blood gas analysers allow measurement of gas PCO_2 directly. The injected gas is analysed in a wet environment, i.e. fully saturated. This method could admittedly lead to absolute values for $\dot{V}CO_2$ being incorrect, but the drawback is outweighed by the knowledge that dead space fractions can be accurately measured.

REFERENCES

Cumming G 1978 In: Kock M A et al (ed) Mechanics of airways obstruction in human respiratory disease. Balkema, Cape Town, p 237

Eriksson L, Wollmer P, Jonson B et al 1985 The diagnosis of pulmonary embolism. Clin Physiol 5 suppl 3: 111–115

Fletcher R 1980 The single breath test for carbon dioxide. MD Thesis, Lund, Sweden. (May be obtained from author.)

Fletcher R 1987 Smoking, age and arterial–endtidal CO_2 difference during anaesthesia. Acta Anaesthesiol Scand 31: 355–356

Fletcher R 1991 The relationship between the arterial to end-tidal PCO_2 difference and hemoglobin saturation in congenital heart disease. Anesthesiology 75: 210–216

Fletcher R 1993 Can one predict arterial PCO_2 from endtidal? Br J Anaesth 71: 316–317P

Fletcher R 1995 In deadspace studies, capnograph and bloodgas analyzer should be cross-calibrated with the same gas. Br J Anaesth 74: 485P

Fletcher R, Jonson B 1981 Prediction of the physiological dead space/tidal volume ratio during anaesthesia/IPPV from simple preoperative tests. Acta Anaesthesiol Scand 25: 58–62.

Fletcher R, Jonson B 1984 Deadspace and the single breath test for CO_2 during anaesthesia/IPPV. Br J Anaesth 56: 109–119

Fletcher R, Larsson A 1986 Gas exchange during atelectasis. Anaesthesia 40: 1186–1188

Fletcher R, Niklason L, Drefeldt B 1986 Gas exchange during controlled ventilation in children with normal and abnormal pulmonary circulation. Anesth Analg 65: 645–652

Folkow B, Pappenheimer I R 1955 Components of the respiratory dead space and their variation with pressure breathing and with bronchoactive drugs. J Appl Physiol 8: 102–110

Fowler K T, Read J 1961 Cardiac oscillations in expired gas tensions, and regional pulmonary blood flow. J Appl Physiol 16: 863–868

Jones N L, Robertson D G, Kane J W 1979 Difference between end-tidal and arterial PCO_2 in exercise. J Appl Physiol 47: 954–960

Malmkvist G, Fletcher R, Nordström L, Werner O 1989 Effects of lung surgery and one-lung ventilation on pulmonary arterial pressure, venous admixture and immediate postoperative lung function. Br J Anaesth 63: 696–701

Michels D B, West J B 1978 Distribution of pulmonary ventilation and perfusion during short periods of weightlessness. J Appl Physiol 45: 987–998

Rehder K, Sessler A D, Rodarte J R 1977 Regional intrapulmonary gas distribution in awake and anesthetized–paralyzed man. J Appl Physiol 42: 391–402

Sames M, Wilkinson D J 1994 Capnography alerts to major breathing system fault. Anaesthesia 49: 167–168

Severinghaus J W, Stupfel M 1957 Alveolar dead space as an index of distribution of blood flow in pulmonary capillaries. J appl Physiol 10: 349–355

Smalhout B, Kalenda Z 1975 An atlas of capnography. Kerckebosch, Zeist, Netherlands.

Stokes M A, Hughes D G, Hutton P 1986 Capnography in small subjects. Br J Anaesth 58: 814P

Otis A B, McKerrow C B, Barlett R A et al 1956 Mechanical factors in distribution of pulmonary ventilation. J Appl Physiol 8: 427–434

Werner O, Malmkvist G, Beckman A, Stahle S, Nordström L 1984a Carbon dioxide elimination from each lung during endobronchial anaesthesia. Br J Anaesth 56: 995–1001

Werner O, Malmkvist G, Beckman A, Stahle S, Nordström L 1984b Gas exchange and haemodynamics during thoracotomy. Br J Anaesth 56: 1343–1349

West J B 1969 Ventilation–perfusion inequality and overall gas exchange in computer models of the lung. Respir Physiol 7: 88–110

West J B 1971 Causes of carbon dioxide retention in lung disease. N Engl J Med 284: 1232–1236

West J B 1974 Respiratory physiology: the essentials. Williams & Wilkins, Baltimore

West J B, Fowler K T, Hugh-Jones P, O'Donnell T V 1957a The measurement of the inequality of ventilation and of perfusion in the lung by analysis of single expirates. Clin Sci 16: 529–545

West J B, Fowler K T, Hugh-Jones P, O'Donnell T V 1957b The measurement of the inequality of ventilation and of perfusion in the lung by analysis of single expirates. Clin Sci 16: 549–564

Yam P C I, Innes P A, Jackson M et al 1994 Variation in the arterial to end-tidal PCO$_2$ difference during one-lung thoracic anaesthesia. Br J Anaesth 72: 21–24

4

The spinal cord and chronic pain

R. Munglani   S. P. Hunt   J. G. Jones

There is now increasing evidence that the spinal cord is not simply a passive route carrying peripheral sensation to the brain but instead the spinal cord may considerably modify incoming information. Thus what is perceived by the brain may bear very little relation to the nature and intensity of the peripheral stimulation. This is often the case in some patients with chronic pain, where seemingly light touch on the skin may give rise to agonizing sensations. In the last decade intensive research has led to increased understanding of these modulatory mechanisms in the spinal cord and some of these are described in this chapter. Potential future therapies for chronic pain based on this work as well as implications for present-day treatment are then outlined.

MODELS AND NEURONAL MECHANISMS OF CENTRAL SENSITIZATION

The dorsal horn of the spinal cord is the site of termination of the majority of primary afferent fibres. It is important to note that there is a distinct difference in the termination sites of nociceptive and non-nociceptive nerve fibres. Thus, the fast-conducting low-threshold Aβ fibres which carry touch and pressure sensations terminate in layers 3 and 4 whilst the high-threshold slower-conducting C and Aδ fibres, which carry pain and temperature information, terminate in layers 1, 2 and 5 (see Fig. 4.1 and Willis & Coggeshall 1991).

In a recent review Woolf (1994) has defined four stimulus-processing states of the dorsal horn of the spinal cord:

1. Control state.
2. Suppressed state.
3. Sensitised state.
4. Reorganized state.

In state 1 – the control or normal state of the dorsal horn – low-intensity stimulation such as touch, brushing and pressure is perceived as innocuous whilst high-intensity stimulation, whether mechanical, chemical or

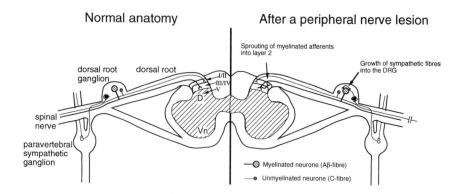

Fig. 4.1 A simplified diagram of primary afferent innervation into the spinal cord. The normal anatomy is shown on the left with the small unmyelinated C fibres which carry pain-innervating layers 1 and 2 (and also layer 5, not shown). The large myelinated Aβ fibre innervates layers 3 and 4. After injury, nerve sprouting and cell death may occur in the spinal cord and the dorsal root ganglia (DRG), which may lead to the setting of chronic pain states. D=dorsal horn of spinal cord; Vn=ventral horn of spinal cord. See text for more details (Adapted from Janig and McLachlan, 1994).

thermal, is perceived as pain. In state 2 – the suppressed state – the spinal cord *fails* to register high-intensity stimulation as painful because of inhibition by a variety of mechanisms, including segmental inhibition by Aβ fibres (Melzack & Wall 1965), counter-irritation or descending inhibition from higher centres (Fields & Basbaum 1994). In state 3, the dorsal horn is sensitized and has an exaggerated response to all types of stimulation. Low-intensity stimulation (transmitted via the Aβ fibres) is now perceived as painful mechanical allodynia,[1] whilst high-intensity stimulation, which is normally painful (transmitted via the C and Aδ fibres), leads to an *exaggerated* pain response known as hyperalgesia.[2] State 3 is commonly seen after surgery, that is, the phenomenon of post-injury hypersensitivity, and also in situations where there is continued high-intensity afferent nerve activity into the spinal cord, e.g. from arthritic joints. State 4, the reorganized state of the dorsal horn, has many of the features of state 3 but is more prolonged in duration and may be associated with structural changes leading to reorganization of the circuitry of the dorsal horn and the dorsal root ganglia (see below).

The model described above treats the spinal cord as a 'black box' and emphasizes the role of the spinal cord in amplification or reduction of the afferent signal. However, a more mechanistic model has to explain the following features that are seen in chronic pain states (from Price et al 1994):

---

[1] Allodynia is clinically defined as the perception of non-nociceptive stimulation such as light touch or pressure as painful.

[2] Hyperalgesia is defined as a leftward shift of the stimulus–response function that relates magnitude of pain to stimulus intensity (Meyer et al 1994).

1. The body area within which pain is experienced often enlarges as the pain intensity increases – this is commonly known as radiation of pain.
2. The perceived pain often outlasts the stimulus that evokes it.
3. Repeated nociceptive stimulation may evoke a slow temporal summation of the perceived pain which is often described in terms of burning, throbbing or aching symptoms. This occurs despite there being no increase in the intensity of the individual nociceptive stimuli.

All three of these features have been shown to depend on central mechanisms, which will be briefly described. Generally speaking, the increasing *intensity* of peripheral stimulus is encoded by a primary afferent nerve fibre as increasing *frequency* of discharge. Further information about a given stimulus on the body is provided by the *number* of primary afferent nerves activated. This is because the area of skin that a single nociceptive primary afferent innervates is small (<1 cm^2) and further increases in intensity of stimulation will tend not to activate more primary afferent fibres. Instead the clinical observation of pain radiating several dermatomes above and below the site of nociceptive stimulation may be explained by the dispersion of the primary afferent input up and down the spinal cord by the propriospinal connections (Yezierski et al 1980). These nerve tracts form interconnections between a number of adjacent segments and are located in layers V–VI of the spinal cord – an area which also contains the neurones of the spinothalamic tracts, including the wide dynamic range (WDR) neurones. The WDR neurone is so called because it can accurately encode a range of afferent stimuli from light touch to intense pain – something that primary afferent neurones cannot do. The receptive field size of the WDR neurones is vast compared to that of the primary afferent neurones and this reflects the degree of convergence of primary afferents and propriospinal tracts upon the WDR neurones. Two observations would help to explain radiation of pain; (1) the receptive field size of a WDR neurone depends on the type of stimulation, being larger for nociceptive stimulation than for light touch; and (2) increasing nociceptive stimulation recruits more WDR neurones. The prolonged responses and temporal summation of pain described earlier may be due to prolonged increases in the activity of the spinothalamic WDR neurones. These long-lived responses of the WDR neurones may occur in response to only brief discharges in C and Aδ fibres. Furthermore, in chronic pain states the usual inhibitory effect of Aβ fibres on C and Aδ activity (state 2 processing) may also be lost on WDR neurones, so that Aβ activity may actually *enhance* the output of the WDR neurones (see Coghill et al 1991).

Woolf (1983) showed that C fibre activation led to prolonged and increased responses in a flexion withdrawal model in the rat. Furthermore this increased excitability was maintained even after inputs from the injured paw were blocked by local anaesthesia. The conclusion was that only central sensitization rather than sensitization of the peripheral neurones could explain this. Another piece of evidence for central sensitization was that of 'wind-up' by nociceptive-specific and WDR neurones within the dorsal horn (Mendell 1966, Davies & Lodge 1987, Dickenson & Sullivan 1987, Dickenson 1994) (see Fig. 4.2). Wind-up is a frequency-dependent phenomenon. Low-frequency (0.1 Hz) C fibre afferent input gives a constant response from the dorsal horn neurones; however stimulation frequencies of 0.5 Hz or above cause a large increase in the response of the dorsal horn neurone. It has been suggested that the slowly increasing intense pain that can be seen in some chronic pain conditions such as neuralgias and reflex sympathetic dystrophy may be related to wind-up. However, direct attribution of chronic pain symptoms to the wind-up phenomenon must be treated with some caution since the increased responsiveness of the neurones only continues for 5 min or so after the initial stimulus and then declines. In the brain, memory formation is accompanied by an electrophysiological event called long-term potentiation (LTP); this has also been demonstrated in dorsal horn neurones of the spinal cord (see Randic et al 1993 and references within). In typical experiments, 3 s episodes of high-frequency input cause a sensitized state to be set up. In this state, lower-intensity afferent stimulation will give rise to an enhanced output from the dorsal horn neurones for up to 60 min or more. It may be that in chronic pain states, a longer-lived wind-up or LTP-type phenomena exist in the spinal cord, or else maintenance of a central sensitized state by further peripheral stimuli is required (see below). The mechanisms so far described

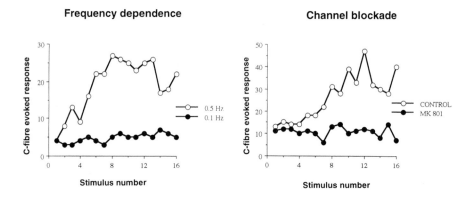

Fig. 4.2   Shows how wind-up in the dorsal horn depends on the frequency of stimulation and can be blocked by NMDA receptor antagonists. In this case MK-801, a non-competitive blocker of the NMDA channel at the PCP site, has been used (see also Fig. 4.3). On the x-axis is shown the number of primary afferent C fibre strength impulses. On the y-axis is shown the response of the dorsal horn neurone to the increasing number of impulses. As the total number of impulses rises, there is an enhanced response from the neurone. Low frequencies of impulse repetition do not induce wind-up. Wind-up can also be blocked by NMDA channel blockade with MK-801. See text for more details. (Adapted from Dickenson 1994, with permission.)

i.e. (1) the presence of the propriospinal system, (2) loss of the Aβ inhibition on nociceptive responses, (3) WDR response and recruitment in the deeper layers of the dorsal horn and (4) LTP and wind-up behaviour shown by dorsal horn neurones, show that the spinal cord has the capacity to amplify responses to nociceptive stimuli. Similar mechanisms probably underlie state 3 processing of the spinal cord.

State 4 processing occurs after degenerative changes alter the highly complex architecture of the dorsal horn. Thus after peripheral nerve injury, there is sprouting of the Aβ fibres in layer 3 of the spinal cord into layers 1–2 the site of termination of the C fibres (Nagy & Hunt 1983, Woolf et al 1992, Shortland & Fitzgerald 1994; see Fig. 4.1). This may give rise to the formation of inappropriate synapses which may allow the low-threshold afferent input to be interpreted as nociceptive input by the spinal cord (Woolf 1994). Furthermore there is a suggestion that there may be sprouting of neurones from the superficial layers to deeper ones, causing the loss of the Aβ inhibitory control from the deeper layers (Cameron et al 1992). Why should peripheral nerve injury cause such a response? Peripheral nerve transection can cause cell atrophy or less commonly cell death of the associated nerve cell body in the dorsal root ganglia and leave vacant synapses associated with that particular primary afferent nerve in the spinal cord. The death or injury of a primary afferent nerve is also accompanied by changes in the dorsal horn levels of some neuropeptides (see below) and perhaps the decreased availability of growth factors and further neuronal cell death in the spinal cord (references below; see also Aldskogius et al 1985, Sugimoto 1991, Lewin & Mendell 1993) which have implications for the stimulus-processing ability of the spinal cord. The neuronal sprouting in response to nerve injury may not only occur in the spinal cord, but also in the dorsal root ganglia, where sympathetic postganglionic nerve fibres grow in between the cell bodies of the primary afferents (McLachlan et al 1993, Chung et al 1993; see Fig. 4.1). These sympathetic nerve fibres may be able to excite the primary afferents directly and give an anatomical basis to sympathetically mediated pain (SMP; see below). Whether these structural changes associated with state 4 processing are permanent or eventually regress is not yet clear; however, what is a more worrying feature is the ease with which some of these changes may be produced. Some studies indicate that simple skin incision (as in minor surgery) may be enough to cause changes in dorsal horn neuropeptide levels (Cliffer et al 1993). On a cautionary note, the changes described above are thought to provide a substrate for chronic pain states; it could be that the same changes may be considered as adaptive responses of the nervous system to injury, reducing the effects of injury.

THE MECHANISMS OF CENTRAL SENSITIZATION

The pharmacology and cellular biology that underlie the above changes in neuronal function will be now described (Coderre et al 1993).

The role of glutamate and the *N*-methyl-D-aspartate (NMDA) receptor in central sensitisation; release of second messengers

It is now clear that the amino acids glutamate and aspartate are excitatory transmitters in the spinal cord (Curtis et al 1959, Willis & Coggeshall 1991, Tolle et al 1993). Glutamate and aspartate have been shown to be present in many types of sensory neurones. The receptors of these excitatory amino acids (EAA) have been divided into four subtypes: (1) NMDA, (2) α-amino-3-hydroxy-5-methyl isoxazole (AMPA), (3) high-affinity kainate receptors and (4) metabotropic glutamate receptors (Seeburg 1993 and references within). Autoradiographic studies, and more recently in situ hybridization studies, reveal the presence of all three types of receptors throughout the mammalian spinal cord, including the dorsal horn (Tolle et al 1993). Non-nociceptive and nociceptive afferent input normally activate the AMPA receptor. However, in situations of sustained nociceptive primary afferent input the NMDA receptor is also activated. The NMDA receptor has unique properties in that the binding of glutamate is inadequate to open the ion channel associated with the receptor, due to ion channel blockade by Mg^{2+} ions. This Mg^{2+} block is only removed when the postsynaptic membrane has been sufficiently depolarized, for example by prior activation of the AMPA channel.

Glutamate has been shown to coexist with a neuropeptide of the tachykinin group called substance P (SP) in some nociceptive neurones (Battaglia & Rustioni 1988). After intense noxious stimulation, SP along with other tachykinins such as neurokinin A may also be released along with glutamate (Radhakrishnan & Henry 1991). These in combination with AMPA receptor activation cause long-lasting postsynaptic depolarization which is enough to cause the removal of the Mg^{2+} block at the NMDA receptor, allowing it to open with the influx of Ca^{2+} ions (Thompson & Woolf 1991). The NMDA channel, once open, remains open for hundreds of milliseconds, leading to long-lasting partial depolarization which lowers the threshold for other subsequent lower-intensity stimuli to generate postsynaptic action potentials. This is part of the mechanism for the increased synaptic efficacy seen in wind-up and spinal cord LTP. Thus both low-intensity mechanical and thermal stimuli are then more likely to result in postsynaptic depolarization (Thompson et al 1993). The NMDA channel can be seen to have unique integrative and amplification properties and the clinical consequence would be the appearance of allodynia and hyperalgesia (Woolf & Doubell 1994; see Fig. 4.3). NMDA receptor activation would also explain the expansion of the receptive fields of WDR neurones, with the clinical consequence of pain radiation and temporal summation of pain. In both inflammatory and neuropathic models, such as induced by constriction of a nerve, NMDA receptor antagonists will markedly delay the onset of the hyperalgesia or allodynia if given preemptively or ameliorate the symptoms if given afterwards (Seltzer et al, 1991, Davar et al 1991, Mao et al 1992b, Ren et al 1992, Yamamoto &

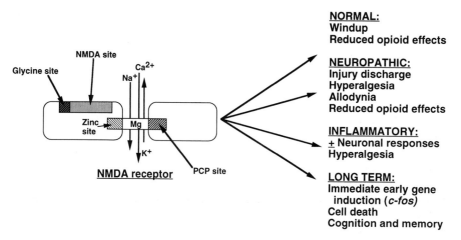

NORMAL:
Windup
Reduced opioid effects

NEUROPATHIC:
Injury discharge
Hyperalgesia
Allodynia
Reduced opioid effects

INFLAMMATORY:
± Neuronal responses
Hyperalgesia

LONG TERM:
Immediate early gene
  induction (*c-fos*)
Cell death
Cognition and memory

Fig. 4.3 Consequences of NMDA receptor activation for pain in the spinal cord. Substance P, neurokinin A and glutamate acting at the NK1, NK2 and AMPA receptor respectively contribute to membrane depolarization, which helps relieve the Mg^{2+} block on the NMDA channel during intense primary afferent stimulation, allowing opening of the channel. The possible consequences of NMDA receptor activation are also shown. Ketamine and MK-801 are two clinically available non-competitive channel blockers at the PCP site. (Adapted from Dickenson 1994, with permission.)

Yaksh 1992, Mao et al 1993, Smith et al 1993, Munglani et al 1994).

NMDA receptor antagonists also reduce the pain behaviour in a model of strychnine-induced allodynia, where there is a loss of Aβ-mediated inhibition of nociceptive input (Yaksh 1989). At a more basic level, NMDA receptor activation has been shown to be essential for the exaggerated flexion reflex (Woolf & Thompson 1991) and for wind-up in neurones and for determining receptive field size of dorsal horn neurones after recovery from nerve injury (Lewin et al 1994).

Following NMDA receptor activation there is an initial increase in intracellular Ca^{2+}, followed by the translocation of protein kinase C (PKC) from the cytosolic to the membrane-bound form (Coderre & Melzack 1987). PKC activation in the spinal cord has been described in both inflammatory and neuropathic models of pain. PKC activation has both pre- and postsynaptic effects since PKC activation has been shown to increase glutamate and aspartate release in a spinal cord preparation (Gerber et al 1989), as well as increasing the responsiveness of neurones to glutamate by reducing Mg^{2+} blockade on the NMDA receptor (Chen & Huang 1992). Stimulators of PKC such as by the phorbol esters increase pain behaviour whilst inhibitors of PKC, such as glycosphingolipid (GM1) have been shown to reduce activation of PKC in the spinal cord as well as prevent or reduce pain behaviour in both neuropathic and inflammatory pain models (Coderre 1992, Hayes et al 1992). This evidence further supports the essential role of the NMDA–Ca^{2+} and the PKC pathway in generation of pain states.

Spinal cord nitric oxide and prostaglandins in chronic pain states

There is increasing evidence that nitric oxide (NO), a small freely diffusible molecule, can act as an intracellular messenger, without requiring synaptic contacts and with a range of action over tens of micrometres (McMahon et al 1993, Meller & Gebhart 1993). NMDA receptor activation seems to be intimately linked to NO production via the Ca^{2+}-activated constitutive enzyme nitric oxide synthase (NOS). NO may then activate guanylate cyclase, producing cGMP. Intrathecal application of NMDA or agents that release NO such as sodium nitroprusside cause hyperalgesia. Furthermore intrathecal NMDA-mediated hyperalgesia is reversed by agents that bind NO (such as free haemoglobin) or inhibitors of NOS or cGMP (Kitto et al 1992, Haley et al 1992). Other NMDA-mediated phenomena such as wind-up and immediate early gene activation have been shown to be critically dependent on NO production (Lee et al 1992). In neuropathic pain models, there seems to be an upregulation of NOS in injured neurones (Fiallos-Estrada et al 1993) and NOS inhibition reduces the hyperalgesia seen in established pain states (Meller et al 1992). However the precise role of NO is not yet clear and it is likely to have both pre- and postsynaptic neuronal sensitizing effects, including the release of the neuropeptides SP and calcitonin gene-related peptide (CGRP; see below) (Garry et al 1994).

The increase in intracellular Ca^{2+} that occurs in the postsynaptic neurone after NMDA activation is essential for a number of other events, including the activation of phospholipase A_2 and subsequently arachidonic acid; this latter compound is converted via the cyclooxygenase (COX) pathway to prostaglandins (PG). PG production in the periphery is well known to contribute to pain production by sensitizing peripheral terminals of primary afferents, but in addition it is now clear that there is production of PG in the spinal cord in inflammatory pain states. The site of production of PG include both neurones and Schwann cells. Inhibitors of COX enzymes like indomethecacin (and other non-steroidal anti-inflammatory compounds; NSAIDS) have been shown to suppress hyperalgesia after intrathecal administration in inflammatory pain states (Malmberg & Yaksh 1992, Chapman & Dickenson 1992a, Eisenach 1993). Furthermore some of the analgesia produce by NSAIDS may be mediated by endogenous opioid systems (Bjorkman et al 1990). It has recently been shown that the COX enzyme can be divided into two forms: COX-1 and COX-2. NSAID inhibition of the constitutive COX-1 form leads to analgesia and the other well-known side effects of NSAIDS such as gastric irritation and renal dysfunction. In contrast, COX-2 is only upregulated in nervous tissue in inflammatory pain. Specific antagonists of COX-2 may have a better side effect profile while having a specific action in inflammatory pain states (Mitchell et al 1993, Vane et al 1994).

Opioid therapy in chronic pain states: synergism with NMDA receptor antagonists

In marked contrast to the panacea-like role of the NMDA receptor antagonists in animal studies, the results of opioid treatment are complex; options are much more effective in preventing central sensitization than treating the established sensitized state (Woolf & Wall 1986). In the case of wind-up studies, 10-fold more opioid is required to treat the heightened neuronal response than to prevent it (Dickenson & Sullivan 1989). One interpretation of this finding is that an established pain state is less opioid sensitive than if the opioid was given pre injury (i.e. pre-emptively; see below). In contrast to the poor effect of opioids post injury, a combination of opioid and an NMDA antagonist has been shown to be a powerful combination in the treatment of a neuropathic chronic pain model (Mao et al 1992b). The combination may be effective as the two agents act at different sites: opioids inhibit the C fibre activation in the dorsal horn, with only moderate inhibitory effects on wind-up; however, the NMDA antagonist, in contrast, has no effect on the C fibre activity reaching the neurones in the dorsal horn, but instead specifically prevents or reduces wind-up (Davies & Lodge 1987, Dickenson & Sullivan 1987). The combination of the two drugs has been shown to be synergistic in preventing wind-up (Chapman & Dickenson 1992b) and in a model of unilateral inflammatory pain (produced by injecting carrageenan into one paw; Yamamoto et al 1993b) intrathecal NMDA antagonist can reduce the hyperalgesia solely in the injured paw without the response of the uninjured paw to painful stimulation. In contrast, morphine effects both paws in parallel, but maintaining the difference in withdrawal latency between the two paws. These results suggest that C fibre activation and pain perception on the one hand and spinal cord sensitization on the other are distinct mechanisms and that NMDA antagonists are not analgesic in the same way as morphine (Dickenson 1994, Price et al 1994).

More recently it has been suggested that NMDA receptor specifically modulates opioid receptor function (Stacey & Watkins 1994 and references within). Thus rats tolerant to morphine who were treated with an NMDA antagonist became opioid sensitive again regardless of concurrent morphine administration (Trujillo & Akil 1991, Tiseo & Inturrisi 1993). The site of action of the NMDA antagonist in this context has been shown to be the spinal cord rather than the brain (Gustein et al 1992). Further work shows that this reversal of opiate tolerance is specific to the μ and κ_1 opioid receptors (Kolesnikov et al 1993a). Interestingly, since NO seems to mediate NMDA receptor action, inhibitors of the enzyme NOS also inhibits tolerance to morphine (Kolesnikov et al 1993b).

Changes in neuropeptides in the dorsal horn in central sensitization

C fibre activation causes the release of a number of neuropeptides, including SP, neurokinin A (NKA) and CGRP in the dorsal horn of the spinal cord (Coderre et al 1993, Hokfelt et al 1994). These neuropeptides and the excitatory amino acids (EAA) such as glutamate coexist in spinal dorsal horn neurones (Battaglia & Rustioni 1988). SP has been shown to synergize with EAAs and causes prolonged excitation of dorsal horn neurones to both noxious and innocuous stimuli (Dougherty & Willis 1991). All three neuropeptides may have presynaptic actions, causing increased EAA release (Kangrga & Randic 1990) as well as perhaps acting as coagonists on the NMDA receptor (Rusin et al 1992, 1993). CGRP has also been shown to inhibit the SP breakdown by endopeptidase (Mao et al 1992a), thereby synergistically enhancing the effect of SP upon glutamate-induced depolarization (Schaible et al 1992). In inflammatory pain states, the increased levels of SP and CGRP at both the peripheral and central terminals of primary afferent fibres may be controlled by the increased production of neurotrophins such as nerve growth factor (NGF) at the site of inflammation (Lewin & Mendell 1993, Lewin et al 1993). It has been suggested that NGF could play a role in signalling the state of the peripheral tissues to the spinal cord (McMahon et al 1993). As might be expected, antagonists at the receptors for SP and NKA (known as NK1 and NK2 receptor antagonists respectively) seem to be effective in blocking central sensitization in inflammatory pain models (see McMahon et al 1993 for references). In contrast to the raised levels of SP and CGRP in the dorsal horn in inflammatory pain states, there are decreases in levels of these peptides after nerve injury (see Hokfelt et al 1994 for references and Fig. 4.4 for an example). In contrast to the decrease in SP and CGRP, levels of vasoactive intestinal peptide (VIP) rise after nerve injury (McGregor et al 1984) and it has been suggested that VIP takes over the excitatory role of SP in these situations. Other neuropeptides such as cholecystokinin, galanin and neuropeptide Y (NPY) also rise in response to nerve injury (see Fig. 4.4). Galanin and NPY both have an analgesic role. Thus intrathecal infusions of galanin antagonize the excitatory effects of SP and reduce pain behaviour, whilst galanin antagonists have the opposite effect (Wiesenfeld-Hallin et al 1992). NPY levels increase in the dorsal horn and DRG in response to nerve injury (Wakisaka et al 1991, 1992) and reduce nerve activity in the dorsal horn (see Colmers & Bleakman 1994 for review); correlations between NPY levels in the dorsal horn and pain behaviour have been found in a neuropathic pain model (Munglani et al 1994a). Cholecystokinin (CCK) on the other hand has been found to antagonize the action of opioids and may explain in part the resistance of patients with neuropathic pain to the action of opioids (Xu et al 1993). CCK_b antagonists will reverse the allodynia produced in some neuropathic models,

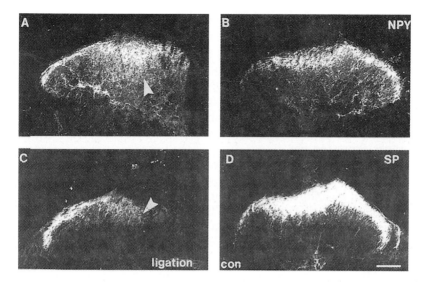

Fig. 4.4 Examples of the changes in the levels of substance P (SP) and neuropeptide Y (NPY) in the dorsal horn of the spinal cord with unilateral sciatic nerve ligation. On the right (B and D) are the control dorsal horns showing much labelling in layers 1 and 2 (cf. Fig. 4.1). With nerve injury there is an increase in layer 3–4 NPY staining in the region of the myelinated Aβ afferents (A) and a decrease in layer 1 and 2 SP in the region of the C and Aδ fibres (C). Bar=100 μm. (Munglani and Hunt, unpublished observations.)

this latter effect in turn can be reversed by naloxone, indicating that endogenous opioid systems may be activated in neuropathic pain states but their effect is masked by the CCK upregulation (Xu et al 1994a). In contrast, in inflammatory pain states there is evidence that endogenous opioid activity is also present, but since there is no nerve injury-mediated upregulation of CCK the opioid system operates unhindered (see Dickenson 1991, Hokfelt et al 1994, Xu et al 1994b for further discussion).

Immediate early genes (IEGs) as markers of nerve cell activity in the spinal cord

IEGs were originally described as a class of genes rapidly and transiently expressed in cells stimulated with growth factors without the requirement for de novo protein synthesis. IEGs such as *c-fos* and *c-jun* have been shown to be transcription factors and are expressed in the central nervous system following specific types of stimulation (Hunt et al 1987, Curran et al 1987, Munglani & Hunt 1994). The proteins Fos and Jun dimerize to form AP1 protein complex, which binds on the AP1 binding site on DNA to effect the transcription of other genes (Curran & Franza 1988).

Recently it was shown that Fos is expressed postsynaptically in dorsal horn neurones of the spinal cord following noxious stimulation (Hunt et al

1987). The protein product appears within 1–2 h post stimulation and then tends to decline rapidly. Fos-positive neurones are restricted to Rexed layers 1 and 2 of the dorsal horn, with some labelling in layer 5 – the same layers that receive the nociceptive primary afferents, the C and Aδ fibres (see Figs 4.1 and 4.5). Non-noxious stimulation is largely ineffective in inducing Fos expression. No Fos expression was seen in the stimulated dorsal root ganglion cells (the cells bodies of the stimulated primary afferents themselves). In other words, only a subset of postsynaptically stimulated neurones expressed Fos.

Using noxious thermal stimulation, Fos protein appears within 30 min and peaks at 2 h in layers 1 and 2 ipsilateral to the injury. However, another peak of Fos expression was seen within the deep layers (5–7 and 10), commencing at 8 h and peaking at 16 h; this second wave of labelling started ipsilaterally and spread to become bilateral. Thermal stimulation activates unmyelinated C fibres which terminate in layers 1, 2 and 5 as previously described. Fos-positive neurones in other layers and at much later time points indicate a polysynaptic mechanism. This second wave of Fos activity was found to be independent of any further impulses from the primary afferent fibres as it was not prevented by local anaesthetic blockade of the injured sciatic nerve. This suggests that continuing primary afferent activity is not required for ongoing Fos activation by neurones in the spinal cord. Instead the system becomes self-sustaining (Williams et al 1989, 1990a, 1990b, 1991). The pattern of Fos activity has also been examined in a model of Freund's adjuvant-induced arthritis (AIA), (Abbadie et al 1992, Abbadie & Besson 1992, 1993a, 1993b). Ten days after the inoculation of the adjuvant, there is a polyarthritis affecting the hind limb joints and behavioural changes appear such as decreased locomotion and hyperalgesia to paw pressure. The symptoms peak at 3 weeks, at which time there is also peaking of the Fos response in layer 5 of the dorsal horn

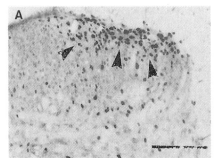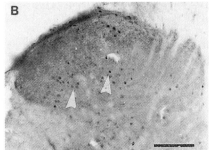

Fig. 4.5 Comparison of different types of Fos labelling in the dorsal horn of the spinal cord after: (A) acute thermal stimulation of C fibre leading to Fos labelling in Rexed layers 1-2, the termination of C fibre primary afferents; (B) in a neuropathic pain model produced by sciatic nerve ligation; there is Fos-increased labelling in layers 3 and 4, which receive predominantly the Aβ myelinateed afferents. Allodynia, which is mediated by the Aβ fibres, is a major feature in this pain model. Bar = 100 μm. (From Williams et al 1991 and Munglani and Hunt, unpublished observations.)

in lumbar segments (corresponding to innervation of the arthritic hind limbs). Treatment of the animals with NSAID has shown that it is much easier to suppress the Fos activity 1 week after the inoculation rather than 3 weeks later. If one accepts the premise that Fos activity represents dorsal horn activity, these results may suggest it is better to treat a chronic pain earlier rather than later.

We have examined Fos expression in a neuropathic model developed by Bennett & Xie (1988). In this chronic constriction injury (CCI) model one sciatic nerve is loosely ligated with chromic catgut and ipsilateral hyperalgesia; allodynia develops over the following 7–10 days and persists for up to 7–8 weeks. After the initial surge in Fos on the ipsilateral side at the time of ligation in layers 1–2 and 5–10 there was a decline in the numbers to control values by 14–28 days, and there is very little Fos expression in the superficial layers; however, there was a persistent increase in Fos-positive cells in layers 3–4 of the spinal cord (Munglani et al 1994b, Munglani & Hunt 1994; see Fig. 4.5). As has been described earlier, layers 3 and 4 are the site of termination of the myelinated afferents (Aβ) and do not usually express Fos (Hunt et al 1987), but will do so after peripheral nerve injury (Herdegen et al 1991, Molander et al 1992). It is increasingly being recognized that the normally innocuous Aβ input may play a large part in the generation of neuropathic states (Woolf & Doubell 1994).

These descriptions of pain-evoked patterns of Fos expression are all very interesting, but does Fos activation mean anything? As described, Fos increases are seen in the dorsal horn in both arthritic and the nerve injury models; similarly, increases in dynorphin (an endogenous opioid acting at the κ receptor) have also been seen in both models (Dubner & Ruda 1992, Hunt et al 1993, Millan 1993 and references within). The increased expression of dynorphin is thought to occur in both local circuit and projection neurones which receive nociceptive afferent input. There is some recent evidence of dynorphin having a tonic analgesic action under both normal and inflammatory conditions (see Stiller et al 1993 and references within). Since the preprodynorphin gene has several AP1-like binding sites and potentially may bind Fos (as a component of the AP1 transcription factor complex) it was tempting to speculate that Fos might directly lead to dynorphin expression. Certainly Fos is expressed in the same dorsal horn cells as those expressing dynorphin following noxious stimulation (Noguchi et al 1991) and in a recent in vitro study (Lucas et al 1993) activation of prodynorphin was completely blocked by an injection of a c-fos antisense DNA (hence blocking DNA transcription). Furthermore it has been shown in a formalin pain model that pre-emptive antisense c-fos administration reduces dynorphin staining and increases the pain behaviour (Woodburn et al 1994). We conclude that these results show that the Fos–preprodynorphin pathway is physiologically important and suggest that Fos activation, as well as being a marker of nerve cell activity, may directly result in the activation of analgesic opioids in the spinal cord.

PERIPHERAL NERVE AND SYMPATHETIC ACTIVITY IN MAINTAINING CENTRAL SENSITIZATION

The role of ongoing nerve activity in the maintenance of a pain state

Much of the evidence presented above suggests that once central sensitization is established by noxious input it is relatively self-sustaining. However, there is evidence that ongoing peripheral activity, both abnormal and normal, can contribute to the maintenance of a pain state. In a notable study Gracely et al (1992) showed that some chronic pain patients have small areas of very highly sensitive skin physically distinct from larger areas of skin which show allodynia and hyperalgesia. Local anaesthetic blockade of the smaller hypersensitive areas not only abolished sensation in these areas but also caused reduction or resolution of the symptoms in the larger areas. This study shows that small foci can maintain abnormal processing in other larger areas. In a neuropathic animal model sciatic nerve injury can cause the appearance of abnormal sensations in the territory of the ipsilateral saphenous nerve as well as in the contralateral sciatic and saphenous nerves (Attal et al 1990, Tal & Bennett 1994). The situation is even more complex as it has been shown that in some situations cutting the adjacent saphenous nerve dramatically reduces the hyperalgesia seen in the territory of the injured sciatic nerve (Kingery et al 1993, Ro & Jacobs 1993). Together, these results indicate that afferent activity from both injured and intact nerves can maintain abnormal sensations in the territories of injured and intact nerves – even on the contralateral side of the body (Bennett 1994).

The mechanisms underlying peripheral maintenance of central sensitization include the following (see Figs 4.1 and 4.6):

1. Sensitization of the peripheral nerves in inflammatory pain states by the 'soup' of PG, bradykinins, cytokines etc. (Heller et al 1994, Rang et al 1994) so that they discharge more readily (Wall & Gutnik 1974, Wall et al 1974), some of them also acquire sensitivity to circulating noradrenaline (Sato & Perl 1991).
2. The expression of abnormally excitable sodium channels at the site of injury and in the dorsal root ganglia after nerve injury causes spontaneous discharges from these nerves into the spinal cord (Wall & Devor 1981, Devor 1994). Furthermore the spontaneous discharges can excite adjacent nerves in the dorsal root ganglia (Devor & Wall 1990), thus increasing the afferent input.
3. Nerve injury also causes the ingrowth of postganglionic sympathetic fibres into the DRG of the injured nerve. Activity of the sympathetic system may increase nerve discharges in the DRG that can feed into the cord (McLachlan et al 1993, Chung et al 1993, Devor et al 1994, Janig & McLachlan 1994).

Mechanisms 1 and 3 may account for the phenomenon of sympathetically mediated pain.

NOVEL THERAPEUTIC STRATEGIES IN CHRONIC PAIN

Many of the above-mentioned findings can be used to suggest new therapies for chronic pain. SP and NKA activation may be important and the antagonists their receptors may be useful, especially in inflammatory pain states. After nerve injury, however, SP levels decline in the spinal cord and VIP increases. Thus VIP antagonists might be of therapeutic value. NPY and galanin agonists have been shown to be analgesic and offer other therapeutic options for further research. After nerve injury the neuropeptide CCK increases to antagonize the endogenous opioid system via action at the CCK_b receptor, and drugs which antagonize the CCK_b receptor may have a significant role in the treatment of neuropathic pain states. The μ opioid receptors have well-known side-effects; more selective κ opioid agonists (in the same group as dynorphin) may be able to deliver the promise of analgesia without potential for respiratory depression, abuse or tolerance (Millan 1993). Increase in intracellular Ca^{2+} is a fundamental step in the production of spinal cord sensitization, and Ca^{2+} antagonists have been shown to synergize with opioids at the spinal level to reduce hyperalgesia (Omote et al 1993). Inhibitors of second messenger systems such as NOS and PKC activation are also potentially very exciting but limited by systemic effects. The role of intrathecal NSAIDs and inhibitors selective for the inducible form of cyclooxygenase (COX-2) have yet to be assessed. The effect of using antisense oligonucleotide to *c-fos* on pain behaviour may mean that highly selective control of the spinal cord response to stimulation may be possible in the future.

PRESENT-DAY PAIN MANAGEMENT STRATEGIES

It has been pointed out by many authors that general anaesthetics have little effect either on inhibiting C fibre input or on preventing central sensitization; indeed many of the studies showing central sensitization including wind-up were done during conventional anaesthesia. It has been suggested that by preventing the input of the C fibre discharge at the time of surgery (ie pre-emptive analgesia) should lead to:

1. Less spinal cord sensitization in the postoperative period and therefore postoperative analgesia requirements.
2. Reduction in the long-term incidence of chronic pain.

Lowered pain perception and analgesia requirements after pre-emptive analgesia have been shown clinically in only a few studies (see Richmond

Peripheral maintenance of central sensitization

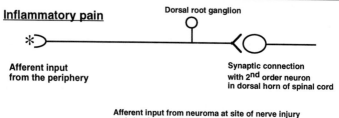

Inflammatory pain

Dorsal root ganglion

Afferent input
from the periphery

Synaptic connection
with 2nd order neuron
in dorsal horn of spinal cord

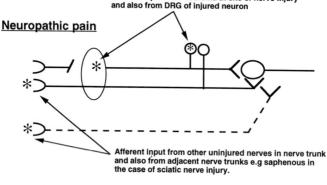

Afferent input from neuroma at site of nerve injury
and also from DRG of injured neuron

Neuropathic pain

Afferent input from other uninjured nerves in nerve trunk
and also from adjacent nerve trunks e.g saphenous in
the case of sciatic nerve injury.

$*$ = site of nerve discharge

Fig. 4.6 In chronic pain states the central sensitization can be maintained by afferent discharge from the periphery in both inflammatory and neuropathic pain stages. Furthermore ectopic nerve discharge from neuromas or from the dorsal root ganglion may contribute to the pain state after nerve injury. Afferent input from adjacent intact primary afferents may also help maintain a state of central sensitization. (Adapted from Woolf & Doubell 1994.)

et al 1993, McQuay 1992, Dahl & Kehlet 1993, Woolf & Chong 1993 for reviews). One factor may be that the inflammatory response associated with wounds lead to a continued afferent barrage that persists long after initial pre-emptive therapy has ceased (Munglani et al 1993, Woolf & Chong 1993). A recent study by Yamamoto et al (1993a) illustrates this point. The authors used the neuropathic pain model of Bennett & Xie (1988), which is produced by constriction of the sciatic nerve. In this model, there is a surge of sciatic nerve activity produced at the time of ligation (the 'injury discharge') which lasted for about 30 s in this study. Within a few days, hyperalgesia developed in the paw with the injured sciatic nerve. In contrast, pre-emptive local anaesthetic applied proximally to the nerve prevented the spinal cord receiving the injury discharge and suppressed the development of hyperalgesia in this model. Interestingly, the hyperalgesia did eventually develop after pre-emptive local anaesthesia, but with a delay in onset of about 2 weeks. Thus the pre-emptive local anaesthetic obviously reduced the sensitization of the spinal cord that immediately followed the nerve injury, without affecting the longer-term outcome. We suggest that the spontaneous discharges from the injured nerves and the DRG along with the changes in spinal cord which have been described may be capable of producing the sensitized state (Fig. 4.6). This may explain why those studies that do show a positive pre-emptive effect reveal only a moderate clinical reduction in analgesia requirements and perhaps longer-lasting pre-emptive regimes are required (Munglani et al 1993).

The second suggestion, that of the relationship of pre-emptive analgesia to the development of chronic pain, is also not clear. Though animal studies indicate that the development of chronic pain is certainly delayed and perhaps prevented (Yamamoto et al 1993a, Seltzer et al 1991a, 1991b, Davar et al 1991, Munglani et 1994a) there have been no adequate trials in humans, though two small studies in post-amputation phantom limb pain indicate there may be some benefit (Bach et al 1988, Fisher et al 1991).

The theoretical basis for using NMDA antagonists in the treatment of chronic pain has been described earlier. Convincing results are seen with NMDA antagonists in animal studies or in anecdotal reports in patients (Stannard & Porter 1993). Not all controlled studies in chronic pain patients are successful (McQuay et al 1994); however, some successful studies report a high incidence of psychomimetic side effects (Eide et al 1994).

Understanding the role of the sympathetic system in maintaining chronic pain after nerve injury has been advanced since the discovery of the increased sympathetic sprouting into DRG after nerve injury (Fig. 4.1). α_2 agonists such as clonidine reduce the sympathetic outflow and recently it has been shown that clonidine may have a very useful role in the treatment of neuropathic pain, especially where a sympathetic component is obvious (Rauck et al 1993). The new sodium channels produced at the site of nerve injury and in the DRG after nerve injury not only discharge more easily but are also four or five times more sensitive than normal sodium channels found in nerves to sodium channel blockers such as lignocaine (Devor et al 1992). Mexilitene, an oral congener of lignocaine, has been found to be a useful adjunct in chronic pain management (Tanelian & Brose 1991, Kamei et al 1992).

WHERE ARE WE IN THE PAIN STORY?

The numerous changes seen in the spinal cord in chronic pain states suggest a bewildering number of therapeutic options. Furthermore, the state of central sensitization is, rather than a fixed entity, probably maintained by further input from the periphery as well as the continued activity of second messengers within the spinal cord, as described above. Whether the system becomes less dependent on peripheral maintenance with time is not clear; certainly the clinical experience is that long-standing pains are more difficult to treat.

The last decade has provided a better understanding of pain mechanisms in the spinal cord and the reasons why acute pain becomes chronic. The next few years will bring into the clinical realm a great number of new therapies and we can look forward to the application of these to prevent and alleviate suffering (see also Dray et al 1994). Until then, modification of anaesthetic and surgical practice should allow effective pre-emptive and continuing postoperative analgesia for most major operations using combinations of opioids, NSAIDS, α_2 agonists and NMDA antagonists (see Kehlet 1994, Tverskoy et al 1994, Budd 1994, Breivik 1994). This type of practice should become the norm rather than the domain of an interested few anaesthetists. Furthermore, we suggest there should be increased availability of pain relief clinics to allow clinicians to treat chronic pain *before* it becomes established, rather than waiting for patients to do the round of other clinics first. This will require education of our colleagues in other specialities as well as increased resources.

ACKNOWLEDGEMENTS

We would like to thank Kerrie Thomas and Tony Dickenson for useful discussion during the writing of this chapter.

REFERENCES

Abbadie C, Besson J M 1992 c-fos expression in rat lumbar spinal cord during the development of adjuvant-induced arthritis. Neuroscience 48: 985–993

Abbadie C, Besson J M 1993a C-fos expression in rat lumbar spinal cord following peripheral stimulation in adjuvant-induced arthritic and normal rates. Brain Res 607: 195–204

Abbadie C, Besson J M 1993b Effects of morphine and naloxone on basal and evoked Foslike immunoreactivity in lumbar spinal cord neurons of arthritic rats. Pain 52: 29–39

Abbadie C, Lombard M C, Morain F, Besson J M 1992 Fos-like immunoreactivity in the rat superficial dorsal horn induced by formalin injection in the forepaw: effects of dorsal rhizotomies. Brain Res 578: 17–25

Aldskogius H, Arvidsson S, Grant G 1985 The reaction of primary sensory neurons to peripheral nerve injury with particular emphasis on transganglionic changes. Brain Res 373: 15–21

Attal N, Jazat F, Kayser V, Guilbaud G 1990 Further evidence of pain related behaviours in a model of unilateral peripheral neuropathy. Pain 41: 235–251

Bach S, Noreng M F, Tjellen N U 1988 Phantom limb pain in amputees during the first 12 months following limb amputation after preoperative lumbar epidural blockade. Pain 33: 297–301

Battaglia G, Rustioni A 1988 Coexistence of glutamate and substance P in dorsal root ganglion cells of the rat and monkey. J Comp Neurol 277: 302–312

Bennett G J 1994 Chronic pain due to peripheral nerve damage: an overview. In: Pharmacological approaches to the treatment of chronic pain: new concepts and critical issues. Seattle, IASP Press, pp.173–188

Bennett G J, Xie Y-K 1988 A peripheral neuropathy in rat that produces disorders of pain sensation like those seen in man. Pain 33: 87–108

Bjorkman R, Hedner J, Hedner T, Henning M 1990 Central, naloxone- reversible antinociception by diclofenac in the rat. Arch Pharmacol 342: 171–176

Breivik H 1994 Pre-emptive analgesia. Curr Opin Anaesthesiol 7: 458–461

Budd K 1994 Prevention or cure. Curr Opin Anaesthesiol 7: 453–457

Cameron A A, Pover C M, Willis W D, Coggeshall R E 1992 Evidence that fine primary afferent axons innervate a wider territory in the superficial dorsal horn following peripheral axotomy. Brain Res 575: 151–154

Chapman V, Dickenson A H (1992a) The combination of NMDA antagonism and morphine produce profound antinociception in the rat dorsal horn. Brain Res 573: 321–323

Chapman V, Dickenson A H 1992b The spinal and peripheral roles of bradykinin and prostaglandins in nociceptive processing in rat. Eur J Pharmacol 219: 427–433

Chen L, Huang L 1992 Protein kinase C reduces Mg^{2+} block NMDA- receptor channels as a mechanism of modulation. Nature 356: 521–523

Chung K, Kim H J K, Park M J, Chung J M 1993 Abnormalities of sympathetic innervation in the area of an injured peripheral nerve in a rat model of neuropathic pain. Neuroscie Lett 162: 85–88

Cliffer K D, Cameron A A, Willis W D 1993 Chronic cutaneous compression causes central changes. 7th World Congress on Pain. IASP Press, Seattle

Coderre T J 1992 Contribution of protein kinase C to central sensitization and persistent pain following tissue injury. Neurosci Lett 140: 181–184

Coderre T, Melzack R 1987 Cutaneous Hyperalgesia: contributions of the peripheral and central nervous systems to the increase in pain sensitivity after injury. Brain Res 404: 95–105

Coderre T, Katz J, Vaccarino A, Melzack R 1993 Contribution of central neuroplasticity to pathological pain: review of clinical and experimental evidence. Pain 52: 259–285

Coghill R C, Price D D, Hayes R, Mayer D J 1991 Spatial distribution of nociceptive processing in the rat spinal cord. J Neurophysiol 65: 133–140

Colmers W F, Bleakman D 1994 The effects of neuropeptide Y on the electrical properties of neurons. Trends Neurosci 17: 373–379

Curran T, Franza B R 1988 Fos and Jun: the AP-1 connection. Cell 55: 315–397

Curran T, Gordon M B, Rubino K L, Sambucetti L C 1987 Isolation and characterization of the c-fos (rat) cDNA and analysis of post-translational modification in vitro. Oncogene 2: 79–84

Curtis D R, Philis J W, Watkins J C 1959 Chemical excitation of spinal neurones. Nature 183: 611–612

Dahl J B, Kehlet H 1993 The value of pre-emptive analgesia in the treatment of postoperative pain. Br J Anaesth 70: 434–439

Davar G, Hama A, Deykin A, Vos B, Maciewicz R 1991 MK-801 blocks the development of thermal hyperalgesia in a rat model of experimental painful neuropathy. Brain Res 553: 327–330

Davies S N, Lodge D 1987 Evidence for involvement of N-methyl-D-aspartate receptors in the 'windup' of class 2 neurons in the dorsal horn of the rat. Brain Res 424: 402–406

Devor M 1994 The pathophysiology of damaged peripheral nerves. In: Melzack R, Wall P D (eds) Textbook of pain (3rd edn). Churchill Livingstone, Edinburgh, pp.79–100

Devor M, Wall P D 1990 Cross-excitation in dorsal root ganglia of nerve-injured and intact rats. J Neurophysiol 64: 1733–1746

Devor M, Wall P D, Catalan N 1992 Systemic lidocaine silences ectopic neuroma and DRG discharge without blocking nerve conduction. Pain 48: 261–268

Devor M, Janig W, Michaelis M 1994 Modulation of activity in dorsal root ganglion neurons by sympathetic activation in nerve injured rats. J Neurophysiol 71: 38–47

Dickenson A H 1991 Recent advances in the physiology and pharmacology of pain: plasticity and its implication for clinical analgesia. J Psychopharmacol 5: 342–351

Dickenson A H 1994 NMDA receptors as analgesics. In: Pharmacological approaches to the treatment of chronic pain: new concepts and critical issues. Seattle, IASP Press, pp 173–188

Dickenson A H, Sullivan A F 1986 Electrophysiological studies on the effects of intrathecal morphine on nociceptive neurones in the rat dorsal horn. Pain 24: 211–222

Dickenson A H, Sullivan A F 1987 Evidence for a role of the NMDA receptor in the frequency dependent potentiation of deep rat dorsal horn nociceptive neurones following c fibre stimulation. Neuropharmacology 26: 1235–1238

Dickenson A H, Sullivan A F 1989 Subcutaneous formalin induced activity of dorsal horn neurones in the rat: differential response to an intrathecal opiate administered pre or post formalin. Pain 30: 349–360

Dougherty P M, Willis W D 1991 Enhancement of spinothalamic neuron responses to chemical and mechanical stimuli following combined microiontophoretic application of N-methyl-D-aspartic acid and substance P. Pain 47: 85–93

Dray A, Urban L, Dickenson A 1994 Pharmacology of chronic pain. Trends Pharmacol Sci 15: 190–197

Dubner R, Ruda M A 1992 Activity dependant neuronal plasticity following tissue injury and inflammation. Trends Neurosci 15: 96–103

Eide P K, Jorum E, Stubhaug A, Bremnes J, Breivik H 1994 Relief of post herpetic neuralgia with the N-methyl-D-aspartate acid receptor antagonist ketamine: a double blind, cross over comparison with morphine and placebo. Pain 58: 347–354

Eisenach J C 1993 Asprin, the miracle drug: spinally, too? Anesthesiology 79: 211–213

Fiallos-Estrada C E, Kummer W, Mayer B, Bravo R, Zimmermann M, Herdegen T 1993 Long-lasting increase of nitric oxide synthase immunoreactivity, NADPH-diaphorase reaction and c-JUN co- expression in rat dorsal root ganglion neurons following sciatic nerve transection. Neurosci Lett 150: 169–173

Fields H L, Basbaum A I 1994 Central nervous system mechanisms of pain modulation. In: Melzack R, Wall P D (eds) Textbook of pain (3rd edn). Churchill Livingstone, Edinburgh, pp 243–260

Fisher A, Meller Y. 1991 Continuous postoperative regional anaesthesia by nerve sheath block for amputation surgery – a pilot study. Anaesth Analg 72: 300–303

Garry M G, Richardson J D, Hargreaves K M 1994 Sodium nitroprusside evokes the release of immunoreactive calcitonin gene-related peptide and substance P from dorsal horn slices via nitric oxide dependent and nitric oxide independent mechanisms. Neurosci 14: 4329–4337

Gerber G, Kangrga I, Ryu P D, Larew J S A, Randic M 1989 Multiple effects of phorbol esters in the rat spinal dorsal horn. J Neurosci 9: 3606–3617

Gracely R, Lych S, Bennett G 1992 Peripheral neuropathy: altered central processing maintained dynamically by peripheral input. Pain 51: 175–194

Gustein H B, Trujillo K A, Akil H 1992 MK-801 inhibits the development of morphine tolerance in the rat at spinal sites. Soc Neurosci Abstracts 18: 369

Haley J E, Dickenson A H, Schacter M 1992 Electrophysiological evidence for a role of nitric oxide in prolonged chemical nociception in the rat. Neuropharmacology 31: 251–258

Hayes R L, Mao J, Price D D et al 1992 Pretreatment with gangliosides reduces abnormal nociceptive responses associated with a rodent peripheral mononeuropathy. Pain 48: 391–396

Heller P H, Green P G, Tanner K D, Miao F J P, Levine J D 1994 Peripheral neural contributions to inflammation. In: Pharmacological approaches to the treatment of chronic pain: new concepts and critical issues. IASP Press, Seattle, pp 31–42

Herdegen T, Kovary K, Leah J, Bravo R 1991 Specific temporal and spatial distribution of JUN, FOS, and KROX-24 proteins in spinal neurons following noxious transsynaptic stimulation. J Comp Neurol 313: 178–191

Hokfelt T, Zhang X, Wiesenfeld-Hallin Z 1994 Messenger plasticity in primary sensory neurons following axotomy and its functional implications. Trends Neurosci 17: 22–30

Hunt S P, Pini A, Evan G 1987 Induction of c-fos like protein in spinal cord neurons following sensory stimulation. Nature 328: 632–634

Hunt S, Smith G, Bond A, Munglani R, Thomas T, Elliot P 1994 Changes in immediate early gene, neuropeptides immunoreactivity and other neuronal markers in the spinal cord and dorsal root ganglion in a rat model of neuropathic pain. In: Schmidt R, Schaible H G (eds) Neuropeptides Nociception Pain. Chapman Hall, p. 329–349

Janig W, McLachlan E M 1994 The role of modifications in noradrenergic peripheral pathways after nerve lesions in the generation of pain. In: Pharmacological approaches to the treatment of chronic pain: new concepts and critical issues. IASP Press, Seattle, pp 173–188

Kehlet H 1994 Postoperative pain relief : what is the issue? Br J Anaesth 72: 375–378

Kamei J, Hitosugi H, Kawashima N, Aoki T, Ohhashi Y, Kasuya Y 1992 Antinociceptive effect of mexiletine in diabetic mice. Res Commun Chem Pathol Pharmacol 77: 245–248

Kangrga I, Randic M 1990 Tachykinins and calcitonin gene-related peptide enhance release of endogenous glutamate and aspartate from the rat spinal dorsal horn slice. J Neurosc 10: 2026–2038

Kingery W S, Castellote J M, Wang E E 1993 A loose ligature induced mononeuropathy hyperalgesia mediated by both the injured sciatic nerve and the adjacent saphenous nerve. Pain 55: 297–304

Kitto F F, Haley J E, Wilcox G L 1992 Involvement of nitric oxide in spinally mediated hyperalgesia in the mouse. Neurosci Lett 148: 1–5

Kolesnikov Y A, Ferkany J, Pasternak J W 1993a Blockade of mu and kappa 1 opioid analgesic tolerance by NPC17742, a novel NMDA antagonist. Life Sci 53: 1489–1494

Kolesnikov Y A, Pick C G, Ciszewska G, Pasternak J W 1993b Blockade of tolerance to morphine but not opioids by a nitric oxide synthetase inhibitor. Proc Nat Acad Sci USA 90: 5162–5166

Lee J, Wilcox G, Beitz A J 1992 Nitric oxide mediates Fos expression in the spinal cord induced by mechanical noxious stimulation. NeuroReport 3: 841–844

Lewin G R, Mendell L M 1993 Nerve growth factor and nociception. Trends Neurosci 16: 353–359

Lewin G R, Ritter A M, Mendell L M 1993 Nerve growth factor induced hyperalgesia in the neonatal and adult rat. J Neurosci 13: 2136–2148

Lewin G R, Mckintosh E, McMahon S B 1994 NMDA receptors and activity-dependent tuning of the receptive fields of spinal cord neurones. Nature 369: 482–485

Lucas J, Mellstrom B, Colado M, Naranjo J 1993 Molecular mechanisms of pain: serotonin 1A receptor agonists trigger transactivation by c-fos of the prodynorphin gene in spinal cord neurons. Neuron 10: 599–611

Malmberg A B, Yaksh T L 1992 Antinociceptive actions of spinal nonsteroidal anti-inflammatory agents on the formalin test in the rat. J Pharmacol Exp Ther 263: 136–146

Mao J, Coghill R C, Kellstein D E, Frenk H, Mayer D J 1992a Calcitonon gene-related peptide enhances substance P-induced behaviours via metabolic inhibition: in vivo evidence for a new mechanism of neuromodulation. Brain Res 574: 157–163

Mao J, Price D D, Mayer D J, Lu J, Hayes R L 1992b Intrathecal MK-801 and local nerve anesthesia synergistically reduce nociceptive behaviors in rats with experimental peripheral mononeuropathy. Brain Res 576: 254–262

Mao J, Price D D Hayes R L, Lu J, Mayer D J, Frenk H 1993 Intrathecal treatment with dextrorphan or ketamine potently reduces pain-related behaviors in a rat model of peripheral mononeuropathy. Brain Res 605: 164–168

McGregor G P, Gibson S J, Sabate I M et al 1984 Effect of peripheral nerve section and nerve crush on spinal cord neuropeptides in the rat: increased VIP and PHI in dorsal horn. Neuroscience 13: 207–216

McLachlan E M, Janig W, Devor M, Michaelis M 1993 Peripheral nerve injury triggers noradrenergic sprouting within dorsal root ganglia. Nature 363: 543–545

McMahon S B, Lewin G R, Wall P D 1993 Central hyperexcitability triggered by noxious inputs. Curr Opin Neurobiol 3: 602–610

McQuay H J 1992 Pre-emptive analgesia. Br J Anaesth 69: 1–3

McQuay H J, Carool D, Jadad A R et al 1994 Dextromethorphan for the treatment of neuropathic pain: a double blind randomised controlled crossover trial with integral n of 1 design. Pain 59: 127–134

Meller S T, Pechman P S, Gebhart G F, Maves T J 1992 Nitric oxide mediates the thermal hyperalgesia produced in a model of neuropathic pain in the rat. Neuroscience 50: 7–10

Meller S T, Gebhart G F 1993 Nitric oxide (NO) and nociceptive processing in the spinal cord. Pain 52: 127–136

Melzack R, Wall P D 1965 Pain mechanisms: a new theory. Science 150: 971–979

Mendell L 1966 Physiological properties of unmyelinated fiber projections to the spinal cord. Exp Neurol 16: 316–322

Meyer A M, Campbell J N, Raja S N 1994 Peripheral neural mechanisms of nociception. In: Wall P D (eds) Textbook of pain (3rd edn). Churchill Livingstone, Edinburgh, pp 101–112

Meyer M, Schreck R, Baeuerle P A 1993 H_2O_2 and antioxidants have opposite effects on activation of NF-csi B and AP-1 in intact cells: AP-1 as secondary antioxidant-responsive factor. Embo J 12: 2005–2015

Millan M J 1993 Multiple opioid systems and chronic pain. In: Herz A Opioids II. Springer-Verlag, Berlin, pp 127–162

Mitchell J A, Akarasereenont P, Thiemermann C, Flower R J, Vane J R 1993 Selectivity of nonsteroidal antiinflammatory drugs as inhibitors of constitutive and inducible cyclooxygenase. Proc Natl Acad Sci USA 90: 11693–11697

Molander C, Hongpaisan J, Grant G 1992 Changing pattern of c-fos expression in spinal cord neuron after electrical stimulation of the chronically injured sciatic nerve in the rat. Neuroscience 50: 223–236

Munglani R, Hunt S 1994 Proto-oncogenes: basic concepts and stimulation induced changes in the spinal cord. In: Wiesenfeld-Hallin S, Sharma N, Nyberg F (eds) Neuropeptides in the spinal cord: fundamental and clinical aspects (in press)

Munglani R, Jones J G, Hunt S 1993 Pre-emptive analgesia: use of immediate early genes expression as markers of neuronal stimulation. Br J Anaesth 71: 458

Munglani R, Bond A, Smith G et al 1994a Changes in neuronal markers in a mononeuropathic rat model: relationship between Neuropeptide Y, pre-emptive drug treatment and long term mechanical hyperalgesia. Pain (In press)

Munglani R, Bond A, Smith G, Elliot P J, Birch P J, Hunt S P 1994b NPY and c-Fos levels in layers 3 and 4 of the spinal cord correlate with mechanical hyperalgesia in a rat model of mononeuropathy. Brain Res Assoc Abstracts 10: 94

Nagy J I, Hunt S P 1983 The termination of primary afferents within the rat dorsal horn: Evidence for rearrangement following capsaicin treatment. J Comp Neuro 218: 145–158

Noguchi K, Kowalski K, Traub R, Solodkin A, Iadarola M J, Ruda M A 1991 Dynorphin depression and Fos-like immunoreactivity following inflammation induced hyperalgesia are colocalized in spinal cord neurons. Mol Brain Res 10: 229–234

Omote K, Sonada H, Kawamata M, Iwasaki H, Namki 1993 Potentiation of antinoceptive effects of morphine by calcium-channel blockers at the level of the spinal cord. Anesthesiology 79: 746–752

Price D D, Mao J, Mayer D J 1994 Central neural mechanisms of normal and abnormal pain states. In: Pharmacological approaches to the treatment of chronic pain: new concepts and critical issues. IASP Press, Seattle, pp 61–84

Radhakrishnan V, Henry J L 1991 Novel substance P antagonist, CP-96,345 blocks responses of spinal dorsal horn neurones to noxious cutaneous stimulation and to substance P. Neurosci Lett 132: 39–43

Randic M, Jiang M C, Cerne R 1993 Long term potentiation and long term depression of primary afferent neurotransmission in the rat spinal cord. J Neurosci 13: 5228–5241

Rang H P, Bevan S, Dray A 1994 Nociceptive peripheral neurons: cellular properties. In: Textbook of pain (3rd edn). Churchill Livingstone, Edinburgh, pp 57–78

Rauck R L, James M D, Eisenach J C, Jackson K, Young L D, Southern J 1993 Epidural clonidine for the treatment of reflex sympathetic dystrophy. Anaesthesiology 79: 1163–1169

Ren K, Hylden J L K, Williams G M, Ruda M A, Dubner R 1992 The effects of a non-competitive NMDA receptor antagonist, MK-801, on behavioural hyperalgesia and dorsal horn neuronal activity in rats with unilateral inflammation. Pain 50: 331–344

Richmond C, Bromley L, Woolf C 1993 Preoperative morphine pre-empts postoperative pain. Lancet 342: 73–75

Ro L S, Jacobs J M 1993 The role of the saphenous nerve in experimental sciatic nerve mononeuropathy produced by loose ligatures: a behavioural study. Pain 52: 359–369

Rusin K I, Ryu P D, Randic M 1992 Modulation of excitatory amino acid responses in rat dorsal horn neurones by tachykinins. J Neurophysiol 68: 265–286

Rusin K I, Jiang M C, Cerne R, Randic M 1993 Interactions between excitatory amino acids and tachykinins in the rat spinal dorsal horn. Brain Res Bull 30: 329–338

Sato J, Perl E R 1991 Adrenergic excitation of cutaneous pain receptors induced by peripheral nerve injury. Science 251: 1608–1610

Schaible H G, Hope P J, Lang C W, Duggan A W 1992 Calcitonin gene-related peptide causes intraspinal spreading of substance P released by peripheral stimulation. Eur J Neurosci 4: 750–757

Seeburg P 1993 The TIPS/TINS lecture: the molecular biology of the mammalian glutamate receptor channels. Trends Pharmacol Sci 14: 297–303

Seltzer Z, Cohn S, Ginzburg R, Beilin B Z 1991 Modulation of neuropathic pain behavior in rats by spinal disinhibition and NMDA receptor blockade of injury discharge. Pain 45: 69–75

Shortland P, Fitzgerald M 1994 Neonatal sciatic nerve section results in a rearrangement of the central terminals of the saphenous and axotomized sciatic nerve afferents in the dorsal horn of the spinal cord of the adult rat. Eur J Neurosc 6: 75–86

Stacey B R, Watkins W D 1994 Mechanisms and modulators of opioid analgesia. Curr Opin Anaesthesiol 7: 343–346

Stannard C F, Porter G E 1993 Ketamine hydrochloride in the treatment of phantom limb pain. Pain: 227–230

Stiller R U, Grubb B D, Schaible H G 1993 Neurophysiological evidence for increased Kappa opioidergic control of spinal cord neurons in rats with unilateral inflammation at the ankle. Eur J Neurosci 5: 1520–1527

Sugimoto T 1991 Transsynaptic degeneration after peripheral nerve injuries: a mini-review with regard to clinical manifestation of neuropathic symptoms. Eur J Pain 12: 93–99

Tal M, Bennett G J 1994 Extra-territorial pain in a peripheral mononeuropathy: mechano-hyperalgesia and mechano-allodynia in the territory of an uninjured nerve. Pain 57: 375–382

Tanelian D L, Brose W G 1991 Neuropathic pain can be relieved by drugs that are use-dependent sodium channel blockers: lidocaine, carbamazepine, and mexiletine. Anesthesiology 74: 949–951

Thompson S W N, Woolf C J 1991 Primary afferent-evoked prolonged potentials in the spinal cord and their central summation : role of the NMDA receptor. Proceedings of the 6th world conference of pain. Elsevier, Amsterdam, pp 291–298

Thompson S W N, Woolf C J, Sivilotti L G 1993 Small-Caliber afferent inputs produce a heterosynaptic facilitation of the synaptic responses evoked by primary afferent A-fibers in the neonatal rat spinal cord in vitro. J Neurophysiol 69: 2116–2128

Tiseo P J, Inturrisi C E 1993 Attenuation and reversal of morphine tolerance by the competitive N-methyl-D-aspartate receptor antagonist, LY274614. J Pharmacol Exp Ther 264: 1090–1096

Tolle T R, Berthle A, Zieglgansberger W, Seeburg P H, Wisden W 1993 The differential expression of 16 NMDA and non-NMDA receptor subunits in the rat spinal cord and periaqueductal gray. J Neurosci 13: 5009–5028

Trujillo K A, Akil H 1991 Inhibition of morphine tolerance and dependence by the NMDA receptor antagonist MK-801. Science 251: 85–87

Tverskoy M, Oz Y, Isakson A, Finger J, Bradley E L, Kissin I 1994 Pre-emptive effect of fentanyl and ketamine on postoperative pain and wound hyperalgesia. Anesth Analg 78: 205–209

Vane J R, Mitchell J A, Appleton I, et al 1994 Inducible isoforms of cyclooxygenase and nitric oxide in inflammation. Proc Nat Acad Sci USA 91: 2046–2050

Wakisaka S, Kajander K C, Bennett G J 1991 Increased neuropeptide Y (NPY)-like immunoreactivity in rat sensory neurons following peripheral axotomy. Neurosci Lett 124: 200–203

Wakisaka S, Kajander K C, Bennett G J 1992 Effects of peripheral nerve injuries and tissue inflammation on the levels of neuropeptide Y-like immunoreactivity in rat primary afferent neurons. Brain Res 598: 349–352

Wall P, Devor M 1981 Sensory afferent impulses originate from the dorsal root ganglia as well as from the periphery in normal and nerve injured rats. Pain 17: 321–339

Wall P, Gutnik M 1974 Properties of afferent nerve impulses originating from a neuroma. Nature 248: 740–743

Wall P D, Waxman S, Basbaum A I 1974 Ongoing activity in peripheral nerve: injury discharge. Exp Neurol 45: 576–586

Wiesenfeld-Hallin Z, Xu X J, Langel U, Bedecs K, Hokfelt T, Bartfai T 1992 Galanin-mediated control of pain: enhanced role after nerve injury. Proc Nat Acad Sci USA 89: 3334–3337

Williams S, Pini A, Evan G, Hunt S P 1989 Molecular events in the spinal cord following sensory stimulation. In: Processing of sensory information in the superficial dorsal horn of the spinal cord. Plenum Press, New York, pp 273–284

Williams S, Evan G, Hunt S 1990a Spinal c-fos indication by sensory stimulation in neonatal rats. Neurosci Lett 109: 309–314

Williams S, Evan G I, Hunt S P 1990b Changing patterns of c-fos induction in spinal neurons following thermal cutaneous stimulation in the rat. Neuroscience 36: 73–81

Williams S, Evan G, Hunt S P 1991 c-fos induction in the spinal cord after peripheral nerve lesion. Eur J Neurosci 3: 887–894

Willis W D, Coggeshall R E 1991 Sensory mechanisms of the spinal cord. Plenum Press, New York

Woodburn V L, Poat J, Hunter J, Pettersson E, Durieux C, Hughes J 1994 c-fos antisense oligodeoxynucleotide increases formalin-induced nociception. Brain Res Assoc Abstract 11: 96

Woolf C 1983 Evidence for a central component of post injury pain. Nature 306: 686–688

Woolf C J 1994 The dorsal horn: state dependent sensory processing and the generation of pain. In: Melzack R, Wall PD (eds) Textbook of Pain (3rd edn). Churchill Livingstone, Edinburgh, pp 101–112

Woolf C J, Chong M 1993 Pre-emptive analgesia: treating postoperative pain by preventing the establishment of central sensitization. Anaesth Analg 77: 362–379

Woolf C J, Doubell T P 1994 The pathophysiology of chronic pain- increased sensitivity to low threshold Ab-fibre inputs. Curr Opin Neurobiol 4: 525–534

Woolf C, Thompson W 1991 The induction and maintenance of central sensitization is dependent on N-methyl-D aspartic acid receptor activation: implications for the treatment of post-injury pain states. Pain 44: 293–299

Woolf C J, Wall P D 1986 Morphine sensitive and morphine insensitive actions of c fibre input on the rat spinal cord. Neurosci Lett 64: 221–225

Xu X J, Puke M, Verge V, Wiesenfeld-Hallin Z, Hughes J, Hokfelt T 1993 Up regulation of cholecystokinin in primary sensory neurons is associated with morphine insensitivity in experimental neuropathic pain in the rat. Neurosci Lett 152: 129–132

Xu X J, Hao J, Seiger A, Hughes J, Hokfelt T, Wiesenfeld-Hallin Z 1994a Chronic pain related behaviours in spinally injured rats: evidence for functional alteration of the endogenous cholecystokinin and opioid system. Pain 56: 271–277

Xu X J, Hughes J, Hokfelt T, Wiesenfeld-Hallin Z 1994b The CCK-B antagonist C 1988 enhances the reflex-depressive effect of morphine in axotomized rats.

Yaksh T L 1989 Behavioral and autonomic correlates of the tactile evoked allodynia produced by spinal glycine inhibition: effects of modulatory receptor systems and excitatory amino acid antagonists. Pain 37: 111–123

Yaksh T, Malmberg A B 1994 Central pharmacology of nociceptive transmission. In: Melzack R, Wall P D (eds) Textbook of Pain (3rd edn). Churchill Livingstone, Edinburgh, pp 165–200

Yamamoto T, Yaksh T L 1992 Studies on the spinal interaction of morphine and the NMDA antagonist MK-801 on the hyperesthesia observed in a rat model of sciatic mononeuropathy. Neurosci Lett 135: 67–70

Yamamoto T, Shimoyama N, Mizuguchi T, 1993a Role of the injury discharge in the development of thermal hyperaesthesia after sciatic nerve constriction in the rat. Anaesthesiology 79: 993–1002.

Yamamoto T, Shimoyama N, Mizuguguchi T 1993b The effect of morphine, MK801, an NMDA antagonist and CP-96, 345, an NK1 antagonist on the hyperaesthesia evoked by carrageenan injection in the rat paw. Anesthesiology 78: 124–133

Yezierski R P, Culberson J L, Brown P B 1980 Cells of origin of propriospinal connections to cat lumbosacral grey as determined with horseradish peroxidase. Exp Neurol 69: 493–512

5

Controversies in pain management

T. Nash

Pain management has recently been recognized as a specialty within anaesthesia. There has also been a surge in interest in postoperative pain. It is not appropriate to consider that acute pain is a different problem from chronic pain. Acute pain can become chronic, and the approach to the control of all pain revolves around the need to assess and reassess the patient, the use of drug control, psychological support or manipulation, counter-stimulation, nerve blockade, and rehabilitation. Chronicity of pain can lead to very marked psychological and behavioural responses, although acute pain problems have their own attending fear and anxiety that need to be addressed. The more chronic the pain, therefore, the more depression the patient may experience, and the greater the psychological management required. The future development of pain management services should embrace both the chronic and acute problems, thus combining knowledge and resources.

EPIDEMIOLOGY

The suggestion that poor postoperative pain control leads to persistent pain (Cousins 1989) has not been supported by any satisfactory studies. Forty-four per cent of post-thoracotomy patients had post-thoracotomy pain lasting more than 6 months (Kalso et al 1992). This incidence was despite the fact that 60% of patients considered their pain control postoperatively to be good, and 38% to be satisfactory. Only 2% considered their pain control to be poor. Perry & Nash (1992) do not consider that persistent pain is common after surgery, but this was based on the frequency of referral to a pain management clinic and is inconclusive.

The full socio-economic impact of chronic pain is not known, though current studies are attempting to define this. A telephone survey of the incidence of pain suggested that 7% of the population in the UK suffer chronic pain (Bowsher et al 1991).

Certain aspects of pain and its management are either misunderstood or are controversial. Some of these aspects are considered in this chapter.

PHYSICIAN ATTITUDES

Pain is such a common symptom that many may wonder why a subspecialty needs to be devoted to the problem. Indeed there is a need for all physicians to know how to treat pain, and more importantly to direct treatment aimed at curing the underlying condition when this can be treated. The World Health Organization's guidelines on cancer pain relief (1986) can produce good pain relief in terminal cancer in nearly 90% of patients (Takeda 1986). This compares with an overall figure in developed countries of 40–80% of cases with unrelieved severe cancer pain (Hillier & Nash 1991).

Education is essential, and its value has been shown in both acute and chronic situations (Evans et al 1993, Gould et al 1992).

As a result of improved awareness of pain as a problem and the possibilities for treatment, there has been an improvement in the confidence of physicians to cope with pain over the last decade or so. Nash (1994) has discussed training for specialists in the field and its effect on the ability of the profession to treat pain. A questionnaire survey, performed in 1985 and repeated in 1990, showed that Finnish physicians had improved their theoretical knowledge relating to the treatment of pain from terminal cancer. Their problems had changed from frustration at their inability to treat the pain to looking to find a suitable preparation and dosage to control the pain (Vainio 1992).

Physicians have had considerable difficulty achieving good pain control for their patients. A considerable improvement can be achieved by appropriate education.

THE PLACEBO EFFECT

The placebo effect is perhaps the most misunderstood aspect of pain therapy. It is generally believed to be a purely psychological manifestation, and only to occur in 'imaginary' pain. Nothing could be further from the truth.

How the placebo effect is mediated is still unknown. It is effective particularly in the presence of organic disease, and its incidence is considerably more variable than the 35% quoted. Beecher's original paper (1955), from which this value was taken, reviewed many series, and the average incidence was 35%. Indeed, it can be as high as 85%, as in the series of patients having placebo surgery for angina pectoris (Cobb et al 1959). These patients showed improvements in a range of measures, including electrocardiography and exercise tolerance.

In chronic pain patients there is a generally lower placebo response rate, and in laboratory-based studies of experimentally induced pain the proportion of placebo responders is also typically well below 35%. The placebo response also has side effects which include drowsiness, nausea, concentration problems, sweating, vomiting, skin rashes and seizure. There have also been cases of apparent placebo dependence, and placebo-induced symptom worsening: the 'nocebo' effect. It is at present impossible to quantify why some people respond to placebo. Indeed, it would appear that this response varies under different circumstances for each individual, at times responding to placebo and at others not responding. Richardson (1994) has reviewed the subject fully.

Sadly, the commonest use of the placebo is to punish 'difficult' and 'undeserving' patients, and to prove that the patient's symptoms were imaginary. Its use was reported as 80% of 300 nurses and physicians admitting recent placebo administration.

Colour and type of placebo (injections or sophisticated equipment) have not been shown to affect the power of the placebo, although the status, attitudes and behaviour of the therapist have. The therapist's interest in the patient, the treatment and results are related to the success of that treatment. The beliefs of therapists may even influence placebo responses in the context of a double-blind trial, even though therapist blindness has been successfully maintained.

ACUTE PAIN CONTROL

It is often believed that good postoperative pain control can only be achieved using high-technology methods such as epidural/spinal administration and patient-controlled analgesia systems. Lessons can be learned from the provision of good analgesia in cancer pain, where the analgesics are given by the clock and by attention to detail (World Health Organization 1986).

This is supported by the work of Gould et al (1992), who found that the most important single factor in improving pain after surgery was the regular assessment of pain and the more frequent use of intramuscular analgesia using an algorithm. Further improvements were made using patient-controlled analgesia systems and spinal techniques, but the most important step was monitoring the pain and making good use of conventional analgesic regimens.

Heath & Thomas (1993) have pointed out that the modern need for, and interest in, postoperative pain control is due to the increasing use of short-acting anaesthetic agents.

PRE-EMPTIVE ANALGESIA

Interest in the possibility of pre-empting the changes, including 'wind-up', that occur in the central nervous system following on nociceptive stimulation was aroused by an editorial by Wall (1988). McQuay (1994) addressed the question 'Do pre-emptive treatments provide better pain control?' At present, there is no good evidence that non-steroidal anti-inflammatory drugs or paracetamol have a pre-emptive effect. The evidence for local anaesthetic blocks is inconclusive, because the negative studies lack power, but positive studies do exist. For opioids, again the evidence is inconclusive but stronger. Better studies are still required.

The surgical stimulus continues after the cessation of surgery, and so pre-emptive analgesic treatment must continue until the stimulus has abated. It is naive to believe that one analgesic or one single technique will solve a complex problem. Most probably a combination of pre-emptive analgesia and multimodal pain therapy will provide the most effective pain alleviation. Efficacy is almost satisfactory at present (using a multimodal approach of opioids, non-steroidal anti-inflammatory drugs, N-methyl-D-aspartate antagonists and local blocks appropriately). The way forward is to find techniques and drugs with fewer side effects (Kehlet 1994).

OPIOID SENSITIVITY

Not all pain responds to opioids – the classic example is trigeminal neuralgia, for which anticonvulsants are the treatment of choice. Arner & Meyerson (1988) showed that there was a very poor response to opioids in a range of neuropathic pain problems. This led to the belief that opioids should not be prescribed for neurogenic pain. Portenoy et al (1990) addressed this issue, and stated that opioids should not be withheld on the assumption that the pain mechanism, or any other factor, precludes a favourable response. McQuay et al (1992) described a method of evaluating opioid sensitivity using patient-controlled analgesia and showed that there was a spectrum of sensitivity that did not relate well to the pain being neuropathic or nociceptive. Five out of 13 patients with neuropathic pain had a good response to opioids, and 5 out of 14 nociceptive pain patients did not respond to opioids. It is therefore appropriate to assess opioid sensitivity in all patients.

In partial opioid insensitivity, a combination of local anaesthetic and morphine infusion intrathecally can be maintained long term and give good analgesia (Goucke 1993).

Midazolam may prolong the effects of morphine by delaying morphine-induced development of tolerance to antinociception.

Should narcotics be used for chronic non-malignant pain?

There is an inappropriate degree of myth, misconception and prejudice surrounding the use of opioid drugs in the treatment of all pain states. The general consensus indicates that opioids are contraindicated in long-term pain syndromes associated with non-terminal disease states. Gourlay (1994) considers that opioids to treat severe pain associated with non-terminal disease states should not be considered as a first-line treatment. Patients should be fully assessed physically and psychologically, and all non-invasive techniques given a reasonable trial. However patients with a predominant nociceptive focus can be considered for long-term opioid therapy if the psychiatric and psychological assessment reveals no drug-seeking behaviour or dependency traits.

Portenoy (1994) has performed a critical review of the literature, and has shown that some of the doctrinaire pronouncements about long-term opioid therapy for non-malignant disease have derived from long-standing misapprehensions about pharmacological outcomes, such as tolerance, physical dependence and persistent side effects. He sets out guidelines for the use of opioids in this situation. Portenoy considers that clinicians who choose to take responsibility for this treatment after careful consideration of the medical issues involved, should feel free to communicate the nature of this judgement to the patient, family, colleagues and regulatory personnel. Ultimately, the decision to implement a therapeutic trial of an opioid drug that takes into account the potential risks and benefits, applies appropriate dosing guidelines and monitoring, and adequately documents outcomes, should garner no more stigma, and no more concern on the part of the clinician, than a trial with any other type of analgesic. Portenoy does, however, temper this by pointing out that neither the medical literature nor clinical experience provides compelling evidence that long-term opioid use would be salutary for more than a very small number of patients with chronic non-malignant pain.

There is a strong pharmacological rationale for the use of opioid drugs such as morphine in severe pain of any origin. These drugs may have a side effect profile that may prove unacceptable to some patients in the long term, and there is some risk of the development of tolerance and dependence, though this is more of a social than a medical problem (Hill 1994).

The rational view would appertain to the use of opioids in all pain states according to well-considered guidelines. To withhold such a potentially useful agent may well be inhumane.

Guidelines for the use of opioids in non-malignant pain:

1. Opioids should only be used when all other attempts to control pain have failed.
2. History of substance abuse and personality disorder are relative contraindictions to their use.
3. One practitioner only should take responsibility for the patient.
4. Patients should give informed consent.
5. Opioid should be administered on a 'round-the-clock' basis.
6. The pain should have been shown to be opioid sensitive.
7. Opioid therapy is complementary to other analgesic and rehabilitation approaches.
8. The regime should be flexible enough to cater for 'bad' days.
9. The patient should be given monthly assessments and prescriptions until stable.

(Portenoy 1994)

If drug control is unsatisfactory, then two main approaches exist: behavioural and interventional. These approaches are often seen as mutually exclusive, and this stems from the traditional view that pain is either somatic or psychological. In the UK, the facility for the behavioural approach is not common, as psychologists, and the funding to provide them, are scarce. Indeed the traditional pain clinic was a nerve block clinic, the first starting in 1947 at University College Hospital, London (Swerdlow 1986). Certain aspects of each approach do tend to exclude the other.

THE PLACE OF THE PAIN MANAGEMENT PROGRAMME

Behavioural therapy may be effective in increasing activity levels and exercise tolerance, and decreasing pain medication, but may not result in a change in pain experience or level.

Admission criteria for pain management programmes frequently cite that the patient should be 'at the end of the line', with part of the contract with the patient being that no further investigation, treatment or cure will be sought. The main outcome measures focus on drug intake, which gives the agenda to reduce analgesic consumption, and activity. It is easy for the programmes to focus on reducing drug consumption per se, to prove the value of the treatment, and lose sight of the main reason for the programme, which is to help the patient with pain. This reduction in analgesic consumption is also considered to enable the patient to take control of their pain more readily. Both the seeking of further investigation and cure, which includes the interventional pain therapies, and the use of analgesics, may be considered to perpetuate the pain behavioural response that the programme is designed to reduce.

Linton et al (1993) have shown the value of early intervention in preventing the development of chronic musculoskeletal pain. For patients with a previous history of pain there was no impact on their recovery from acute musculoskeletal pain but for those with no previous history the risk of developing chronic pain was reduced by more than eight-fold.

Linton's work suggests that the behavioural approach may be valuable at an early stage, before the pain has developed into a chronic problem.

Thus, it may be that behavioural management would be even more effective if used before the chronic pain syndrome develops, and if reduction in analgesic consumption is not considered to be a prime aim of treatment.

THE PLACE OF INTERVENTIONAL TREATMENT

Are the results just placebo effects?

The biggest problem that has faced the interventionalists is to convince their doubters that interventional therapy is effective, and not just due to a placebo effect. Several placebo-controlled randomized studies have now been performed that show the value of radiofrequency denervation procedures in low back pain (Gallagher et al 1994) and cervical dorsal root ganglion thermocoagulation for cervical pain (Kleef 1994). Gallagher et al showed the value of facet joint denervation in a double-blind, placebo-controlled trial in patients who have a good though brief response to local anaesthetic blockade. North et al (1994) have shown that results are maintained at long-term follow-up (3 years) following facet joint denervation for low back pain.

Facet joint pain does not seem to involve an inflammatory aspect within the joint (Nash 1990, Marks et al 1992).

Lesioning does therefore have an effect that is not placebo.

Are lesioning techniques safe?

Percutaneous cordotomy in experienced hands is relatively safe and effective. Lipton (1989) obtained complete analgesia in 86% of 710 patients, 24% requiring a second procedure to achieve this. Mortality was 6%, all within the first week, but the selection of patients was anyone presenting with intractable pain and a minimum life expectancy of 2 weeks. All 6% were due to respiratory dysfunction in patients with carcinoma, and the majority with carcinoma of the lung. The main long-term complication was paresis (2%).

A case of possible spinal coning within minutes of an intrathecal injection of 10% phenol in glycerol at T9–10 for pain at T4 from carcinoma of the lung, producing paraplegia, is described by Morgan & Steller (1994). Spinal secondaries can usually be suspected from the history, and are often obvious on spinal X-ray. The risk of paresis and paraplegia with intrathecal neurolysis in the presence of spinal secondaries is known to be high. This case highlights the dangers of intrathecal injection in the presence of pre-existing spinal secondaries, and the need for proper evaluation of the pain problem. The author well remembers discussing this possibility with one patient with a spinal secondary. Six months after the intrathecal block she developed paraplegia, and blamed the block! This highlights the problem of informed consent, which is discussed later.

Coeliac plexus ablation remains one of the most successful treatments for upper abdominal pain of visceral origin (Petriccione di Vadi & Wedley 1990).

Gasserian thermocoagulation for trigeminal neuralgia remains a useful way to control the pain of trigeminal neuralgia. A personal unpublished series (26 patients) has shown that all cases of trigeminal neuralgia in which a lesion was successfully performed had excellent relief, but 30% had to be repeated. No permanent sequelae, other than mild sensory loss in the treated area, occurred. New developments in imaging techniques have shown that vascular compression of the trigeminal rootlets is commonly present, and suggests that vascular decompression may be the treatment of choice. This requires a craniotomy, and resources and morbidity may not enable this treatment to become standard for some time.

The most serious complication of dorsal root ganglion thermocoagulation is reported to be paraplegia due to hyperaemia in the foramen ovale producing hypoxia of the cord by a 'steal' effect (Koning et al 1991). The intervertebral foramina are of critical value in the blood supply of the spinal cord (Dommisse 1980). The author is now aware of two cases where ischaemia of the conus medullaris produced cauda equinus lesions following low thoracic ganglion thermocoagulation, probably due to damage to the artery of Adamkiewicz.

Permanence of lesioning depends on site of lesion more than type of lesion. Lesions of the sensory ganglia can produce permanent nerve damage (Nash 1986). Lesions elsewhere will allow the nerve axons to regenerate, and this may lead to neuroma formation and dysaesthesias. Cryotherapy does not destroy the axon sheaths, and thus allows total neuronal regeneration without the dysaesthesias and neuromata formation. This is a possible advantage over other neurodestructive techniques that needs to be evaluated.

Neurodestructive techniques do carry a risk, but if performed by an experienced practitioner this risk is minimized (Nash 1986, Niv & Chayen 1992). Training in these techniques is therefore imperative.

LONG-TERM INTRASPINAL OPIATES

It is generally believed that neurodestructive procedures carry more risk than intraspinal opiates. The risk of neurodestructive lesions performed by experienced therapists is small and this may well outweigh the disadvantage of continued supervision of an implanted reservoir system, and the risk of meningitis developing. Chrubasik et al (1992) state that almost all patients receiving long-term spinal opiates had some sort of side effects or complications, including urinary retention, pruritus, pain from bolus injection, and perspiration, as well as dose-dependent opiate effects such as sedation, nausea/emesis, dysphoria, euphoria, respiratory depression, hypotension and constipation. The intrathecal route can also produce cerebrospinal fluid leakage or persistent fistulae with spinal headache. Such systems also fail by leaking, kinking or disconnecting. The relative cost–benefits of the two approaches have not been fully evaluated.

INFORMED CONSENT

The value of informed consent in all therapies is being increasingly appreciated. The need for consent when prescribing long-term narcotics for non-malignant pain has been mentioned above. A case of opiate dependence in chronic pain recently won a negligence settlement of £50 000.

The recent media hype over epidural depomedrone (methylprednisolone acetate) injection, and pending court cases, illustrates the need to point out that many drugs used by varying routes for pain control are not being used according to the data sheet published by the pharmaceutical companies. Such drugs include anticonvulsants and antidepressants. Epidural steroid injection for lumbo-sciatica has been used for 25 years, and an extensive search of the literature has not been able to show any long-term sequelae (Walsh 1992). Nelson (1993) points out the theoretical danger of intrathecal injection, and reviews the literature which includes series of arachnoiditis following the use of methylprednisolone acetate to treat or attempt to prevent the development of arachnoiditis following myelography! No series focused on epidural methylprednisolone, only on intraspinal and/ or epidural injection. If the problem exists it would appear to be small, and this was the decision of the working party of the National Health and Medical Research Council in Australia (1994). The value of steroid in the injectate in the alleviation of sciatica was shown by Rogers et al (1992).

It is imperative that the patient is informed when the use of an agent is contrary to that specified in its product licence.

The use of narcotics for spinal administration, both epidural and intrathecal, is again not within the product licence of the drugs. The potential risk of arachnoiditis in this situation must also be considered and the patient warned that a product licence does not exist for use in this way.

CONCLUSION

This discussion has only focused on a few aspects of pain management. The tendency to see pain as a disease that can be cured has been responsible for the pursuit of single modalities of treatment. The need to research the comparative value of individual treatments has also obviated against the multimodal approach. Pain itself is not a disease. It is amenable to control, and may often require an approach that balances a number of therapeutic modalities which revolve around the need to assess and reassess the patient, and the use of drug control, psychological support or manipulation, counter-stimulation, nerve blockade and rehabilitation.

REFERENCES

Arner S, Meyerson B A 1988 Lack of analgesic effect of opioids on neuropathic and idiopathic forms of pain. Pain 33: 11–23
Beecher H K 1955 The powerful placebo. JAMA 159: 1602–1606
Bowsher D, Rigge M, Sopp L 1991 Prevalence of chronic pain in the British population: a telephone survey of 1037 households. Pain Clin 4: 223–230
Chrubasik J, Chrubasik S, Friedrich G et al 1992 Long-term treatment of pain by spinal opiates: an update. Pain Clin 5: 147–156
Cobb L A, Thomas G I, Dillard D H et al 1959 An evaluation of internal mammary artery ligation by a double blind technique. N Engl J Med 260: 1115–1118
Cousins M 1989 Acute and post-operative pain. In: Wall P D, Melzack R (eds). Textbook of pain (2nd edn). Churchill Livingstone, Edinburgh, pp 284–305
Dommisse G F 1980 The arteries, arterioles and capillaries of the spinal cord. Ann R Coll Surg 62: 369–375

Evans R J, Watson C P N, Kuch K 1993 Chronic pain tuition at the University of Toronto Smythe Pain Clin, Toronto Hospital (General). Pain Clin 6: 39–48

Gallagher J, Petriccione di Vadi P L, Wedley J R et al 1994 Radio-frequency facet joint denervation in the treatment of low back pain: a prospective controlled double-blind study to assess its efficacy. Pain Clin 7: 193–198

Goodwin J S, Goodwin J M, Vogel J M 1979 Knowledge and use of placebo by house officers and nurses. Ann Intern Med 91: 106–110

Goucke R 1993 Continuous intrathecal analgesia with opioid/local anaesthetic mixture for cancer pain. Anaesth Intensive Care 21: 222–223

Gould T H, Crosby D L, Harmer M et al 1992 Policy for controlling pain after surgery: effect of sequential changes in management. Br Med J 305: 1187–1193

Gourlay G K 1994 Long-term use of opioids in chronic pain patients with non-terminal disease states. Pain Rev 1: 62–76

Heath M L, Thomas V J 1993 Patient-controlled analgesia: confidence in postoperative pain control. Oxford University Press, Oxford

Hill R G 1994 Pharmacological considerations in the use of opioids in the management of pain associated with non-terminal disease states. Pain Rev 1: 47–61

Hillier R, Nash T P 1991 Pain management. Med Int 93: 3894–3899

Kalso E, Perttunen K, Kaasinen S 1992 Pain after thoracic surgery. Acta Anaesthesiol Scand 36: 96–100

Kehlet H 1994 Postoperative pain relief: what is the issue? Br J Anaesth 72: 375–378

Kleef M van 1994 Personal communication

Koning H M, Koster H G, Niemeijer P E 1991 Ischaemic spinal cord lesion following percutaneous radiofrequency spinal rhizotomy. Pain 45: 161–166

Linton S J, Hellsing A L, Andersson D 1993 A controlled study of the effects of an early intervention on acute musculoskeletal pain problems. Pain 54: 353–359

Lipton S 1989 Percutaneous cordotomy. In: Wall PD, Melzack R (eds) Textbook of pain (2nd edn). Churchill Livingstone, Edinburgh, pp 832–839

Marks R C, Houston T, Thulbourne T 1992 Facet joint injection and facet nerve block: a randomised comparison of 96 patients with chronic low back pain. Pain 49: 325–328

McQuay H J 1994 Do pre-emptive treatments provide better pain control? In: Gebhart G F, Hammond D L, Jensen T S (eds) Proceedings of the 7th World Congress on Pain, Progress in Pain Research and Management, Vol. 2. IASP Press, Seattle, pp 702–723

McQuay H J, Jadad A R, Carroll D et al 1992 Opioid sensitivity of chronic pain: a patient-controlled analgesia method. Anaesthesia 47: 757–767

Medical Defence Union 1993 Iatrogenic opiate dependence. J Med Defence Union 9: 93–94

Morgan R J, Steller P H 1994 Acute paraplegia following intrathecal phenol block in the presence of occult epidural malignancy. Anaesthesia 49: 142–144

Nash T P 1986 Percutaneous radiofrequency lesioning of dorsal root ganglia for intractable pain. Pain 24: 67–73

Nash T P 1990 Facet joints: intra-articular steroids or nerve block? Pain Clin 3: 77–82

Nash T P 1994 Education of a pain specialist. In: Prithvi Raj P (ed) Proceedings of the Sixth International Congress , 'The pain clinic'. Monduzzi Editore, Bologna (in press)

National Health and Medical Research Council 1994 Epidural use of steroids in the management of back pain and sciatica of spinal origin. NHMRC, Canberra

Nelson D A 1993 Intraspinal therapy using methylprednisolone acetate: twenty-three years of clinical controversy. Spine 18: 278–286

Niv D, Chayen M S 1992 Reduction of localized cancer pain by percutaneous dorsal root ganglia lesions. Pain Clin 5: 229–234

North R B, Han M, Zahurak M et al 1994 Radiofrequency lumbar facet denervation: analysis of prognostic factors. NVBPijnbulletin 14(2): 15

Perry H, Nash T P 1992 Scar neuromata. Pain Clin 5: 3–7

Petriccione di Vadi P, Wedley J R 1990 The use of coeliac plexus block in abdominal cancer pain: a review. Pain Clin 3: 223–227

Portenoy R K 1994 Opioid therapy for chronic nonmalignant pain: current status. In: Fields H L, Liebrskind J C (eds) Pharmacological approaches to the treatment of chronic pain: new concepts and critical issues. IASP, Seattle, pp 247–287

Portenoy R, Foley K, Inturrisi K 1990 The nature of opioid responsiveness and its implications for neuropathic pain: new hypotheses derived from studies of opioid infusions. Pain 43: 273–286

Richardson P H 1994 Placebo effects in pain management. Pain Rev 1: 15–32

Rogers P, Nash T P, Schiller D et al 1992 Epidural steroid injections for sciatica. Pain Clin 5: 67–72

Swerdlow M 1986 A preliminary history of pain relief clinics in Europe. Pain Clin 1: 77–82

Takeda F 1986 Results of field-testing in Japan of the WHO draft interim guide-line on relief of cancer pain. Pain Clin 1: 83–89

Tejwani G A, Rattan A K, Sribanditmongkol P et al 1993 Inhibition of morphine-induced tolerance and dependence by a benzodiazepine receptor agonist midazolam in the rat. Anesth Analg 76: 1052–1060

Vainio A 1992 Treatment of terminal cancer pain in Finland: a second look. Acta Anaesthesiol Scand 36: 89–95

Wall P D 1988 The prevention of postoperative pain. Pain 33: 289–290

Walsh E M 1992 Steroid epidurals for low back pain and sciatica: Still safe and effective after all these years? J Pain Soc 10: 21–24

World Health Organization 1986 Cancer pain relief. World Health Organization, Geneva

6

Transdermal drug administration

C. S. Reilly

The concept of delivering drugs across the skin is not new. Although the skin is a relatively impermeable waterproof layer, drugs can permeate it down a diffusion gradient and be absorbed subsequently into the systemic circulation. This has been noted as an adverse effect of topically administered drugs which are used principally in dermatology. For example, the systemic side effects of topically administered steroids have been well described. In recent years attention has focused on utilization of the transdermal route as a method for delivering drugs therapeutically. A number of potential advantages for this route have been described and in practice a number have been shown to be beneficial (Berner & John 1994). These include:

1. The avoidance of first-pass metabolism.
2. A method of continuous administration of drug which avoids the peak and trough effect of oral or parenteral routes and achieves a steady-state concentration as a result of a fixed delivery rate.
3. A prolonged duration of action.
4. With some systems, delivery of a drug to the appropriate plasma concentration to produce the desired effect without producing some of the adverse systemic effects associated with higher concentrations.

A number of drugs have been studied clinically for administration transdermally. These include hyoscine for motion sickness, nitroglycerine for angina treatment, fentanyl for postoperative and chronic pain relief, antihypertensive therapy using clonidine, timolol and bupranolol, hormone replacement using testosterone, oestradiol and oestradiol/norethisterone and finally nicotine as an anti-smoking aid. Not all of these products have been introduced fully into clinical practice. This chapter will first discuss the principles involved in the delivery of drugs transdermally, then describe the clinical use of the systems currently available, with particular emphasis on those that have direct or indirect relevance to anaesthetic practice. Finally, the developments which are likely to occur in the near future using these systems will be discussed.

PRINCIPLES OF ACTION OF TRANSDERMAL SYSTEMS

The determinants for effective delivery of drugs transdermally are the nature of the skin site and the nature of the drug to be delivered.

Skin

Skin is a very effective barrier to the absorption of water. The principal barrier is the stratum cornium, which has a relatively high lipid content. Drugs can pass across this membrane by diffusion. The thickness of the skin layer varies around the body and ranges from 20 to 80 μM. It has a good underlying blood supply which facilitates absorption of the drug.

A number of factors will influence the effectiveness of drug absorption across the skin and the rate at which this occurs (Shaw & Chandrasekaran 1981). These include the skin thickness, skin temperature and blood flow.

Skin thickness

The thickness of skin varies with site and is on average 40 μM thick. Age, gender and race also produce variations in skin thickness. Using an in vitro model it has been estimated that the peak concentration achieved over 20 μM thick skin would be three times that achieved over 60 μM thick skin (Gupta et al 1992). The effect of a disrupted skin layer would markedly increase drug absorption and it is important that transdermal patches are not placed over broken or diseased skin areas.

Temperature

The temperature at which this process occurs can influence the amount of drug absorbed, with higher temperatures producing a greater uptake. Using fentanyl in an in vitro system, it has been estimated that over the range 32–37°C drugs flux was approximately doubled (Gupta et al 1992). The skin temperature may vary at different sites on the body, with the thigh being the coolest and the postauricular area the warmest. However, there was only a 2.5–3°C difference between these sites.

Blood flow

Blood flow, theoretically, plays a role in the rate of absorption of a drug in that, as the drug crosses the stratum cornium, it will be absorbed into vessels. This washout effect will serve to maintain a concentration gradient. However, in normal circumstances the blood flow to the skin is considerably higher than that which would be a limit to the rapid uptake of drug. Therefore, in clinical practice the permeability of the drug across the skin is the determinant of the rate of uptake.

Drug

Not all drugs are appropriate for administration by the transdermal route (Shaw & Urquhart 1981). To allow adequate transfer across the skin it is desirable that the drug has a molecular weight of <1000 and has adequate lipophilicity and hydrophilicity. It is important that the drug is potent so that only a small amount of drug needs to be transported to produce the desired effect. It is also essential that it has a high partition coefficient between skin and water. This allows a concentration gradient to be created from the drug reservoir to the skin. In choosing a drug for transdermal delivery it is also important that the drug does not produce irritation of the skin, is not extensively bound in skin and undergoes minimal metabolism in skin.

The importance of these physical chemical properties in the transfer of drugs across the skin is well illustrated in a review comparing the physico-chemical properties of morphine and fentanyl (Lehman & Zech 1992). The two drugs are of similar molecular weight but fentanyl is less water soluble and considerably more lipid soluble than morphine. This results in fentanyl having an estimated partition coefficient between skin and water (i.e. skin and drug reservoir) 400 times that of morphine. Although the diffusion coefficients across the skin are fairly similar the above properties lead to fentanyl having a skin flux (g/cm^2/per hour) approximately 160 times that of morphine.

Design of systems

The pharmacology and pharmacokinetics of transdermal drug delivery and their relevence to the design of delivery systems have been reviewed recently (Berner & John 1994, Wester & Maibach 1992).

As can be seen from the above description the obvious rate-limiting step for absorption of a drug is the rate at which it would cross the stratum cornium. The simplest system therefore would be application of the drug directly to the skin – for example, in the use of nitroglycerine for the control of angina. This can be applied as a paste to the skin and absorption occurs into the systemic circulation. The rate and amount of drug absorbed will be determined by the amount of drug present and the surface area that it covers. The amount of drug will determine the diffusion gradient and the surface area covered will obviously influence the total amount of drug absorbed. Indeed, the absorptive capacity of the skin for a drug can be described in units per square centimetre of skin covered. A slightly more complicated system would involve the drug being placed in a matrix which is then applied directly to the skin under an occlusive dressing. Again with this system the rate of absorption would be determined by the gradient across the skin. If the rate of absorption per unit area of skin covered can be determined, the next step in the designs of a transdermal system would be the introduction of a membrane which limited the release of drug on to the skin surface. This would mean that different doses of the same drug could be administered by varying the size (surface area) or capacity (drug reservoir) of this rate-limiting membrane. Therefore a patch could be designed to deliver a fixed amount of drug to the skin surface which would then be taken up into the systemic circulation. This would apply only if the amount of drug released did not exceed the capacity of the skin to transfer the drug.

A transdermal system would therefore have a number (Fig. 6.1) of components starting with an adhesive area that applies to the skin, then a controlled-release membrane or rate-limiting membrane, a reservoir of the drug in an appropriate matrix and finally an overall occlusive backing to protect the system. In some systems a loading dose of drug is included in the adhesive layer to speed up the rate of achieving a steady-state concentration.

FENTANYL

Fentanyl is an appropriate drug for administration transdermally. It is of suitable molecular weight and has a high lipophility which allows diffusion across the skin.

The structure of the transdermal fentanyl patch is similar to the general description given above in that it has an occlusive backing, a drug reservoir, a rate-limiting membrane and an adhesive membrane. The reservoir contains fentanyl 0.25 mg/cm^2 surface area, ethanol and water in a hydroxyethylcellulose gel. There are four sizes of patch releasing 25, 50, 75 and 100 µg/h of fentanyl. The variation in delivery is achieved by proportional changes in the amount in the drug reservoir and the surface area which is available for drug exchange. These patches release 25 µg/h per 10 cm^2 surface area from a reservoir of 2.5 mg fentanyl per 25 µg/h. For example, the 50 µg/h patch has an active surface area of 20 cm^2 and a reservoir of 5 mg of fentanyl. Initial studies applied the patch for only 24 h. However, as can be seen from the amount of drug present in the reservoir, there is potential for longer application. Subsequent studies have used 72 h application.

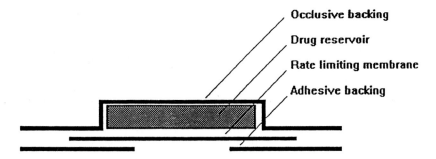

Fig. 6.1 Schematic diagram of a transdermal patch. In some systems the adhesive layer contains a loading dose of drug.

Pharmacokinetics

There is an initial delay in achieving any measurable fentanyl concentrations in plasma as the drug has to pass initially through the skin before absorption into the bloodstream. It frequently takes over 2 h to achieve measurable plasma concentrations of fentanyl. The concentration then rises steadily and achieves a relative plateau level at 6–8 h. The concentration achieved is similar to that which would be achieved by an intravenous infusion at the same rate (Duthie et al 1988, Holley & van Steennis 1988). However, there is lag time of 2–3 h in achieving a concentration similar to that which would result from intravenous infusion at the same rate. There is a proportional increase in the plasma concentration achieved by increasing size of patch (Fig. 6.2). There is however, the same degree of inter-individual variability in concentration achieved as would be found with intravenous infusion. With prolonged application i.e. 72 h application, a steady-state concentration is usually achieved by 24 h. This will normally stay stable until removal of patch at 72 h although some studies have noted a small decline in concentration towards the end of the 72 h application (Broome et al 1995). When the patch is removed some investigators have noted a small increase in the fentanyl concentration over the first hour and have attributed this to changes in the gradient across the skin produced by removing the patch. However, this has not been a consistent finding across the studies. There is then a steady decline in plasma concentration. It has been noted, however, that while the clearance of fentanyl relative to intra-

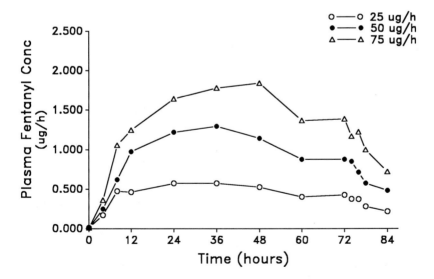

Fig. 6.2 Plasma fentanyl concentrations achieved during 72 hour application of 25, 50 or 75 µg/h transdermal systems in a group of patients undergoing abdominal hysterectomy (Based on Broome et al 1995).

venous clearance is not changed there is a marked prolongation of the half-life to some 15–18 h. This is thought to be due to the reservoir effect within the skin.

It is obvious from the kinetic description that use in the perioperative period would require that the patch was put on several hours before the operation. An alternative is to give a bolus dose of fentanyl at the start of the operation which raises the concentration towards the desired level. This is well illustrated in the study by Duthie and colleagues (1988), who supplemented a 100 µg/h fentanyl patch with 100 or 200 µg bolus doses. This was compared with a continuous intravenous infusion of fentanyl at 100 µg/h. Similar plasma concentrations were achieved in all three groups by 12 h.

Clinical use

The majority of initial studies of transdermal fentanyl were directed at its use in acute pain, particularly for postoperative analgesia (Sandler 1992). These studies, in general, applied the transdermal patch 2 h before surgery and peroperative supplementation with fentanyl or some other opioid was included. The efficacy of pain relief was assessed in most of the studies by pain scores and by the reduction in supplementary analgesia requested, usually PCA morphine. Early studies such as those of Duthie and colleagues (1988) and Holley & van Steennis (1988) demonstrated that plasma concentrations of fentanyl within the analgesic range were achieved by the end of the operation when a bolus dose was given peroperatively. This technique was used in subsequent control studies and shown to provide reasonable analgesia (Rowbotham et al 1989). A consistent finding across all the studies, however, was that supplementary analgesia was required to achieve adequate pain control (Table 6.1). However, significant reduction in the amount of morphine required was demonstrated in all studies. The

Table 6.1 Mean morphine usage during the first 24 h postoperatively in studies comparing fentanyl patches (25, 50, 75 or 100 µg/h) with placebo.

Study	Surgery	No.	Placebo	25 µg/h	50 µg/h	75 µg/h	100 µg/h
Plezia et al (1988)	Ortho/ abdom	43	24			12	
Caplan et al (1989)	Ortho	42	30			18	
Rowbotham et al (1989)	Upper abdom	40	49				33
McLeskey et al (1989)	Lower abdom	54	29			10	
Sandler et al (1991)	Abdom hyst	36	36		24	9	
Broome et al (1995)	Abdom hyst	81	44	38	33	31	

Ortho = orthopaedic; abdom = abdominal; abdom hyst = abdominal hysterectomy; No. = number of patients studied.

incidence of nausea and vomiting within these study groups was relatively high, varying from 30% to 70% (Sandler 1992). Potentially the most serious adverse effect is respiratory depression. While the incidence of this is low, it has been noted in several studies in which patients were withdrawn because of low respiratory rates (<8 beats/min), usually occurring during sleep (Sandler 1992). The later studies of postoperative analgesia kept the patch in place for 72 h and the reduced supplementary analgesic dose effect was noted throughout the study period. The incidence of postoperative respiratory depression, which is probably less than 2%, the inability to titrate the dose of fentanyl and the requirement for supplementary opioid analgesia would suggest that transdermal fentanyl on its own is not a particularly useful method for providing postoperative analgesia.

The second area of clinical application of transdermal fentanyl has been its use in cancer pain. The use of a system which will deliver an opioid continuously while avoiding the oral route and the effects of first-pass metabolism, minimizes alterations in gastric motility and avoids intramuscular or subcutaneous administration is an attractive alternative in this group of patients. A number of studies have now been conducted looking at the efficacy of transdermal fentanyl in cancer pain patients (Simmonds & Richenbacher 1992). The initial studies looked at 24 h application but subsequent studies have looked at 72 h application of each patch. These have, in general, shown this to be a useful and efficacious route for administering an opioid analgesic to these patients. The initial problem to be addressed in converting a patient from oral morphine preparations to transdermal fentanyl is the dose equivalence. The findings of the initial studies were that for every 120 mg morphine taken orally per day a 25 μg/h patch was applied (Simmonds & Richenbacher 1992). Therefore, for example, a patient taking 200 mg morphine orally per day would start with a 50 μg/h patch. In general, this was found to be effective. However, in some of the studies withdrawal symptoms were noted in the patients and many required supplementary oral morphine during the transition period. However, the majority of patients in these studies have found this to be an effective way of delivering analgesia and the use of multiple patches has been shown to be effective. At the end of these studies the patients were given the option of continuing with the patches and many opted to continue this form of treatment.

One of the major benefits that appears to accrue from this method of treatment is improvement in measures of quality of life. An example of this can be seen in a recent study where 40 patients were transferred to transdermal fentanyl from a stable oral morphine therapy (Ahmedzai et al 1994). The quality of pain relief provided by the two methods was similar and supplemental morphine was required in about only 50% of the patients. However, there were significant improvements in a number of quality of life measurements, including, sleep quality, morning vigilance, nausea, vomiting and constipation. These findings are consistent with other studies in patients with cancer pain and together suggest that this is a further treatment option for these patients. It is interesting to note that 60% of the patients in the study described above took up the option to continue with fentanyl patches at the end of the study period.

Summary

It has been shown that fentanyl can be delivered transdermally to achieve concentrations in the plasma that are appropriate for pain relief. Patches have been shown to be effective for up to 72 h. The main adverse effects noted have been respiratory depression in <3% of patients and nausea in around 30%.

The requirement for supplementary analgesia in the acute pain studies suggests that this is not an appropriate sole method for postoperative analgesia. However, a consistent reduction in the amount of morphine required was demonstrated in all the studies. The initial studies with its use in cancer pain suggest that this is a much more appropriate technique for these patients. In addition to providing analgesia a number of studies have shown improvement in quality of life.

NITROGLYCERINE

Nitrates have been used for many years in the treatment of angina. The pharmacological action is to produce vasodilatation in the coronary vessels and in the peripheral vessels. The effect on the peripheral vessels is dose related, with venodilatation occurring at lower concentrations and arteriolar dilatation occurring at higher concentrations. The beneficial effects on the myocardium are therefore threefold: improved coronary perfusion and a reduction in preload and afterload. Nitroglycerine was administered originally as a tablet placed under the tongue, giving rapid buccal absorption. When given orally little or no nitroglycerine reaches the systemic circulation due to extensive first-pass metabolism. In the 1970s nitroglycerine paste was developed for administration across the skin. This was shown to be effective and was extensively used for a number of years. However, it required application several times a day and there was low patient compliance with its use. Transdermal patches were developed in the early 1980s and have gained wide acceptance in clinical practice. There are a number of proprietary preparations available.

There is variation in the structure of various patches available, with some able to deliver a constant rate per hour on application, others which have a higher release, initially, and some which have a phased release with a large amount being released in the first 12 h and small percentage (<15%) in the second 12 h of application (Todd et al 1990). All have been shown to be effective at delivering therapeutic concentrations of nitroglycerine to the circulation. However, as with other transdermal drugs there is considerable inter-individual variation in the plasma concentration achieved.

Pharmacokinetics

Nitroglycerine is rapidly metabolized in the body by glutathione nitrate reductase, which is found in the liver, vascular smooth muscle and red blood cells. The elimination half-life has been estimated to be <3 min. There is a large apparent volume of distribution and a very large total body clearance (Bogaert 1987). The majority of studies of the kinetics of nitro-glycerine patches have demonstrated measurable concentrations in plasma within the first hour, with achievement of steady-state levels (with the constant rate release patches) around 2 h (Todd et al 1990). The total bio-availability of nitroglycerine from the patches is usually greater than 75%. When the patch is removed the drug is cleared rapidly from the plasma and is not detectable within 1 h. There is considerable inter-individual variation in the plasma concentrations achieved by nitroglycerine patches. This may be explained in part by the difficulty encountered in accurate measurement of plasma concentrations as the drug continues to be metabolized in whole blood after a sample has been taken.

Clinical use

The major clinical use for transdermal nitroglycerine has been in the treatment of stable angina. The concept of continuously administering a vaso-dilator to decrease the incidence and severity of angina attacks is an attractive one. Following placement of a transdermal nitrogen patch many studies have demonstrated an initial improvement in angina symptoms and improvement in exercise tolerance (Scardi et al 1985). However, with continuous administration this is not sustained and it would appear that tolerance to continuously administered nitroglycerine occurs quite quickly (Abrams 1988). The problem of tolerance has been noted not only with transdermal administration but also with sustained-release oral preparations. It would appear that the maximum response to application of a patch occurs between 3 and 6 h (usually measured by exercise testing to onset of angina). This initial effect appears markedly decreased by 24 h of continuous administration.

The development of tolerance has led to the development of the strategy of intermittent use, thus allowing a patch-free period during each day, usually overnight. This method of administration has been shown to have advantages over continuous administration in the maintenance of the improvement produced by the patch. It is now accepted that treatment with transdermal patches of nitroglycerine should include a patch-free period. Attempts have been made to use phased-release patches which will give the majority of the dose (about 75%) in the first 12 h.

A further clinical use of nitroglycerine patches has been in therapy for congestive cardiac failure (Lindvall et al 1988). The rationale for using this is to decrease preload and afterload by vasodilatation and arteriolar dilatation. Transdermal nitroglycerine has been shown to produce an initial improvement in haemodynamic measures, including improvement in cardiac index and a decrease in pulmonary capillary wedge pressure while maintaining arterial pressure. The pattern of improvement is similar to that found in angina, which reaches a maximum within 6 h but then loss of effect occurs with continued application as a result of development of tolerance. This would suggest that continuous treatment of congestive cardiac failure with transdermal nitroglycerine will not be effective. The role of intermittent treatment with patches needs further evaluation. Transdermal nitroglycerine has been used in unstable angina and also following acute myocardial infarction. The number of studies conducted in these areas do not allow any conclusion to be drawn (Todd et al 1990).

An interesting potential therapeutic use has been described of placing transdermal nitroglycerine patches near the site of intravenous cannulation (Wright et al 1985, Khawaja et al 1989). This has resulted in prolongation of the viability of an infusion and decreased need for resiting of intravenous access. Both studies have shown a marked reduction in the infusion failure rate and prolongation of the mean survival of an intravenous infusion site by up to 50 h.

The potential application in anaesthesia of transdermal nitroglycerine patches is in the role of preventing perioperative myocardial ischaemia. There are few published studies of the use of transdermal nitrogen patches in this period. However, evidence from studies using continuous infusion of nitroglycerine in the perioperative period would suggest that little benefit accrues from continuous administration. This would support the view that transdermal nitroglycerine patches are not a specific preventative measure for perioperative ischaemia. However, their acute use in episodes of ischaemia may be of value.

Summary

Nitroglycerine administered transdermally has been shown to achieve appropriate plasma concentrations rapidly. It is of clinical use in the treatment of stable angina when used intermittently. However, continuous use leads rapidly to tolerance. It may be of some use in treatment of congestive cardiac failure. Its role in prevention of perioperative myocardial ischaemia is probably limited.

HYOSCINE

Hyoscine is a competitive antagonist at muscarinic cholinergic receptors. It has similar actions to those of atroprine, to which it is structurally similar. The major difference in action between atropine and hyoscine is that hyoscine has a depressant action on the central nervous system at normal therapeutic doses, producing drowsiness, amnesia and fatigue. At low dose, which avoids some of the excitatory effects noted at higher doses, it has a central antiemetic effect by blocking impulses from the vestibular nuclei to higher centres and to the vomiting centre. It is of particular use in motion sickness.

Hyoscine was the first drug to be administered with a transdermal system (Price et al 1981). The hyoscine is dissolved in the mineral oil within a polymeric gel. The system contains about 1.5 g of hyoscine and a rate control membrane releases the drug at approximately 5 μg/h. The rate of release is used to achieve a plasma concentration which will produce antiemetic effects but will minimize the unwanted sedative effects.

Pharmacokinetics

The pharmacokinetics of hyoscine are poorly described. It is a difficult drug to assay in plasma. The few reported studies of hyoscine pharmacokinetics suggest that it has a relatively rapid (5 min) distribution half-life and an elimination half-life of between 2 and 5 h. It has a relatively rapid clearance (800–1000 ml/min) and an apparent distribution volume of around 1 litre/kg. The oral bioavailability is variable between 10 and 50%. The principal use for transdermal hyoscine has been in the prevention of motion sickness, which has been shown to be effective (Dahl et al 1984). Plasma concentrations achieved by transdermal administration of hyoscine are low but it appears that the antiemetic effects of hyoscine are achieved at very low plasma concentrations. Indeed, the concentrations achieved may be below the sensitivity of the assay methods used and several authors have used the urinary excretion rate of hyoscine as a measure of the amount of drug present (Shaw & Chandrasekaran 1981). Using this, antiemetic effects have been shown to occur at urinary excretion rates lower than that found in patients complaining of mouth dryness and which in turn were lower than in those complaining of drowsiness and again lower than those in whom tachycardia was noted. These three effects are, in descending order, the most common side effects noted with the use of transdermal hyoscine.

Transdermal hyoscine has also been used in a number of studies to treat postoperative nausea and vomiting (Rowbotham 1992). The outcome of these studies has been variable, with some studies showing significant improvements over placebo treatment with hyoscine and others showing no difference. Studies in which the hyoscine patch was placed well before surgery had, in general, a better outcome. This would be in keeping with the findings from other patch systems where a lag time in achieving appropriate plasma concentrations has been well demonstrated.

CLONIDINE

Clonidine is a partial agonist at α_2 adrenergic receptors. Its principal site of action is in the central nervous system acting at postsynaptic α_2 receptors and producing a decrease in sympathetic outflow. This has led to its therapeutic use for control of blood pressure. Clonidine is a suitable drug for transdermal administration and its clinical use in control of blood pressure in hypertensive patients has been evaluated. A transdermal system for the administration of clonidine is available in the USA and a similar system is being evaluated in Europe and Japan.

The system consists of a backing layer, a drug reservoir which contains the clonidine in a polymer base, a rate-limiting membrane and finally an adhesive layer which contains a loading dose of clonidine. The loading dose is intended to achieve more rapid plasma concentrations of clonidine in the early part of treatment and the reservoir then provides a sustained release to maintain a constant plasma concentration. As with other drug systems the amount of drug in the reservoir greatly exceeds that required and also the rate of release is directly related to the surface area of the patch. Three sizes are available containing 2.5, 5 and 7.5 mg of clonidine with respective surface areas of 3.5, 7 and 10.5 cm^2. These systems deliver clonidine at a rate of 0.1, 0.2 and 0.3 mg per day.

Pharmacokinetics

Measurable concentrations of clonidine are achieved within 12 h but steady-state concentration is not reached until between 2 and 3 days (MacGregor et al 1985). However, thereafter a steady concentration was maintained until 7 days, when the patch is removed. There is, in general, good correlation between the size of patch applied and the plasma concentration achieved. On removal of the patch, the clonidine concentration falls to zero over the next 3–4 days. The system is designed to be in place for 7 days and, if left in place longer than that, concentrations start to fall after 9 days.

Clinical use

In normotensive patients application of a clonidine patch produces a 5–10% fall in both systolic and diastolic pressure over a period of 2 days (Langley & Heel 1988). This decrease was maintained over the period of application of the patch and returned to normal over 2–3 days following removal of the patch. In hypertensive patients there is a dose-related decrease in systolic and diastolic pressure with systems releasing 0.2–0.3 mg per day producing a 15–20% fall in systolic and diastolic pressure (Popli et al 1986). As would be expected the effect on diastolic pressure was more marked. There was little effect on heart rate with any of the systems. During treatment with transdermal clonidine plasma noradrenaline concentrations are reduced. When treatment is discontinued the noradrenaline levels returned to their pretreatment levels but did not exhibit rebound to higher concentrations (Klein et al 1985). A number of studies have shown a decrease in circulating plasma renin concentrations particularly with higher doses and a decrease in urinary aldosterone excretion (Weber et al 1984).

Clonidine has been shown to be of clinical therapeutic use in mild to moderate hypertension, often in combination with an oral diuretic. It has been used for long-term treatment and shows good patient compliance in that the majority of patients found it an acceptable form of treatment. Longer-term treatment appears to suggest that once an appropriate rate of administration is achieved further increases in the dose are not usually required over a prolonged period of treatment (Hollifield 1986, Burris 1993). The treatment regime will require doses of 0.1–0.6 mg per day. Rebound hypertension has been demonstrated following stopping oral clonidine administration. However, this is unlikely to happen with transdermal administration as the plasma concentrations decline over a longer period. A further clinical use has been suggested in a study of patients with reflex sympathetic dystrophy (Davis et al 1991). Topical application of clonidine relieved the hyperalgesia in the region of patch application, suggesting a local rather than central action on adrenergic receptors.

OESTRADIOL

Supplemental oestrogens have been used to prevent the effects of the menopause in perimenopausal and postmenopausal women. This has been used to prevent the effects such has hot flushes, mood changes and sleep disturbances which may occur during the menopause. Oral oestrogens have been used to prevent these effects, as have subcutaneous implants and intramuscular depot injections. Oestradiol can be given transdermally at a low dose, which avoids first-pass metabolism, thus achieving concentrations appropriate for prevention of the systemic effects of the menopause.

Pharmacokinetics

Three patch sizes are available which deliver 0.025, 0.05 and 0.1 mg per 24 h. Maximum plasma concentrations are achieved quickly, in less than 8 h, and remain constant over the 4-day period that they are designed to be applied for. There is a dose-related increase plasma oestradiol concentration from 25 to 75 ng/litre with the above patch sizes (Powers et al 1985). Oestradiol levels return to pretreatment level within 24 h of removal of the patch.

Clinical use

This method has been shown in a number of studies to be effective in reducing menopausal symptoms (Balfour & Heel 1990). The aim of therapy is to achieve oestradiol levels similar to those observed in premenopausal women in early to mid-cycle. In addition to the symptomatic improvements, bone resorption is inhibited (Stevenson et al 1990). However, lipid and lipoprotein metabolism does not appear to be altered by this treatment.

It is possible that transdermal oestradiol combined with progestagen could be appropriate for contraception.

The incidence of erythema and itching at the patch site is higher than found with other transdermal systems (Balfour & Heel 1990). This may be as high as 40%, but is severe in less than 10%. Systemic adverse effects are relatively rare but include breakthrough bleeding, fatigue, depression and other symptoms typical of oestrogen effects. A combined patch delivering oestradiol and norethisterone transdermally is also available.

The dose of oestrogen used is much lower than that in oral contraceptives but the risk of thromboembolism must be considered a contraindication to the use of transdermal oestradiol. Discontinuation of therapy should be considered in a patient presenting for a procedure for which there is a high risk of thromboembolism.

NICOTINE

Nicotine is thought to be the addictive component of cigarette smoke. It acts on nicotinic cholinergic receptors in the peripheral and central nervous system. Its action in the central nervous system is thought to be important in the development of addiction. The administration of nicotine on its own has been used as part of treatment for patients wishing to stop smoking. A number of routes of administration have been tried, including chewing gum, lozenges, nasal sprays and aerosols. The use of a transdermal system would be logical in this situation in that a steady plasma concentration of nicotine could be achieved throughout the day.

A number of systems have been evaluated and shown to provide appropriate plasma concentrations of nicotine. These concentrations are approximately half of those achieved by regular smoking. The aim is to alleviate symptoms of withdrawal while not producing systemic effects from nicotine. These effects would include neurological, cardiovascular, endocrine and metabolic effects (Palmer et al 1992).

A number of clinical studies have shown that the abstinence rate produced by the use of transdermal systems is initially approximately double that produced when nicotine replacement therapy is not used (Palmer et al 1992). However, follow-up on these patients after completing a 6-week course suggests that, in the long term, abstinence rate declines to the same as no active treatment. Both the initial and long-term response can be improved if supportive therapy (behavioural therapy) is given at the same time.

There are a number of systems available, some of which are rate controlled and are designed to deliver between 5 and 22 mg per 24 h. The systems are in general well tolerated with few adverse effects, although disturbances of sleep and gastrointestinal upsets have been reported (Hughes 1993). It is recommended that the transdermal nicotine should only be used with caution in patients with cardiovascular disease.

FUTURE DEVELOPMENTS

While the continuous delivery of drugs across the skin to achieve a steady-state concentration has many advantages there are also some inherent disadvantages to the system. The principal ones are the initial delay in achieving a therapeutic plasma concentration and the inability to vary the concentration when the patch is in place. Both these factors are being addressed in the future developments of patch systems: First by use of absorption enhancers and secondly by the use of iontophoresis. The aim of these developments is not only to improve the therapeutic efficacy of systems already in use but to increase the range of drugs and substances which could be delivered transdermally.

Enhancers

It has been noted that the addition of other substances to the adhesive layer of the matrix of the drug reservoir can augment the rate and amount of drug absorbed. This can be well illustrated by the inclusion of alcohol in the oestradiol patches. This considerably augments the absorption of oestradiol, allowing a more rapid increase in plasma concentrations than would be achieved in the absence of the alcohol. Other substances such as dimethylsulphoxide and dimethylformamide have been shown to enhance the uptake of drugs.

A second method is to alter the pH of the area of the patch in contact with the skin. The pH of skin is around 4; this may lead to ionization of some drugs and will decrease the rate of absorption. Adjustment of the pH to a more appropriate level for absorption of the drug will enhance its absorption.

Iontophoresis

This technique involves the production of a small electric current across the skin. This acts to enhance the delivery of drugs, particularly charged compounds, across the skin. The technique involves placement of the ionic form of the drug under the active electrode of a pair of electrodes and the passing of a small direct or pulsed current between the two electrodes. The charged drug is then repelled by the appropriate electrode and pushed across the skin (Singh & Maibach 1994). Such a system would theoretically have all the advantages of a transdermal system for delivering drugs at a constant rate and in addition have the potential advantages of achieving an appropriate plasma concentration more rapidly and the potential to give bolus as well as continuous dosage. The majority of systems currently available or under development are of a continuous direct current but some pulsed current models are being developed.

The other potential advantage of such a system is that it would allow a greater variety of compounds to be transported across the skin. This would include proteins and peptides and offers the potential of being able to deliver hormones such as insulin, growth hormone and luteinizing hormone releasing hormone (Singh & Maibach 1994). These systems are as yet at an early stage of development but would be a significant advance in therapy if they could be made to function reliably.

The potential to deliver drugs using a pulsatile current opens up the prospect of drugs being given as a constant infusion with additional bolus doses on request. This offers the potential of delivering drugs postoperatively for analgesia by this route. Such a system is currently under development for the delivery of fentanyl.

The potential of such systems is an exciting development for the future use of the transdermal route for administration of drugs.

REFERENCES

Abrams J 1988 A reappraisal of nitrate therapy. JAMA 259: 396–401
Ahmedzai S, Allan E, Fallon M et al 1994 Transdermal fentanyl in cancer pain. J Drug Dev 6: 93–97
Balfour J A, Heel R C 1990 Transdermal oestradiol: a review of its pharmacodynamic and pharmacokinetic properties, and therapeutic efficacy in the treatment of menopausal complaints. Drugs 40: 561–582
Berner B, John V A 1994 Pharmacokinetic characterisation of transdermal delivery systems. Clin Pharmacokinet 26: 121–134
Bogaert M G 1987 Clinical pharmacokinetics of glyceryl trinitrate following the use of systemic and topical preparations. Clin Pharmacokinet 12: 1–11
Broome I J, Wright B, Bower S et al 1995 The efficacy of different dose regimens of transdermal fentanyl for relief of pain after lower abdominal surgery. Anaesthesia 50: 300–303
Burris J F 1993 The USA experience with the clonidine transdermal therapeutic system. Clin Auton Res 3(6): 391–396
Dahl E, Offer-Ohlsen D, Lillevold P E et al 1984 Transdermal scopolamine, oral meclizine and placebo in motion sickness. Clin Pharmacol Ther 36: 116–120
Davis K D, Treede R D, Raja S N et al 1991 Topical application of clonidine relieves hyperalgesia in patients with sympathetically maintained pain. Pain 47: 309–317
Duthie D J R, Rowbotham D J, Wyld R et al 1988 Plasma fentanyl concentrations during transdermal delivery of fentanyl to surgical patients. Br J Anaesth 60: 614–618
Gupta S K, Southam M, Gale R et al 1992 System functionality and physicochemical model of fentanyl transdermal system. J Pain Symp Man 7: S17–S26
Holley F O, Van Steennis C 1988 Postoperative analgesia with fentanyl: pharmacokinetics and pharmacodynamics of constant-rate I.V. and transdermal delivery. Br J Anaesth 60: 608–613
Hollifield J 1986 Clinical acceptability of transdermal clonidine: a large-scale evaluation by practitioners. Am Heart J 112: 900–906
Hughes J R 1993 Risk-benefit assessment of nicotine preparations in smoking cessation. Drug Safety 8: 49–56
Khawaja H T, O'Brien B J, Buxton M J et al 1989 Costs minimisation study of transdermal glyceryl trinitrate in reducing failures of peripheral intravenous infusion. Br Med J 299: 97–98
Klein C, Morton N, Kelley S 1985 Transdermal clonidine therapy in elderly mild hypertensives: effects on blood pressure, plasma norepinephrine and fasting plasma glucose. J Hypertension 3: S81–S84
Langley M S, Heel R C 1988 Transdermal clonidine: a preliminary review of its pharmacodynamic properties and therapeutic efficacy. Drugs 35: 123–142
Lehmann K A, Zech D 1992 Transdermal fentanyl: clinical pharmacology. J Pain Symp Man 7: SS16

Lindvall E, Erikksson S V, Langerstrand L et al 1988 Efficacy and tolerability of transdermal nitroglycerin in heart failure. Eur Heart J 9: 373–379

MacGregor T R, Matzek K M, Keirns J J et al 1985 Pharmacokinetics of transdermally delivered clonidine. Clin Pharmacokinet Ther 38: 278–284

Palmer K J, Buckley M M, Faulds D 1992 Transdermal nicotine. Drugs 44: 498–529

Popli S, Daugirdas J T, Neubauer J A et al 1986 Transdermal clonidine in mild hypertension: a randomised, double-blind, placebo-controlled trial. Arch Intern Med 146: 2140–2144

Powers M S, Schenkel L, Darley P E 1985 Pharmacokinetics and pharmacodynamics of transdermal dosage forms of 17β-oestradiol: comparison with conventional oral estrogens used for hormone replacement. Am J Obstet Gynecol 152: 1099–1106

Price N M, Schmitt L G, McGuire J et al 1981 Transdermal scopolamine in the prevention of motion sickness at sea. Clin Pharmacol Ther 29: 414–419

Rowbotham D J 1992 Current management of postoperative nausea and vomiting. Br J Anaesth 69: 46S–59S

Rowbotham D J, Wyld R, Peacock J E et al 1989 Transdermal fentanyl for the relief of pain after upper abdominal surgery. Br J Anaesth 63: 56–59

Sandler A 1992 Transdermal fentanyl: acute analgesic clinical studies. J Pain Symp Man 7: S27–S35

Scardi S, Pivotti F, Fonda F et al 1985 Effect of a new transdermal therapeutic system containing nitroglycerin on exercise capacity in patients with angina pectoris. Am Heart J 110: 546–551

Shaw J E, Chandrasekaran S K 1981 Transdermal therapeutic systems. In: Prescott L F, Nimmo W S (eds). Drug absorption. Proceedings of international conference on drug absorption, Edinburgh. ADIS Press, Balgowlash, Australia, pp 186–193

Shaw J E, Urquhart J 1981 Transdermal drug administration: a nuisance becomes an opportunity. Br Med J 283: 875

Simmonds M A, Richenbacher J 1992 Transdermal fentanyl: long-term analgesic studies. J Pain Symp Man 7: S36–S39

Singh P, Maibach H I 1994 Transdermal ionotophoresis: pharmacokinetic considerations. Clin Pharmacokinet 26: 327–334

Stevenson J C, Cust M P, Gangar K F et al 1990 Effects of transdermal versus oral hormone replacement therapy on bone density in spine and proximal femur in postmenopausal women. Lancet 335: 265–269

Todd P A, Goa K L, Langtry H D 1990 Transdermal nitroglycerin (glyceryl trinitrate): a review of its pharmacology and therapeutic use. Drugs 40: 880–902

Weber M A, Drayer J I M, Brewer D D 1984 Transdermal continuous antihypertensive therapy. Lancet i: 9–11

Wester R C, Maibach H I 1992 Percutaneous absorption of drugs. Clin Pharmacokinet 23: 253–266

Wright A, Hecker J F, Lewis G B H 1985 Use of transdermal glyceryl trinitrate to reduce failure of intravenous infusion due to phlebitis and extravasation. Lancet ii: 1148–1150

7

Infusion techniques in anaesthesia

N. P. Sutcliffe   T. M. Akthar   G. N. C. Kenny

Modern anaesthesia has evolved over the last century into a safe form of medical practice, using a combination of drugs employed in a balanced method to provide the triad of hypnosis, analgesia and muscle relaxation. Traditionally induction of anaesthesia is achieved with an intravenous (i.v.) bolus of hypnotic agent, and maintained by inhalation of a volatile agent in an oxygen and nitrous oxide mixture. Muscle relaxation is achieved most commonly by intermittent bolus doses and analgesia, by either inhalation of nitrous oxide, intermittent i.v. bolus doses of opioids, a regional technique or any combination of these.

An alternative technique is to use total intravenous anaesthesia (TIVA) during which the same agent is used for induction and maintenance of anaesthesia via a continuous i.v. infusion. Muscle relaxation and analgesia can likewise be provided by continuous infusions, thus avoiding the peaks and troughs of drug concentration which are inherent in the bolus technique. There are a number of potential advantages in the use of TIVA (Table 7.1). However, the technique has not become widespread, and inhalational agents have remained the routine choice for maintenance of anaesthesia in spite of the development of new i.v. drugs. One of the prin-

Table 7.1 Advantages of TIVA versus inhalational anaesthesia

---

1. Lack of pollution
    Local (Halsey 1991)
    Global (Dale & Dale 1991)
2. Toxicity
    N_2O (Nunn 1987)
    Fluoride ions (Cook et al 1978, Brown 1991, Smith et al 1992b)
3. Access to airway
    Bronchoscopy
    Laryngoscopy
4. Preservation of hypoxic pulmonary vasoconstriction reflex (Van Keer et al 1989, Spies et al 1991)
5. Safe in malignant hyperpyrexia (Cartwright 1989)
6. Reduced incidence of postoperative nausea and vomiting (Van Hemelrijck et al 1991, Raftery & Sherry 1992)
7. Rapid increase in depth of anaesthesia
8. Rapidity of awakening from anaesthesia

---

cipal reasons is the availability of sophisticated delivery systems for volatile anaesthetics, which have been developed over many decades and which remain simple to use, yet allow the anaesthetist a fine degree of control of the concentration administered to the patient. In addition, all anaesthetists have been trained to administer volatile agents but most are not familiar with the use of i.v. drugs to maintain anaesthesia.

Until recently, the i.v. drugs and delivery equipment available to the anaesthetist have not been particularly suitable for TIVA, which has meant that the technique has only been practised by enthusiasts. However, over the last decade, the availability of new i.v. anaesthetic agents and our increased knowledge of the pharmacokinetics of these agents, together with the increasing sophistication of i.v. delivery systems, has allowed TIVA to rival the traditional techniques in terms of simplicity and efficacy.

PHARMACOKINETICS OF INTRAVENOUS DRUG ADMINISTRATION

When a drug is administered intravenously, it undergoes metabolism and distribution to other tissues of the body. The concentration of the drug in the blood and other tissues can be described by a pharmacokinetic model. For many drugs a three-compartment model can be used to describe the relationship between the dose administered and drug concentrations measured within the blood (Fig. 7.1). This model is a mathematical concept and the individual compartments do not represent any specific tissue. The model is constructed by measuring the drug concentration in blood samples taken at known times after the drug has been administered since the blood is considered to reflect the concentration within the central compartment.

The administration of a single dose of drug causes a peak blood concentration which then decreases rapidly with time. This can result in an excessive blood concentration at the time of achieving the peak, with possible toxic effects (Fig. 7.2). Repeated single doses can be given to maintain drug effect, but this will result in alternating peak and trough drug concentrations within the central compartment, with the potential for both toxic and subtherapeutic effects (Fig. 7.3). The degree to which this is undesirable will depend on the therapeutic window of individual drugs. When using drugs with a wide therapeutic window and low toxicity, this is not a major problem and intermittent bolus dosing can be an appropriate delivery method. However, this is not an appropriate delivery method for drugs with a narrow therapeutic window and clinically significant toxicity.

When drugs are administered by infusion at a constant rate, a considerable period of four to five times the distribution half-life would be required to achieve a steady-state concentration (Fig. 7.4). An alternative strategy is to load the central compartment by administering a single bolus dose and starting a continuous infusion at the same time. This results in a high blood

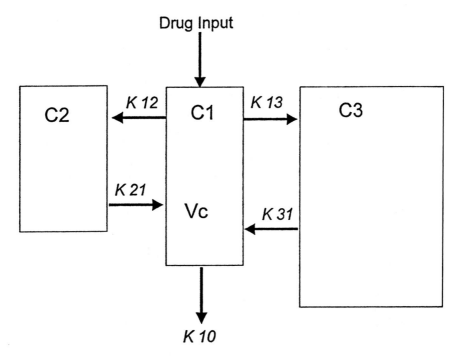

Fig. 7.1   Three-compartment pharmacokinetic model describing the distribution and elimination of an intravenous drug.

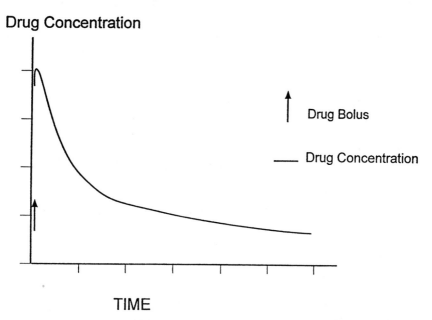

Fig. 7.2   Changes in drug concentration with time within the blood following a single bolus dose of drug.

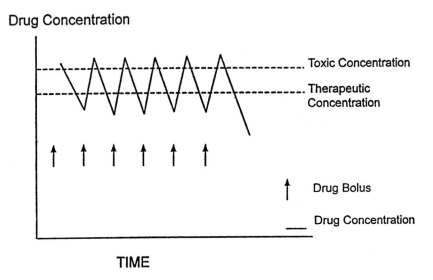

Fig. 7.3   Changes in drug concentration with time within the blood during repeated bolus dosing of drug.

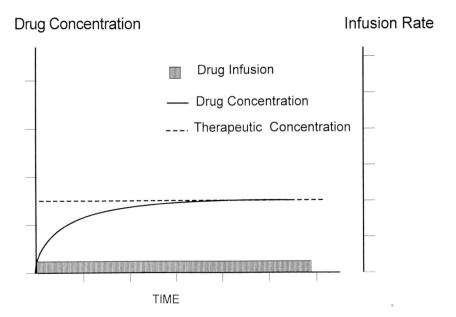

Fig. 7.4   Changes in drug concentration with time within the blood during a zero order infusion of drug.

concentration following the bolus dose which may be associated with toxic effects, followed by a reduced concentration which gradually increases towards steady state (Fig. 7.5), during which time subtherapeutic drug concentration may be present. It is possible to design a simplified stepped infusion regimen based on an approximation to a computer-generated infusion regimen which can be designed to achieve and maintain a fixed drug concentration within the central compartment. However, such regimens do not offer the flexibility of changing the infusion in response to a perceived need for a change in level of drug effect.

Clearly, the optimal infusion regimen would produce a bolus designed to achieve rapidly the desired drug concentration followed by a continuously adjusting infusion rate calculated to maintain this 'target' drug concentration, and allow this target concentration to be reduced or increased as appropriate. Such regimens are available (White & Kenny 1990) but require specialized computer-controlled infusion equipment not generally available at present. One further degree of sophistication would be a system designed to change the target concentration in response to some form of measure of drug effect. If a suitable measurement were available for a particular drug effect, then it would be possible to 'close the loop' and design a system which would control the delivery of a drug so as to maintain a constant drug effect. Again, such systems do exist but are at present limited to research tools (Kenny et al 1992). Examples of all these delivery methods will be discussed.

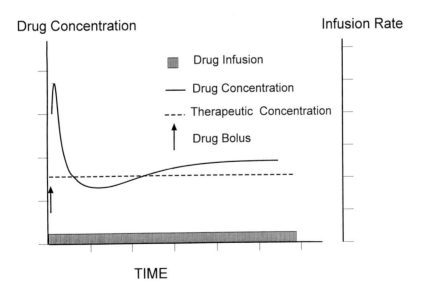

Fig. 7.5 Changes in drug concentration with time within the blood following a single bolus dose followed by a continuous infusion of drug.

In general, drugs which are most suited for delivery by infusion are those with a rapid offset of action once the infusion is stopped. This property is usually described in the literature by the elimination half-life of the drug in question. However, it must be appreciated that the speed of elimination of an infused drug from the central compartment will vary with the duration of that infusion. The longer the duration of infusion before cessation, then the longer will be the time taken for the drug concentration within the central compartment to decrease. This can be illustrated by referring to Figure 7.1; the longer the infusion of a drug continues, the more compartments C2 and C3 become filled with drug. On cessation of the infusion, as drug is eliminated from the central compartment (C1) there will be a degree of refilling from the other compartments, which will prolong the half-time for the drug infusion concerned. Hughes and colleagues have referred to this time dependence of elimination of infused drugs as 'context-sensitive half-time' (Hughes et al 1992). The factors which determine this context-sensitive half-time are the duration of infusion (thus the quantity of drug within the various compartments), the clearance of the drug and the speed of refilling of the central compartment from the other compartments, which depends on the rate constants $K21$, $K12$, $K13$, $K31$ (Fig. 7.6). This time dependence of the context-sensitive half-time is less apparent for drugs with a high clearance.

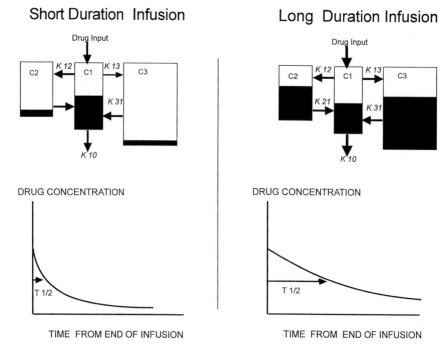

Fig. 7.6 Schematic representation of the concentration of drug within the various compartments during a short and a prolonged infusion of drug, and the effect on context sensitive half-time.

INTRAVENOUS HYPNOTIC AGENTS

Several drugs have been used to provide TIVA, including propanidid and althesin, which are no longer available for use. Etomidate has also been investigated for TIVA but has been found to interfere with steroid synthesis and should not be used for maintenance of anaesthesia. When ketamine is used as a single agent for anaesthesia, it can lead to dysphoria in the recovery phase, but has been reported to be successful when combined with midazolam (Restall et al 1988) or propofol (Schüttler et al 1991). Benzodiazepines appear to act in synergism with opioids (Ben Shlomo et al 1990) and midazolam has been used successfully when combined with fentanyl (Theil et al 1993) or alfentanil (Nilsson et al 1988). However, recovery from midazolam may be prolonged after infusion because of its low clearance (Table 7.2).

Methohexitone and thiopentone have also been used to provide TIVA (Schwilden et al 1987, Crankshaw & Karasawa 1989) but these agents also prolong recovery after infusion due to low clearance (Table 7.2). Propofol has a satisfactory pharmacokinetic profile for the maintenance of anaesthesia (Marsh et al 1991) and, in addition, it has been shown to have a specific antiemetic action (McCollum et al 1988, Borgeat et al 1992). Unlike volatile agents, there appears to be no adverse effect on the hypoxic pulmonary vasoconstriction reflex with propofol (Van Keer et al 1989, Spies et al 1991) and it may be a preferable agent for neuroanaesthesia in patients with decreased intracranial compliance (Fischer et al 1992). Eltanolone (pregnanolone) is a naturally occurring metabolite of progesterone and is the latest steroid anaesthetic to be investigated. It is insoluble in water and is formulated as an 0.4% emulsion in 10% Intralipid. Eltanolone is approximately three times as potent as propofol but is associated with less pain on injection. A reduced frequency of apnoea has been reported compared with propofol in one study (Gray et al 1992), but the degree of cardiovascular and respiratory depression appeared similar to propofol in another report (Van Hemelrijck et al 1994).

Currently, propofol is the agent most suited to be given by i.v. infusion for the maintenance of anaesthesia because of its short elimination half-life and high clearance (Table 7.2). For very short surgical procedures in healthy patients, a single dose of the drug may suffice. Longer procedures may be

Table 7.2 Pharmacokinetic variables of i.v. hypnotic agents

	V_{dss} (l/kg)	Clearance (ml/kg per minute)	$t_{1/2\beta}$ (h)	Prot. bind. (%)
Propofol	2.8	59.4	0.9	97
Midazolam	1.1	7.5	2.7	94
Etomidate	2.5	17.9	2.9	77
Ketamine	3.1	19.1	3.1	12
Methohexital	2.2	10.9	3.98	73
Thiopental	2.3	3.4	12.0	83

(V_{dss} = volume of distribution at steady state)

performed whilst the patient is anaesthetized with repeated bolus doses of propofol. However, this will produce a drug concentration profile as described in Figure 7.3. This may cause cardiorespiratory depression at the time of peak concentrations and inadequate anaesthesia during trough concentrations. Several manual infusion schemes have been proposed for infusion rates of propofol which have been developed empirically to maintain anaesthesia (de Grood et al 1985, Turtle et al 1987). A stepped infusion regimen based on approximations to a computer-generated infusion profile has been designed to achieve and maintain a blood propofol concentration of 3 µg/ml (Table 7.3) (Roberts et al 1988) and others have also been described (Sear et al 1989). Such regimens do not allow the flexibility of altering the targeted blood propofol concentration, and must be supplemented to avoid the possibility of awareness. The technique described by Roberts and colleagues targeted a relatively low blood concentration of propofol and supplemented this with nitrous oxide. Using this regimen, with an opiate premedication 25% of patients studied also required supplementation with a volatile agent (Tackley et al 1989).

Target-controlled infusions

The pharmacokinetic parameters describing the distribution and elimination of propofol have been incorporated into infusion systems which are designed to achieve and maintain the desired target blood concentration of propofol appropriate for any individual patient and level of surgical stimulation at any time (Glass et al 1989, White & Kenny 1990). These systems deliver variable infusion schemes based on the complex mathematical solution to the pharmacokinetic model. The weight and age of the patient and a target blood propofol concentration are entered into the system, which then calculates and delivers a drug bolus designed to achieve this target concentration. The bolus is then followed by a constantly adjusting infusion regimen calculated to maintain this target concentration. A new target concentration can be selected at any stage. If a higher target concentration is

Table 7.3   Published propofol infusion regimens*

Infusion regimen one (Sear et al 1989)	
1. Bolus	2.5 mg/kg
2. Infusion rate 1	12 mg/kg per hour for 30 min
3. Infusion rate 2	9 mg/kg per hour for 30 min
4. Infusion rate 3	6 mg/kg until the end of the surgery
Infusion regimen two (Roberts et al 1988)	
1. Bolus	1 mg/kg
2. Infusion rate 1	10 mg/kg per hour for 10 min
3. Infusion rate 2	8 mg/kg per hour for 10 min
4. Infusion rate 3	6 mg/kg until the end of the surgery

* Both regimens described were supplemented with nitrous oxide

chosen, the system will deliver a further bolus or, if a lower concentration is chosen, the control software will stop infusing until it has calculated that the new target concentration has been achieved, after which the system will commence an adjusted infusion regimen to maintain the new target concentration. What this means to the anaesthetist is that changing the depth of anaesthesia is as simple as selecting a new target concentration, much like selecting a particular percentage of inspired volatile agent on a vaporizer. Figure 7.7 shows target blood propofol concentrations in an individual patient receiving a target-controlled infusion of propofol, together with the infusion rate profile delivered by the system in order to achieve these concentrations. Such systems should be available commercially during 1996. Target-controlled infusions have been shown to be superior to manually adjusted regimens in respect of cardiovascular stability during anaesthesia and ease of use with propofol (Chaudhri et al 1992b). By selecting a lower target concentration of propofol these systems can be used to provide sedation for endoscopy (Church et al 1991) and surgery under regional blockade (Skipsey et al 1993) or for patients in the intensive therapy unit (ITU). In fact, target-controlled infusion of propofol is particularly suitable for operative procedures requiring postoperative sedation in the ITU, since at the end of surgery a target concentration of propofol suitable for sedation can be selected to provide seamless drug delivery into the postoperative period.

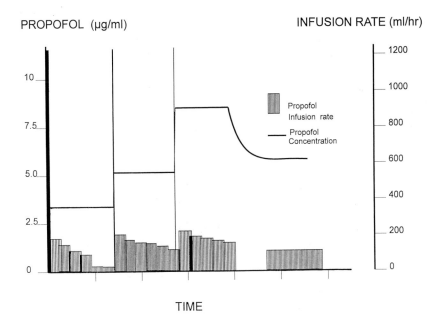

Fig. 7.7   Predicted blood propofol concentration and the concurrent infusion regimen during a target-controlled infusion of propofol.

Closed-loop anaesthesia

In spite of the sophistication of target-controlled drug delivery, the anaesthetist still has to rely on judgement to assess the depth of anaesthesia and alter the target concentration as appropriate. The whole process could be automated (closed-loop anaesthesia) if there were a reliable measurement of depth of anaesthesia. Considerable efforts have been made over the years to develop a reliable index of anaesthetic depth. Most attempts have been based on some form of processed EEG (Arden et al 1986, Schwilden et al 1989), although changes in R–R interval of the ECG (Pomfrett et al 1994) and changes in lower oesophageal contraction (Evans & Davies 1984, Sessler et al 1989) have also been proposed. However, none of these techniques has proven reliable enough for routine clinical use.

The auditory evoked potential (AEP) has been investigated as an alternative measure of the depth of anaesthesia. It is obtained by delivering auditory stimuli in the form of clicks to earphones at a frequency of 6–12 Hz. The EEG activity is recorded after each click from three electrodes placed on the scalp and a total of between several hundred and several thousand EEG sweeps are filtered and averaged to produce the AEP. The AEP appears to provide a reproducible guide to the level of anaesthesia obtained with a wide variety of different anaesthetic agents and to respond appropriately to different levels of surgical stimulation (Thornton et al 1988). A single parameter derived from the AEP has been used to control the delivery of propofol in patients breathing spontaneously during surgery (Kenny et al 1992). There was no occurrence of awareness during the surgical procedures in any patient. The last memory all patients had before loss of consciousness was the clicks being played through the earphones but none of the patients were concerned by the clicks and all were prepared to have the same anaesthetic in the future. It is unlikely that closed-loop control of anaesthesia will become a routine part of anaesthetic practice in the immediate future, but it offers the possibility of providing a valuable and unbiased assessment technique to examine the effects of supplementary drugs and to compare equipotent doses of different i.v. and volatile agents.

NEUROMUSCULAR BLOCKING AGENTS

Muscle relaxation for surgical operations of medium to long duration can be achieved by intermittent bolus dosing. The newer agents have low toxicity and a wide therapeutic window, which negates some of the potential problems of the intermittent bolus technique. However, these newer agents with a rapid offset of action are also eminently suitable for infusion. The advantage of an infusion technique is that a constant level of paralysis can be maintained throughout surgery; this is particularly important for certain types of surgery such as retinal and spinal cord surgery. A number of infusion regimens will be described. However, it is important to stress that these offer guidance on initial dosing and infusion rates, and that neuro-muscular blockade should be monitored with a peripheral nerve stimulator to provide fine control of the infusion regimen.

The short duration of action and Hoffman degradation of *atracurium* make it a suitable agent for continuous infusion. A loading dose of atracurium 0.25 mg/kg, followed by a continuous infusion at the rate of 5.0 µg/kg per minute for up to 206 min, does not cause accumulation (Martineau et al 1992). An alternative approach is to give a larger initial bolus of 0.5 mg/kg to facilitate rapid intubation followed by an infusion commenced 15–20 min later at a rate of 5.0 µg/kg per minute. Delaying the infusion has no effect on steady-state concentration and avoids the pos-sibility of having a profound degree of neuromuscular blockade if the planned surgery is curtailed. When suxamethonium (1 mg/kg) is used to facilitate tracheal intubation this reduces the maintenance requirement of atracurium by 30% (Olkkola & Schwilden 1990). The use of an inhalation agent further reduces the requirement of atracurium by 2 µg/kg per minute for each increase in MAC (Beattie et al 1992).

The rate of neuromuscular recovery from a fixed-bolus loading dose is related to the most appropriate initial infusion rate of atracurium required to maintain adequate neuromuscular blockade (Beemer et al 1990). Simpson and colleagues have exploited this fact and described a simple dose guidance graph or 'ready reckoner' (Fig. 7.8) for atracurium infu-sions (Simpson & Souter 1990). A loading dose of 35 mg is followed by an

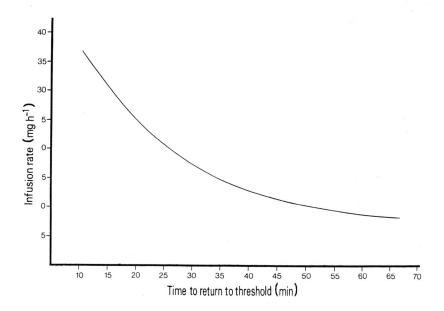

Fig. 7.8 "Guidance graph" of atracurium infusion requirements following an intubating dose of 35 mg. (From Simpson & Souter, 1990.)

infusion rate predicted by the graph in milligrams per hour. The advantage of this simple and practical system is that a knowledge of the patient's weight is not necessary. It also eliminates need for calculations of milligrams per kilogram, unusual dilutions and doses. However, this approach is unsuitable for children and the initial bolus dose may be inadequate for rapid intubation in larger patients.

It is possible to predict accurately the infusion dose of *vecuronium* required to achieve a predetermined degree of neuromuscular blockade from the duration of action of one or two test doses (Harrison 1990). However, the requirement for vecuronium decreases with the duration of the infusion. A loading dose of vecuronium of 0.05 mg/kg, followed by a prolonged infusion at 1.0 µg/kg per minute, may result in accumulation of vecuronium (Martineau et al 1992), thus emphasizing the need to monitor neuromuscular function.

Mivacurium has a short duration of action due to its rapid elimination by plasma cholinesterase and it does not accumulate significantly, rendering it suitable for continuous infusion. An initial bolus of 0.15 mg/kg is required to facilitate endotracheal intubation. Maintenance of neuromuscular blockade requires an infusion at a rate of 6–10 µg/kg per minute. The duration of mivacurium block is prolonged by 50% in end-stage chronic renal failure (Phillips & Hunter 1992) and cirrhotic patients (Devlin et al 1993).

Target-controlled infusions

As with i.v. anaesthetic agents, target-controlled infusion systems for atracurium and vecuronium have been designed. These systems are designed to achieve and maintain a selected drug concentration. However, because of the ease of monitoring neuromuscular function and the wide therapeutic window of muscle relaxants, we have not found such techniques to offer a major clinical advantage.

Closed-loop infusion

The degree of neuromuscular blockade can be accurately and rapidly assessed by measurement of the electromyograph or the muscle force generated following an electrical stimulus. This measurement, or an index of it, can then be used to provide negative feedback control of the infusion of a

Table 7.4 Infusion regimens for muscle relaxant

Drug	Initial bolus (mg/kg)	Maintenance (µg/kg per minute)
Atracurium	0.5	4–8
Vecuronium	0.1	0.4–1
Mivacurium	0.15	6–10

neuromuscular blocking agent in a closed-loop system. Assef and colleagues have described a computer-controlled, closed-loop system for continuous infusion of atracurium or vecuronium to achieve any desired degree of neuromuscular blockade (Assef et al 1993). The control algorithm rapidly induced the selected level of neuromuscular blockade and maintained this level of blockade at steady state with minimal oscillation. Ebeling and colleagues found vecuronium requirement was significantly lower when administered by a model-based adaptive feedback system (Ebeling et al 1991). A computerized closed-loop system for mivacurium infusion has also been described (Meretoja & Olkkola 1993).

VASOACTIVE DRUGS

The anaesthetist is sometimes required to manipulate the cardiovascular system pharmacologically in order to provide optimum operating conditions or to provide support or protection for the myocardium. Many vasoactive drugs are metabolized rapidly and have a very short half-life within the circulation (Table 7.5), which means that infusion is the only suitable delivery method. Drugs such as dobutamine, with a half-life of 2–3 min (even in patients with cardiac failure), achieve steady-state concentration so rapidly with a zero-order infusion that a loading bolus dose is not required. Enoximone, on the other hand, with a half-life of 1–2 h (up to 24 h in cardiac failure) requires a bolus dose to load the central compartment followed by an infusion. Vasoactive drugs can be divided into four broad categories: inotropes, vasodilators, vasoconstrictors and negative inotropes, although a number of drugs have mixed effects.

Most commonly the anaesthetist is asked to provide control of systemic blood pressure either to facilitate surgical technique or protect suture lines

Table 7.5 Dosing guidelines, classification and half-lives for commonly used vasoactive drugs

Drug	Classification	Bolus (mg/kg)	Infusion rate (µg/kg per minute)	$t_{1/2\beta}$ (min)
Adrenaline	Inotrope*	–	0.05–2[†]	2–4
Dopamine	Inotrope*	–	2–20[†]	2–4
Dobutamine	Inotrope*	–	2–30[†]	2–4
Enoximone	Inotrope/vasodilator	0.5–1	5–20	60–120[‡]
Esmolol	Negative inotrope	0.25–0.5	50–300	9–10
Glyceryl Trinitrate	Vasodilator	–	0.15–3	
Labetolol	Negative inotrope/ vasodilator	0.25–1	2–20	120–180
Sodium nitroprusside	Vasodilator	–	0.2–8	

[*] Mixed effect according to dose. [†] Dose requirement highly variable.
[‡] Prolonged in heart failure.

and vital organs from the effects of hypertension. This control can be effected by vasodilatation or a reduction in cardiac output. In general, vasodilatation is the preferred method of providing controlled hypotension since cardiac output and thus tissue blood flow are preserved. However, when hypertension is due to increased sympathetic activity then negatively inotropic drugs such as beta-blocking agents may be more appropriate. Table 7.5 shows those vasoactive drugs most commonly used in anaesthesia, with dosing guidelines. The rapidity of onset and offset of action of many of these drugs makes titrating the infusion to drug effect relatively simple, so that target-controlled infusion techniques are generally unnecessary. However, the quality of control achieved over the cardiovascular system, with drugs such as enoximone that have an intermediate half-life may be improved by using target-controlled infusion systems. To date no such system has been described for a vasoactive agent.

Closed-loop control of blood pressure

Hypertension may occur after coronary artery bypass surgery and can cause serious complications. Several groups have developed closed-loop control systems which use the arterial pressure as the input signal to alter automatically the infusion of a vasodilator (Ruiz et al 1993, Reid & Kenny 1987). These systems have demonstrated that improved quality of blood pressure control can be achieved compared with manual control of the infusion rate, following cardiac surgery (Murchie & Kenny 1989).

Chaudhri and colleagues (1992a) compared closed-loop induction of controlled systemic hypotension using sodium nitroprusside with the performance of experienced anaesthetists using a manual system. They found that the anaesthetist performed as well as the closed-loop system when able to devote full attention to the control of blood pressure.

It is essential in any closed-loop system that the input or controlling signal is accurate and free from artefacts. Errors in measurement will lead to inappropriate drug delivery, with potentially deleterious results. Attention must be paid to details such as regular re-zeroing, particularly when the patient's position is changed or the height of the bed is altered. Artefact rejection algorithms are required within the controlling software and this can only be achieved by analysing the raw arterial waveform for consistency and accuracy (Colvin & Kenny 1989). In addition to providing improved quality of control of arterial pressure, these systems have been used successfully to compare different vasodilators in an unbiased manner (Chaudhri & Kenny 1990).

INFUSIONS OF ANALGESIC SUPPLEMENTS

Opioids are commonly used to provide the analgesic component of balanced anaesthesia or sedation in the ITU since, with the exception of ketamine, hypnotic drugs used for the maintenance of anaesthesia have no appreciable analgesic effect. They also reduce the requirements for hypnotic agents during the maintenance of anaesthesia. Large doses can be used to provide anaesthesia, usually in combination with other agents (Howie et al 1991). Traditionally bolus doses of long-acting drugs such as morphine are used in the perioperative period. In general, even in large doses, opioids have little adverse effect on cardiovascular stability, which makes them eminently suitable for use during general anaesthesia with controlled ventilation. However, the high peak concentrations associated with intermittent bolus dosing will produce varying degrees of analgesia, and the potential for respiratory depression in spontaneously breathing patients. Newer synthetic opioids, such as fentanyl, alfentanil and remifentanil, have a rapid onset and offset of action, making them particularly suitable for infusion (see Table 7.6). Opioid infusions with such agents offer the potential for a stable level of analgesia throughout surgery, and the flexibility of titration against adverse drug effects in spontaneously breathing and awake patients. A study by Smith and co-workers showed that during propofol anaesthesia the response to skin incision was decreased when patients received an infusion of fentanyl (Smith et al 1992a). Alfentanil has a rapid onset of action but has a short duration when administered as a bolus (Murray et al 1989). It can be delivered as an infusion to supplement the hypnotic effect of propofol (Jenstrup et al 1990). Alfentanil and propofol can be mixed together without loss of effect (Taylor et al 1992). However, this reduces the flexibility of the regimen to respond to the variations in anaesthetic requirements of patients breathing spontaneously during surgery.

Ketamine does not cause the cardiovascular and respiratory depression found with opioid analgesics and may have a valuable role as the analgesic component of TIVA. Schüttler and his colleagues have reported the use of propofol and ketamine for TIVA, both by conventional administration with bolus doses and manually controlled infusions (Schüttler et al 1991). They commented that cardiovascular stability was satisfactory and that the propofol component prevented the emergence phenomena associated with ketamine. This combination resulted in a rapid return to normal respiratory function within a few minutes of the end of surgery. A comparison of

Table 7.6 Pharmacokinetic parameters of opioids

Drug	V_{dss} (l/kg)	Clearance (ml/min per kg)	$t_{1/2\beta}$ (h)
Morphine	3.4	2.3	1.7
Fentanyl	4.0	12.6	3.6
Alfentanil	0.7	5.1	1.6
Remifentanil	0.4	65	0.25

V_{dss} = Volume of distribution at steady state

propofol and ketamine with propofol and fentanyl by Guit and his colleagues (1991) demonstrated that the ketamine combination resulted in improved haemodynamics during surgery and that propofol appeared to prevent the psychotomimetic emergence effects of a subanaesthetic dose of ketamine, although recovery was more prolonged in the ketamine group.

Remifentanil is a new synthetic opioid under investigation in several centres which has a rapid onset of action, but the drug is unique in that it is metabolized rapidly by plasma and tissue esterases, resulting in an extremely short duration of action (Westmoreland et al 1993). It appears to be slightly less potent than fentanyl in the dog (Salmenpera et al 1992), and 20–30 times more potent than alfentanil in man (Glass et al 1993). The rapid elimination of remifentanil (Egan et al 1992) may be of considerable benefit in TIVA, where adequate infusion rates could be administered to ensure a high degree of intraoperative analgesia but with a rapid reversal of respiratory depression at the end of surgery.

Target-controlled analgesic infusions

Target-controlled infusions of alfentanil have been used successfully both intraoperatively and to provide postoperative analgesia (Ausems et al 1988, Davies et al 1992). They have been shown to provide better cardiovascular stability with fentanyl (Alvis et al 1985) and alfentanil (Ausems et al 1988), compared to intermittent bolus doses and manually adjusted infusions. The administration of ketamine via a target-controlled infusion has been described, and was reported to improve the control of the drug administration (Schüttler et al 1991).

Closed-loop analgesic infusions

The efficacy of analgesia can only be adequately assessed by the individual receiving the analgesia. Therefore the control signal in a closed-loop analgesia system must come from the patient's own degree of satisfaction with his pain control. There are a number of systems which offer patient-controlled analgesia. This is usually provided in the form of a bolus of i.v. opioid in response to a button press by the patient. Such systems have been shown to be superior to intermittent intramuscular morphine in respect of quality of analgesia (Wasylak et al 1990, Kenady et al 1992) and nursing satisfaction (Aitken & Kenny 1990). However, problems with this approach are that patients require an initial bolus in order to achieve therapeutic effect and that, secondly, the system can never keep the patient pain free since the patient will only initiate a bolus when he is in pain. One way to overcome these problems is to programme into the system an initial bolus dose and a background continuous infusion. However, with drugs such as morphine this can lead to accumulation and respiratory depression. An alternative approach was adopted by Davies and colleagues (1992).

They described a target-controlled infusion of alfentanil, which rapidly achieved the required level of analgesia due to the rapid onset of action of the drug. The target level was then altered by nursing staff in response to patient request. This nurse-controlled system has been modified so that the target concentration of alfentanil is increased in response to button presses by the patient (Checketts et al 1995). The system will also slowly reduce the target concentration over a period of time if the patient does not press his button. An added safety feature is that the system can be linked to a pulse oximeter so that if the oxygen saturation falls below a predefined limit the infusion will be rapidly reduced by the control software until the saturation rises above the preset value.

CONCLUSION

The i.v. route of drug administration has long been recognized as a convenient method of rapidly achieving a desired drug effect. Anaesthetists routinely use the i.v. route for induction of anaesthesia, because of the speed and efficacy of this route. However, the pharmacokinetics of drugs infused during anaesthesia are complex. Thus complicated infusion regimens are required for maintenance of anaesthesia, muscle relaxation and analgesia. This has resulted in many anaesthetists continuing to use the traditional methods of delivering anaesthesia.

The potential benefits of i.v. infusions in terms of a constant smooth level of drug effect are sometimes outweighed by the attention the anaesthetist has to pay to the drug infusion regimen, thus distracting him from patient care. The advent of target-controlled infusion and closed-loop drug delivery, with the inherent ease of use of such systems, has the potential to revolutionize the delivery of anaesthesia.

REFERENCES

Aitken H A, Kenny G N 1990 Use of patient-controlled analgesia in postoperative cardiac surgical patients: a survey of ward staff attitudes. Intensive Care Nursing 6: 74–78
Alvis J M, Reves J G, Govier A V et al 1985 Computer-assisted continuous infusions of fentanyl during cardiac anesthesia: comparison with a manual method. Anesthesiology 63: 41–49
Arden J R, Holley F O, Stanski D R 1986 Increased sensitivity to etomidate in the elderly: initial distribution versus altered brain response. Anesthesiology 65: 19–27
Assef S J, Lennon R L, Jones K A et al 1993 A versatile, computer-controlled, closed-loop system for continuous infusion of muscle relaxants. Mayo Clin Proc 68: 1074–1080
Ausems M E, Vuyk J, Hug C C, Jr. et al 1988 Comparison of a computer-assisted infusion versus intermittent bolus administration of alfentanil as a supplement to nitrous oxide for lower abdominal surgery. Anesthesiology 68: 851–861
Beattie W S, Buckley D N, Forrest J B 1992 Continuous infusions of atracurium and vecuronium, compared with intermittent boluses of pancuronium: dose requirements and reversal. Can J Anaesth 39: 925–931
Beemer G H, Bjorksten A R, Crankshaw D P 1990 Pharmacokinetics of atracurium

during continuous infusion. Br J Anaesth 65: 668–674

Ben Shlomo I, abd el Khalim H, Ezry J et al 1990 Midazolam acts synergistically with fentanyl for induction of anaesthesia. Br J Anaesth 64: 45–47

Borgeat A, Wilder Smith O H, Wilder Smith C H et al 1992 Adjuvant propofol for refractory cisplatin-associated nausea and vomiting (letter). Lancet 340: 679–680

Brown B R 1991 Inhalational anaesthetics and hepatotoxicity: an update. Anaesthesiol Scand 35: 42–43

Cartwright D P 1989 Propofol in patients susceptible to malignant hyperpyrexia. Anaesthesia 44: 173

Chaudhri S, Kenny G N 1990 Nitroprusside-sparing effects of enoximone. Cardiology 77 (Suppl 3): 46–50

Chaudhri S, Colvin J R, Todd J G et al 1992a Evaluation of closed loop control of arterial pressure during hypotensive anaesthesia for local resection of intraocular melanoma. Br J Anaesth 69: 607–610

Chaudhri S, White M, Kenny G N 1992b Induction of anaesthesia with propofol using a target-controlled infusion system. Anaesthesia 47: 551–553

Checketts M R, Gilhooly C J, Kenny G N 1995 Patient-maintained analgesia with alfentanil after after cardiac surgery: a comparison with morphine PCA. Br J Anaesth 74 (Suppl): 133–134

Church J A, Stanton P D, Kenny G N et al 1991 Propofol for sedation during endoscopy: assessment of a computer-controlled infusion system. Gastrointest Endosc 37: 175–179

Colvin J R, Kenny G N 1989 Microcomputer-controlled administration of vasodilators following cardiac surgery: technical considerations. J Cardiothorac Anesth 3: 10–15

Cook T L, Smith M, Starkweather J A et al 1978 Behavioral effects of trace and subanesthetic halothane and nitrous oxide in man. Anesthesiology 49: 419–424

Crankshaw D P, Karasawa F 1989 A method for implementing programmed infusion of thiopentone and methohexitone with a simple infusion pump. Anaesth Intensive Care 17: 496–499

Dale O, Dale T 1991 Anesthetic gases, the ozone layer and the greenhouse effect: how harmful are the anesthetic emissions for the global environment? Tidsskr Nor Laegeforen 111: 2115–2117

Davies F W, White M, Kenny G N 1992 Postoperative analgesia using a computerised infusion of alfentanil following aortic bifurcation graft surgery. Int J Clin Monit Comput 9: 207–212

de Grood P M, Ruys A H, van Egmond J et al 1985 Propofol ('Diprivan') emulsion for total intravenous anaesthesia. Postgrad Med J 61 (Suppl 3): 65–69

Devlin J C, Head-Rapson A G, Parker C J et al 1993 Pharmacodynamics of mivacurium chloride in patients with hepatic cirrhosis. Br J Anaesth 71: 227–231

Ebeling B J, Muller W, Tonner P et al 1991 Adaptive feedback-controlled infusion versus repetitive injections of vecuronium in patients during isoflurane anesthesia. J Clin Anesth 3: 181–185

Egan T D, Lemmens H J, Fiset P et al 1992 The pharmacokinetics and pharmacodynamics of GI87084B. Anesthesiology 77: A369

Evans, J M, Davies W L 1984 Monitoring anesthesia. In: Sear J W (ed) Clinics in anesthesiology. Saunders, Philadelphia, pp 242–262

Fischer M, Moskopp D, Nadstawek J et al 1992 Total intervaneous anesthesia using propofol and alfentanil as compared to combined inhalation anesthesia reduces the flow velocity in the middle cerebral artery: a Doppler sonographic study. Anaesthesist. 41: 15–20

Glass P S, Markham K, Ginsberg B et al 1989 Propofol concentrations required for surgery. Anesthesiology 71: A273

Glass P S, Hardman D, Kamiyama Y et al 1993 Preliminary pharmacokinetics and pharmacodynamics of an ultra-short-acting opioid: remifentanil (GI87084B). Anesth Analg 77: 1031–1040

Gray H S, Holt B L, Whitaker D K et al 1992 Preliminary study of a pregnanolone emulsion (Kabi 2213) for i.v. induction of general anaesthesia. Br J Anaesth 68: 272–276

Guit J B, Koning H M, Coster M L et al 1991 Ketamine as analgesic for total intravenous anaesthesia with propofol. Anaesthesia 46: 20–24

Halsey M J 1991 Occupational health and pollution from anaesthetics: a report of a seminar. Anaesthesia 46: 486–488

Harrison M J 1990 Prediction of infusion rates: validation of a computer simulation using vecuronium. Br J Anaesth 64: 287–293

Howie M B, Smith D F, Reilley T E et al 1991 Postoperative course after sufentanil or fentanyl anesthesia for coronary artery surgery. J Cardiothorac Vasc Anesth 5: 485–489

Hughes M A, Glass P S, Jacobs J R 1992 Context-sensitive half-time in multicompartment pharmacokinetic models for intravenous anesthetic drugs. Anesthesiology 76: 334–341

Jenstrup M, Nielsen J, Fruergard K et al 1990 Total i.v. anaesthesia with propofol–alfentanil or propofol–fentanyl. Br J Anaesth 64: 717–722

Kenady D E, Wilson J F, Schwartz R W et al 1992 A randomized comparison of patient-controlled versus standard analgesic requirements in patients undergoing cholecystectomy. Surg Gynecol Obstet 174: 216–220

Kenny G N, McFadzean W A, Mantzaridis H et al 1992 Closed-loop control of anesthesia. Anesthesiology 77: A328

Marsh B J, White M, Morton N et al 1991 Pharmacokinetic model driven infusion of propofol in children. Br J Anaesth 67: 41–48

Martineau R J, St.-Jean B, Kitts J B et al 1992 Cumulation and reversal with prolonged infusions of atracurium and vecuronium. Can J Anaesth 39: 670–676

McCollum J S, Milligan K R, Dundee J W 1988 The antiemetic action of propofol. Anaesthesia 43: 239–240

Meretoja O A, Olkkola K T 1993 Pharmacodynamics of mivacurium in children using a computer-controlled infusion. Br J Anaesth 71: 232–237

Murchie C J, Kenny G N 1989 Comparison among manual, computer-assisted, and closed-loop control of blood pressure after cardiac surgery. J Cardiothorac Anesth 3: 16–19

Murray A W, Brockway M S, Kenny G N 1989 Comparison of the cardiorespiratory effects of ketorolac and alfentanil during propofol anaesthesia. Br J Anaesth 63: 601–603

Nilsson A, Persson M P, Hartvig P et al 1988 Effect of total intravenous anaesthesia with midazolam/alfentanil on the adrenocortical and hyperglycaemic response to abdominal surgery. Acta Anaesthesiol Scand 32: 379–382

Nunn J F 1987 Clinical aspects of the interaction between nitrous oxide and vitamin B12. Br J Anaesth 59: 3–13

Olkkola K T, Schwilden H 1990 Quantitation of the interaction between atracurium and succinylcholine using closed-loop feedback control of infusion of atracurium. Anesthesiology 73: 614–618

Phillips B J Hunter J M 1992 Use of mivacurium chloride by constant infusion in the anephric patient. Br J Anaesth 68: 492–498

Pomfrett C J, Sneyd J R, Barrie J R et al 1994 Respiratory sinus arrhythmia: comparison with EEG indices during isoflurane anaesthesia at 0.65 and 1.2 MAC. Br J Anaesth 72: 397–402

Raftery S, Sherry E 1992 Total intervanous anaesthesia with propofol and alfentanil protects against postoperative nausea and vomiting. Can J Anaesth 39: 37–40

Reid J A, Kenny G N 1987 Evaluation of closed-loop control of arterial pressure after cardiopulmonary bypass. Br J Anaesth 59: 247–255

Restall J, Tully A M, Ward P J et al 1988 Total intervaneous anaesthesia for military surgery: a technique using ketamine, midazolam and vecuronium. Anaesthesia 43: 46–49

Roberts F L, Dixon J, Lewis G T et al 1988 Induction and maintenance of propofol anaesthesia: a manual infusion scheme. Anaesthesia 43 (Suppl): 14–17

Ruiz R, Borches D, Gonzalez A et al 1993 A new sodium-nitroprusside-infusion control-ler for the regulation of arterial blood pressure. Biomed Instrum Technol 27: 244–251

Salmenpera M, Wilson D, Szlam F et al 1992 Anesthetic potency of the opioid GI87084B, in dogs. Anesthesiology 77: A368

Schüttler J, Schüttler M, Kloos S et al 1991 Optimal dosage strategies in total intrave-nous anesthesia using propofol and ketamine. Anaesthesist 40: 199–204

Schwilden H, Schüttler J, Stoeckel H 1987 Closed-loop feedback control of methohexital anaesthesia by quantitative EEG analysis in humans. Anesthesiology 67: 341–347

Schwilden H, Stoeckel H, Schüttler J 1989 Closed-loop feedback control of propofol anaesthesia by quantitative EEG analysis in humans. Br J Anaesth 62: 290–296

Sear J W, Shaw I, Wolf A et al 1989 Infusions of propofol to supplement nitrous oxide-oxygen for maintenance of anaesthesia: a comparison with halothane. J Clin Anesth 1: 272–276

Sessler D I, Stoen R, Olofsson C I et al 1989 Lower esophageal contractility predicts movement during skin incision in patients anesthetised with halothane but not with nitrous oxide and alfentanil. Anesthesiology 70: 42–46

Simpson D S, Souter A J 1990 A computer designed graph for administration of atracurium by i.v. infusion. Br J Anaesth 65: 770–778

Skipsey I G, Colvin J R, Mackenzie N et al 1993 Sedation with propofol during surgery under local blockade: assessment of a target-controlled infusion system. Anaesthesia 48: 210–213

Smith C, McEwan A I, Jhaveri R 1992a Reduction of propofol Cp50 by fentanyl. Anesthesiology 77: A340

Smith I, Ding Y, White P F 1992b Comparison of induction, maintenance, and recovery characteristics of sevoflurane–N$_2$O and propofol–sevoflurane–N$_2$O with propofol–isoflurane–N$_2$O anesthesia. Anesth Analg 74: 253–259

Spies C, Zaune U, Pauli M H et al 1991 A comparison of enflurane and propofol in thoracic surgery. Anaesthesist 40: 14–18

Tackley R M, Lewis G T, Prys Roberts C et al 1989 Computer controlled infusion of propofol. Br J Anaesth 62: 46–53

Taylor I N, Kenny G N, Glen J B 1992 Pharmacodynamic stability of a mixture of propofol and alfentanil. Br J Anaesth 69: 168–171

Theil D R, Stanley T E, White W D et al 1993 Midazolam and fentanyl continuous infusion anesthesia for cardiac surgery: a comparison of computer-assisted versus manual infusion systems. J Cardiothorac Vasc Anesth 7: 300–306

Thornton C, Konieczko K, Jones J G et al 1988 Effect of surgical stimulation on the auditory evoked response. Br J Anaesth 60: 372–378

Turtle M J, Cullen P, Prys Roberts C et al 1987 Dose requirements of propofol by infusion during nitrous oxide anaesthesia in man. II: Patients premedicated with lorazepam. Br J Anaesth 59: 283–287

Van Hemelrijck J, Smith I, White P F 1991 Use of desflurane for outpatient anesthesia: a comparison with propofol and nitrous oxide. Anesthesiology 75: 197–203

Van Hemelrijck J, Muller P, Van Aken H et al 1994 Relative potency of eltanolone, propofol, and thiopental for induction of anesthesia. Anesthesiology 80: 36–41

Van Keer L, Van Aken H, Vandermeersch E et al 1989 Propofol does not inhibit hypoxic pulmonary vasoconstriction in humans. J Clin Anesth 1: 284–288

Wasylak T J, Abbott F V, English M J M et al 1990 Reduction of post-operative morbidity following patient-controlled morphine. Can J Anaesth 37: 726–731

Westmoreland C L, Hoke J F, Sebel P S et al 1993 Pharmacokinetics of remifentanil (GI87084B) and its major metabolite (GI90291) in patients undergoing elective inpatient surgery. Anesthesiology 79: 893–903

White M, Kenny G N 1990 Intravenous propofol anaesthesia using a computerised infusion system. Anaesthesia 45: 204–209

8

Postoperative analgesia in children

A. R. Lloyd-Thomas

Over the last 10 years there has been a complete change of approach to the treatment of pain in children. Children undergoing major surgery received minimal pain relief (Beyer et al 1983) with the result that many were found to be in pain postoperatively (Mather & Mackie 1983). In younger patients, anxieties relating to opiate medication in both neonates and infants meant that they often received no analgesia following surgery (Purcell-Jones et al 1988). In part this change in attitude has been brought about by contributions from paediatric anaesthetists and other paediatric specialists (Anand & Hickey 1987, Anand et al 1987, Arthur & McNicol 1986, Murat et al 1987, Yaster & Deshpande 1988, Anand et al 1988, Tyler & Crane 1990, Anand & Hickey 1992). Analgesic techniques, routinely employed for adult patients, e.g. extradurals, patient-controlled analgesia (PCA), have been adapted for use in children by attention to differences in the pharmacodynamics and levels of ability associated with age. As a result children are much less frequently faced with the sole option of on-demand intramuscular opiate analgesia or weak oral analgesics – a pattern of pain relief which historically has been so inadequate.

PATHOPHYSIOLOGY OF PAIN IN CHILDREN

Immaturity of the newborn nervous system and the not infrequent extensor response to stimuli was wrongly interpreted as implying that nociceptive transmission to the cortex did not occur (Anand & Hickey 1987). Indeed nociceptive information can be shown to reach the cortex by 30 weeks post-conceptual age; moreover a biochemical stress response can be measured as early as 23 weeks post-conceptual age during fetal intrahepatic vein needling (Gianna–Koulopoulos et al 1994). Although caution is required in interpreting biochemical stress data as measures of pain, because a response may be present despite adequate analgesia (Wolf 1994), there is evidence that immature nociceptive signal processing may lead to a hypersensitivity state with enhanced pain transmission (Andrews & Fitzgerald 1994). Furthermore, it appears that untreated severe pain as a neonate may result in an increase in the degree of pain experienced during further medical procedures undertaken in infancy (Taddio et al 1995). We have yet to see if this heightened response is retained throughout childhood and adult life.

Although it is now widely accepted that neonates can transmit nociceptive stimuli it is wrong to assume that children are mini adults. There are probable differences in the development of opioid receptors (Lesley et al 1982) and hence differences in the ability to modulate pain transmission (Andrews & Fitzgerald 1994). The neonate and infants (to 6 months of age) have reduced plasma protein levels (especially α_1-acid glycoprotein) (Morselli et al 1980), which will alter drug binding and may result in more free drug being available to cross the blood-brain barrier. Hepatic enzyme systems are immature in neonates (Koren et al 1985), which may result in a prolonged opioid half-life. Furthermore, differences in the ratio of glucuronide production (morphine-3-glucuronide to morphine-6-glucuronide; M-3-G : M-6-G) may result in relative over-production of M-6-G which is a highly potent agonist at the mu receptor (Bhat et al 1992, Choonara et al 1993). There are also large inter-individual differences, with some young patients having a very immature response to narcotics while others are almost normal. Nor does it appear possible to predict on clinical grounds which patient will respond in what fashion. Unpredictable response to narcotics, in particular unpredictable respiratory depression, remains a considerable concern when treating newborns with opioids (Purcell-Jones et al 1987) and is a potent argument for careful patient assessment before and during treatment. All of these factors mean that it is inappropriate to manage infants and neonates as small adults.

PAIN ASSESSMENT

The successful provision of analgesia for children requires that the entire medical episode is planned so as to avoid unnecessary painful interventions. As part of a programme of pain relief, an adequate system of pain assessment needs to be established. Any pain assessment device must be able reliably to (1) detect the presence of pain, (2) estimate its severity and (3) determine the effectiveness of interventions (Porter 1993). Compared to preverbal infants, older children do not present such a challenge as they are able to say if they are in pain, provided that they do not think that this admission will result in an intramuscular injection (Mather & Mackie 1983). They are also able to cooperate with self-report scales (Bieri et al 1990). These should be used hourly when awake, but it is important for the child to understand that pain is to be reported and not just general feelings. Asking about pain on movement can reveal inadequate analgesia (Kehlet 1994) and is a better test of pain control. But it is the younger preverbal children (neonates, infants and toddlers) who present the most difficulty for pain assessment and in whom there is the greatest risk of under-treatment. In these patients some form of behavioural or physiological patient observation is required to assess pain. Of the behavioural methods, facial expression has been systematically coded and validated for neonates, except in the very premature (Grunau 1987). But other measures, for example body posture, have been found to be non-specific. Crying also is too non-specific for reliable pain assessment.

Physiological assessments fall into two categories; immediate feedback and those needing delayed interpretation. Cardiovascular parameters (heart rate and blood pressure) are the most useful immediate measures in term neonates and infants but not in the premature (Porter et al 1988). Delayed interpretation measures (e.g. the biochemical stress response), require careful assessment when used as proxies of pain, because they may be present despite adequate analgesia (Wolf 1994). Overall the clinician is left with a confusing choice of assessment parameters, many of which are age or procedure specific. Progress is being made (for example PAIN, the Pain Assessment Inventory for Neonates; Johnson 1987). But the choice is often between a complex scoring system (for example the Canadian Hospital of Eastern Ontario Pain Scale (CHEOPS) (McGrath et al 1985), which is validated for a reasonably wide age range in the postoperative setting (Tyler et al 1993) or a simple intuitive pain and sedation score (Morton 1993, Lloyd-Thomas & Howard 1994). In the busy ward setting a complex score may be impractical. Although not so accurate, the simple clinical score may be more effective because it is regularly used (Lloyd-Thomas & Howard 1994). A sedation score should be an integral part of postoperative patient assessment as somnolence often precedes respiratory depression. The hourly pain and sedation score should be combined with an assessment of respiratory rate and the volume of drug infused (Lloyd-Thomas & Howard 1994). Many may wish to employ continuous pulse oximetry in children receiving opioid infusions (Morton 1993, Fell 1993).

A PAEDIATRIC PAIN SERVICE

The complexity of modern analgesia demands that a coordinating service is established to organize the safe delivery of pain relief in the hospital. Ready et al (1988) established the concept of an acute pain service; this approach was endorsed by the Royal Colleges (Pain after Surgery 1990) and has been introduced into paediatric practice (Lloyd-Thomas & Howard 1994). Effective yet safe pain control in the ordinary ward is the core aim of a paediatric pain service. Nurses who are familiar with drug techniques and equipment build confidence on the ward that contributes to both the safety and success of pain relief. Clinical nurse specialists are vital, especially in the education and training of ward nurses. Pain service clinicians must also be concerned with the advance of analgesia by research and the identication of side effects by audit. The most important contribution a pain service can offer is the development and supervision of clear protocols for balanced analgesia which are followed by medical and nursing staff throughout the hospital.

BALANCED ANALGESIA FOR CHILDREN

Analgesia for children should provide subjective comfort by inhibition of trauma-induced nociception, thereby also minimizing autonomic and somatic reflex responses to pain. This should allow earlier restoration of normal life. Kehlet (1989) has emphasized that after major surgery sufficient pain relief cannot be achieved by any single analgesic on its own, without incurring side effects. A multi-modal approach with simultaneous administration of analgesics which work by different mechanisms has the advantage of attenuating nociceptive impulses at various sites, thereby allowing the use of smaller doses of each drug and minimizing side effects (Maunuksela et al 1992a, Kehlet 1994). Any pain service for children should plan combination analgesic regimens, tailored both to the individual patient and the operation proposed.

The timing of analgesic medication has been the subject of much discussion, with experimental studies suggesting that a repetitive C fibre firing may lead to pain hypersensitivity by spinal cord 'wind-up' (Coderre et al 1993). Although the concept of pre-emptive medication is an attractive theoretical proposal, there has been little clinical evidence that the administration of analgesics before the surgical incision confers any significant postoperative benefit (Holthusen et al 1994, Kehlet 1994).

Minor analgesics

There can be very few operations in children for which the quality of analgesia provided by either opiates or local anaesthesia is not enhanced by the concomitant use of paracetamol with or without a non-steroidal anti-inflammatory drug (NSAID). Any multi-modal pain relief programme for children should include these drugs (Table 8.1). For day care surgery they may be the sole analgesic or may be combined with local anaesthetic blocks. For more major surgery they can be used synergistically with parenteral opiates or continuous postoperative regional analgesia.

Paracetamol is presented in a wide range of formulations, many of which children find acceptable. It's antipyretic properties are useful in controlling postoperative malaise due to temperature, for which a dose of 10 mg/kg is quite adequate. But for analgesia a higher dose needs to be given and 15 mg/kg per 6 h is effective. As indicated above, paracetamol may be given in combination with NSAIDs, local anaesthesia and opiates. Jaundiced neonates should only be given a dose of 5 mg/kg per 6 h. Suppositories are an increasingly popular route for minor analgesic medication in children, especially when starting these drugs as part of balanced analgesia, whilst the patient is under general anaesthesia. The use of suppositories should

Table 8.1   Dosing schedule for minor analgesics in children.

		Dose (mg/kg)	Dose interval (h)
Paracetamol			
Oral	Antipyretic	10	6
	Analgesic	15	
Rectal	Antipyretic	15	6
	Analgesic	20	
		NB: jaundiced neonates, max. 5 mg/kg	
Ibuprofen[*]			
Oral		5 mg/kg	6
Diclofenac[†]			
Oral		1 mg/kg	8–12
Rectal		1 mg/kg	8–12
		(from 1 year)	
Ketorolac[†]			
Intravenous		0.2–0.5 mg/kg	6
		(from 1 year)	(max. 8 doses)

[*] Ibuprofen is licensed for analgesia in children over 1 year.
[†] Diclofenac and ketorolac are not licensed for postoperative analgesia in children.

always be discussed beforehand with the parents. When paracetamol is given by the rectal route the dose should be increased to 20 mg/kg per 6 h for effective analgesia (Gaudreault et al 1988).

Non-steroidal anti-inflammatory drugs

In practice there are three NSAIDs which are useful in paediatric post-operative analgesia: ibuprofen, diclofenac and ketorolac. Only the suspension of ibuprofen is licensed for pain relief in children (over the age of 1 year) but all three are commonly used for postoperative analgesia. Little data exist on the pharmacokinetics of NSAIDs in infants, though from the age of 3 months they are probably the same as in adults (Kauffman & Nelson 1992). Nor is it known whether infants and children are at greater or lesser risk of gastric irritation and bleeding, or fluid retention and renal toxicity. Many of these side effects are seen in adults with pre-existing disorders who receive NSAIDs, however, concurrent illness is infrequent in children, apart from asthma. The syndrome of nasal polyposis, asthma and aspirin hypersensitivity is very rare in children. NSAIDs may be used in children with asthma; however, if there is any deterioration in respiratory status they must be stopped immediately. Parents should be advised of this. If other pre-existing pathology is present, NSAIDs should be used with great caution or withheld altogether. NSAIDs should be given in the minimum effective dose, but data on this are scarce in children. For ketorolac, there appears to be no difference in the quality of analgesia achieved by a dose of either 0.2 mg/kg or 0.5 mg/kg (Maunuksela et al

1992b). The slow onset of NSAID analgesia (even intravenous ketorolac) (Maunuksela et al 1992b) suggests that they are better used as prophylactic medication given regularly for a fixed period, rather than as acute analgesics – a role to which opioids are better suited.

Opioids

There is now a wide experience of using opioids to treat moderate and severe pain in children of all ages. Although many narcotics have been tried in children, the extensive experience with and knowledge of morphine means that it remains the opioid of choice for postoperative analgesia in most children following major surgery. If an opioid is required to supplement paracetamol and NSAIDs for less severe pain, then codeine phosphate (elixir 5 mg/ml) in a dose of 0.5–1 mg/kg per 8 h is effective (Houck et al 1994) and has a low incidence of nausea and vomiting, which is especially useful in day care surgery.

Morphine and neonates

The physiological differences between neonates and older children outlined above mean that morphine should only be given to neonates who are closely monitored (HDU/ICU nursing, apnoea mattress, ECG, blood pressure and saturation monitoring). For much of the surgery performed in neonates, analgesia can be provided by the use of local analgesia (see below) and this may be a better choice provided there is sufficient expertise available. In neonates, if opioids are used, morphine is best given by intravenous infusion. The dosage should be titrated against clinical effect, as there is a large inter-patient variability in both the response to and excretion of morphine (Yaster and Maxwell 1993). In neonates receiving ventilatory support, a loading dose of 100 µg/kg may be given over 20–30 min, followed by an infusion of 5–15 µg/kg per hour (Koren et al 1985). Higher infusion rates should be avoided because of the risk of convulsions (Koren et al 1985). But in the acutely ill neonate and in the premature, morphine handling patterns may be even more variable (Bhat et al 1992). Although glucuronidation is the main metabolic pathway for the excretion of morphine in neonates – not sulphation as originally proposed – a larger proportion of free drug is cleared by the kidney. In adults the normal ratio of M-3-G to M-6-G is 10:1, but this may be as little at 3:1 in neonates (Bhat et al 1992, Choonara et al 1993). As M-6-G has very significant analgesic properties (Osborne et al 1988), variation in its production may account for the uncertain response in some neonates and the wide range of effective plasma levels seen in some studies (Chay et al 1992). This underlines the need for careful observation of patient response. A rapid infusion may result in significant accumulation in these patients, who may be better managed by intermittent boluses of 5 µg/kg, titrated against clinical effect. Similarly, in spontaneously breathing neonates a maximum infusion rate of 5 µg/kg per hour should be chosen with, if required, nurse-controlled bolus doses of 5 µg/kg should analgesia be inadequate (Lloyd-Thomas & Howard 1994).

Morphine in infants and children

Plasma half-life and clearance approach adult levels at 1 month (Lynn & Slattery 1987). By the age of 6 months, both clearance (McRorie et al 1992) and protein binding are at adult levels (Morselli et al 1980), allowing the use of greater infusion rates, 10–30 µg/kg per hour even in spontaneously ventilating patients. However, although continuous infusions permit the maintenance of steady plasma concentrations, postoperative pain is not constant. Pain will vary for example with movement, with the type of surgery, on a diurnal basis (night-time often being worse), with the stage of recovery and with the persona of the child. Therefore constant infusions will result in periods of over- and under-treatment, but because of the pharmacokinetics of infusions, rate adjustments will have too slow an effect to allow titration to patient requirement. Developments in electronic pumps have allowed the introduction of PCA (Berde et al 1991) and nurse-controlled analgesia (NCA) for infants (Lloyd-Thomas & Howard 1994). Here boluses of morphine are given on patient or nurse demand, titrating analgesic administration against pain.

NCA essentially adds flexibility to a morphine infusion (Table 8.2). A maintenance infusion (10–20 µg/kg per hour) is given with nurse administered boluses of 10–20 µg/kg but the patient is protected by a long lockout interval (30 min) (Lloyd-Thomas & Howard 1994). If the pump has the facility, a 4 h dose limit of 400 µg/kg should be set. Although early reports suggested that parents could administer morphine boluses (Rodgers et al 1988), it is very unwise to allow this, as it removes the safeguards of nurse observation before dosing and parents are too emotionally involved to make objective pain assessments. Parents should always be actively involved in pain management but the decision to give supplementary doses

Table 8.2 Dosing schedule for NCA/PCA morphine infusion. For intravenous use, dilute body weight of morphine in milligrams (e.g. 10 kg child: 10 mg morphine) to 50 ml with dextrose 5% (1 ml=20 µg/kg). For subcutaneous use, dilute body weight of morphine in milligrams to 20 ml with 0.9% saline (0.4 ml=20 µg/kg)

	Bolus dose (µg/kg)	Constant infusion (µg/kg per hour)	Lockout interval (min)
Nurse-controlled analgesia	10–20	10–20	30
Patient-controlled analgesia	20	4	5
Alternative for younger patients			
Day of operation	20	10	20
1st postoperative day	20	4	5

remains the sole province of the nurse in NCA infusions (Lloyd-Thomas & Howard 1994). At Great Ormond Street Hospital for Children NHS Trust, NCA has proved very successful, with high patient satisfaction and a very low incidence of complications in over 1500 continuous infusions given in the last 3 years.

Adult PCA regimens do not translate into paediatric practice. PCA may be used from the age of 5 years, but at this age patients require considerable preoperative preparation and postoperative support (Lloyd-Thomas 1993).The failure rate may still be high and conversion to NCA programming should be undertaken if there is doubt as to the competence of a younger patient. Indeed we have had some success with combined NCA/PCA programming for the younger patient. On the day of operation a higher background infusion is used (8–10 µg/kg per hour) but the patient is protected from over-administration by a longer lockout interval (15–20 min) (Table 8.2). On the first postoperative day when the child is awake and cooperative, it can be changed to standard PCA programming (Lloyd-Thomas & Howard 1994).

Patients of 7 years and above can usually manage PCA without difficulty, but standard bolus dose-only programmes which are used for adults do not give optimal analgesia. A background infusion should be used, not a high-rate infusion (20 µg/kg per hour) as this does not improve pain scores but does result in a higher incidence of side effects (Doyle et al 1993a). An infusion of 4 µg/kg per hour is the best, giving better pain scores than no infusion and a lower incidence of side effects than either none or 10 µg/kg per hour (Doyle et al 1993b). By contrast, small bolus doses are associated with poor pain control during movement and an increase in the incidence of hypoxaemic episodes (Doyle et al 1994b). Bolus doses should be 20 µg/kg with a lockout interval of 5 mins. As with NCA, parents should not give doses on their child's behalf: the only potentially serious case of PCA respiratory depression seen at Great Ormond Street Hospital occurred when a parent did just this. Parents may hold the button, but the patient should be the only person to press it.

To avoid inadvertent bolus dosing, when other drugs are injected, PCA/NCA morphine is given via a dedicated intravenous line. If this is not possible then it is attached to the patient giving set using an anti-reflux valve.The pump must be positioned at the same level as the patient and an anti-siphon valve should be used (Southern & Reed 1994).

Morphine may also be given using a subcutaneous cannula, which must be centrally sited (deltoid, thorax or abdomen) (Fig. 8.1) (Lloyd-Thomas 1990, McNicol 1993). Indeed both PCA (Doyle et al 1994c) and NCA (Lloyd-Thomas & Howard 1994) may be given by this route, with the feedback from feeling the subcutaneous injection resulting in more consistent and reliable use of PCA.The subcutaneous route also gives a dedicated opiate line without using further veins.

When supervised by a pain service both NCA and PCA are associated with a very low incidence of respiratory slowing (1% and 0% respectively)

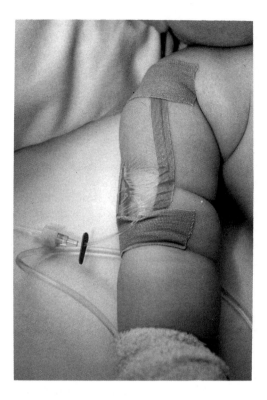

Fig. 8.1

(Lloyd-Thomas & Howard 1994). Postoperative nausea and vomiting (PONV) is, however, a major disadvantage of morphine analgesia. Although the incidence of PONV is low in young patients (2% in infants), it rises to 50% in children over 10 years of age (Lloyd-Thomas & Howard 1994). Nausea reduces the patient's perception of the quality of pain relief. Indeed some children limit their use of morphine preferring to have discomfort rather than feel nauseated, otherwise described as 'patient-controlled side effects' (Notcutt WG, personal communication). Using balanced analgesia to reduce morphine requirements, hence side-effects, is a constructive approach but many patients still require an antiemetic. Ondansetron appears to be highly effective in controlling opiate-induced PONV. A dose of 50 µg/kg has been shown to be as effective in paediatric ambulatory surgery as the previous recommendation of 100–150 µg/kg, which was based upon control of chemotherapy-induced emesis (Watcha et al 1995). Trials are needed to establish a minimum effective dose in children receiving PCA. An alternative approach described by Doyle and co-workers (1994a) is to use hyoscine patches placed behind the ear. One hundred and forty micrograms of hyoscine is released on application, followed by 5 µg/h whilst the patch is in place. It was effective in controlling PONV at the expense of an increase in sedation and dry mouth (Doyle et al 1994a). The quality of analgesia afforded by NCA/PCA means that opioids should always have a place in balanced analgesia. But opioid-induced PONV and the risk of respiratory depression in neonates remind us that balanced analgesia is not complete without the use of local anaesthesia where possible.

Local anaesthesia

A combination of general and local anaesthesia has been a feature of paediatric anaesthetic practice for many years (Arthur & McNicol 1986, Yaster & Maxwell 1989, Dalens 1989). The success of paediatric day care surgery is founded upon adequate analgesia from local anaesthetic blocks. Moreover, simple wound infiltration by the surgeon can improve pain scores in patients having PCA after major surgery (Wright 1993). But developments in extradural analgesia for major surgery have enhanced the role of this method of pain relief in children.

Extradural analgesia

Local anaesthesia

Single-shot caudal extradural analgesia has been widely used in paediatric anaesthesia for many years with the dosage regimen described by Armitage (1979). Using plain bupivacaine 0.25%, 0.5 ml/kg is given for low lumbar and sacral blocks, whilst 1 ml/kg is given for low thoracic blocks. If the volume of bupivacaine rises above 20 ml it should be diluted to 0.19% using saline. Local anaesthetic toxicity is rare in single-shot caudals but for safety short bevelled needles should be used, as these are less likely to puncture epidural veins (long bevel 10.6%, short bevel 1.6%) (Dalens & Hasanoui 1989). Even with this type of needle there is a 0.8% rate of undetected extradural vein cannulation (Dalens & Hasanaoui 1989). More recently paediatric caudal extradural blocks have been performed using ordinary intravenous cannulae but this does not guarantee against accidental intravascular placement, despite negative aspiration tests (Guinard & Borboen 1993). Moreover, unlike in adults, test doses of local anaesthetic with adrenaline (15 μg) do not produce consistent rises in heart rate in anaesthetised children (Desparmet et al 1990). Therefore until more specific markers for intravascular placement are investigated, such as isoprenaline (Perillo et al 1993), the total dose of local anaesthetic should be administered slowly in small increments.

Single-shot blocks are short lived and cannot provide long-term postoperative analgesia. Extradural catheterization and infusion of local anaesthetics are now possible thanks to advances in the equipment available to paediatric anaesthetists. Identification of the extradural space is by a loss of resistance technique (LOR). There are advocates for both air and saline as the marker for LOR in children but the latter is probably the safest. Two case reports of venous air embolism (Guinard & Borboen 1993, Schwartz & Eisenkraft 1993) and a retrospective multicentre survey of accidents following extradural analgesia (Flandin-Blety & Barrier 1995) are testaments to the potential hazards of loss of resistance to air in children. The author supports Sethna & Berde (1993), who strongly advocate LOR to saline in children.

Intraoperative and postoperative analgesia using local anaesthetics alone is a valuable technique for neonates and infants (Murrell et al 1993, Peutrell & Hughes 1993, Wolf & Hughes 1993, Wolf et al 1993, Webster et al 1993). Indeed its use has provided pain relief after major surgery in high-risk infants with pre-existing respiratory disease (Meignier et al 1983). For satisfactory analgesia when using local anaesthetics alone, the tip of the extradural catheter must be sited adjacent to the spinal levels innervating the dermatomes involved in the surgery (Berde 1994). Dilute solutions of local anaesthetics (which avoid the motor block that older children find distressing) infused in caudal or lumbar catheters will not afford adequate analgesia for thoracic or upper abdominal surgery. Clinicians have attempted to overcome poor-quality analgesia, from catheters that were not ideally sited, by increasing the rate of bupivacaine infusion. This can result in local anaesthetic toxicity manifesting as convulsions (Agarwal et al 1992, McCloskey et al 1992) or cardiac dysrhythmias (Maxwell et al 1994). Catheters should be appropriately sited and bupivacaine dosage should not exceed: loading dose 2–2.5 mg/kg, infusion 0.2–0.25 mg/kg per hour for neonates and 0.4–0.5 mg/kg per hour for infants and older children (Berde 1992). If satisfactory analgesia cannot be achieved with a maximal bupivacaine infusion, an opioid should be added to the infusate and the bupivacaine infusion rate reduced (Berde 1994). Thoracic extradural puncture in children should be restricted to anaesthetists with considerable experience, but in neonates and infants it is possible to thread a catheter from a caudal puncture to thoracic levels (Bosenberg et al 1988). Lack of sedation is a feature of postoperative extradural analgesia with local anaesthesia alone, which may make postoperative nursing for the older infant and toddler quite difficult. It is the author's opinion that local anaesthetic extradural infusions via caudal catheters advanced to thoracic level are excellent for neonates and infants less than 3 months of age (Wilson & Lloyd-Thomas 1993). Thereafter paediatric patients having extradural infusions are better managed by a combination of local anaesthesia and opioid.

Extradural opioids

Opioids may be divided into lipophilic (e.g. fentanyl) and hydrophilic (e.g. morphine) and the choice of extradural remove opioid needs to be directed by the site of catheter placement (Berde 1994). Lipophilic opioids injected at an extradural level away from the spinal dermatomes to be blocked will not result in effective segmental analgesia (Campbell et al 1992). By contrast hydrophilic opioids injected at a remote extradural site will provide segmental analgesia (Krane et al 1987, Wolf et al 1990). Whilst extradural opioid infusions provide effective analgesia, they do so at the price of a high incidence of side-effects, namely pruritus, urinary retention, nausea and vomiting (Wilson & Lloyd-Thomas 1993, Lloyd-Thomas & Howard 1994). In patients who do not have a urinary catheter for their surgery, urinary retention is seen in 18% of infants, rising to 63% of 10- to 17-year-old children when diamorphine is used as the extradural opioid (Lloyd-Thomas & Howard 1994). Infants can have their bladders emptied by the Crede manoeuvre, but up to 40% of children receiving extradural diamorphine fail to respond to naloxone and require urinary catheterization (Lloyd-Thomas & Howard 1994). Urinary retention may be less frequent with extradural fentanyl (7–20%) (Caudle et al 1993, Lejus et al 1994, Wood 1994), but the author agrees with Berde (1994) who states that extradural opioids should be limited to infants whose bladders can be expressed and those older patients who require a urinary catheter as part of their surgical management.

Extradural fentanyl may result in less nausea and vomiting and pruritus (Lejus 1994, Wood et al 1994) than morphine or diamorphine (Lloyd-Thomas & Howard 1994), but pruritus usually responds to naloxone (up to 2 μg/kg intravenously) and the incidence of nausea and vomiting is less than with intravenous morphine via NCA or PCA. Respiratory depression is a concern when opioids are added to extradural infusions, but provided that opiate dosing is restricted to less than 5 μg/kg per hour of morphine (Berde 1994) and fentanyl less than 0.4 μg/kg per hour then respiratory depression is extremely rare. Adequate observation is mandatory. Increasing somnolence indicates that the infusion should be halted for a period.

Technical complications with extradural catheters, mainly the fine catheters with a single end hole, are common and demand considerable pain service time to resolve (Lloyd-Thomas & Howard 1994, Wood et al 1994). Infection is rare with short-term use (Berde 1994).

In summary, extradural analgesia for children can offer excellent pain relief but side effects and technical problems are common. These are time consuming for pain service personnel. Controlled trials are needed to show that the quality of analgesia achieved is measurably superior to that of intravenous opioids.

PAEDIATRIC ANALGESIA: THE FUTURE?

Balanced analgesia for children has so far encompassed minor analgesics, opioids and local anaesthetics, but other transmitters are important in nociception. α-Agonists or NMDA antagonists may have a role to play in the future of paediatric analgesia. Lee & Rubin (1994) have shown that extradural clonidine prolongs the analgesia provided by a caudal bupivacaine block in paediatric orthopaedic surgery. The involvement of other drugs for other nociceptive pathways offers the prospect of further improvements in paediatric analgesia.

ACKNOWLEDGEMENT

The author wishes to extend his appreciation to Teresa Quinn for her patience and tenacity.

REFERENCES

Agarwal R, Gutlobe D, Lockhart C 1992 Seizures occurring in paediatric patients receiving continuous infusions of bupivacaine. Anesth Analg 75: 284–286

Anand K J S, Hickey P R 1987 Pain and its effect in the human neonate and fetus. N Engl J Med 317: 1321–1329

Anand K J S, Hickey P R 1992 Halothane, morphine compared with highdose sufentanil for anaesthesia and post-operative analgesia in neonatal cardiac surgery. N Engl J Med 326: 1–9

Anand K J S, Sippell W G, Aynsley-Green A 1987 Randomised trial of fentanyl anaesthesia in preterm babies undergoing surgery: effects on the stress response. Lancet i: 62–66

Anand K J S, Sippell W G, Schofield N M, Aynsley-Green A 1988. Does halothane anaesthesia decrease the metabolic and endocrine stress responses of newborn infants undergoing operation? Br Med J 296: 668–672

Andrews K, Fitzgerald M 1994 The cutaneous withdrawal reflex in human neonates: sensitisation, receptive fields, and the effects of contralateral stimulation. Pain 56: 95–102

Armitage E N 1979 Caudal block in children. Anaesthesia 34: 396

Arthur D S, McNicol L R 1986 Local anaesthetic techniques in paediatric surgery. Br J Anaesth 58: 760–778

Berde C 1992 Convulsions associated with paediatric regional anaesthesia. Anesth Analg 75: 164–166

Berde C 1994 Epidural analgesia in children. Can J Anaesth 41: 555–560

Berde C B, Lehn B N, Yee J D, Sethna N, Russo D 1991 Patient controlled analgesia in children and adolescents: a randomised prospective comparison with intramuscular morphine for postoperative analgesia. J Pediatr 118: 460–466

Beyer J E, DeGood D E, Ashley L C, Russel G A 1983 Patterns of postoperative analgesic use with adults and children following cardiac surgery. Pain 17: 17–81

Bhat R, Abu-Harb M, Chari G, Gulati A 1992 Morphine metabolism in acutely ill preterm newborn infants. J Pediatr 120: 795–799

Bieri D, Reeve R A, Champion G D, Addicoat A L, Ziegler J B 1990 The faces and pain scale for the self assessment of severity of pain experiences by children: development, initial validation and preliminary investigation for ratio scale properties. Pain 41: 139–150

Bosenberg A, Bland B, Schulte-Steinberg O, Downing J 1988 Thoracic epidural anaesthesia via the caudal route in infants. Anesthesiology 69: 265–269

Campbell F, Yentis S, Fear D, Bissonette B 1992 Analgesic efficacy and safety of a caudal bupivacaine fentanyl mixture in children. Can J Anaesth 39: 661–664

Caudle C L, Freid E B, Bailey A G, Valley R D, Lish M C, Azizkhan R G 1993 Epidural fentanyl infusion with patient controlled epidural analgesia for postoperative analgesia in children. J Pediatr Surg 28: 554–559

Chay P C W, Duffy B J, Walker S J 1992 Pharacokinetic-pharacodynamic relationships of morphine in neonates. Clin Pharmacol Ther 51: 334–342

Choonara I, Lawrence A, Michalkiewicz A, Bowhay A, Ratcliffe J 1993 Morphine metabolism in neonates and infants. Br J Clin Pharmacol 34: 434–437

Coderre T J, Katz J, Vaccarino A L, Melzack R 1993 Contribution of central neuroplasticity to pathological pain: preview of clinical and experimental evidence. Pain 52: 259–285

Dalens B 1989 Regional anaesthesia in children. Anesth Analg 68: 654–672

Dalens B, Hasanaoui A 1989 Caudal anaesthesia in paediatric surgery: success rate and adverse events in 750 consecutive patients. Anesth Analg 68: 83–89

Desparmet J, Mateo J, Ecoffey C, Mazoit X 1990 Efficacy of an epidural test dose in children anesthetised with halothane. Anesthesiology 72: 249–251

Doyle E, Robinson D, Morton N S 1993a Comparison of patient controlled analgesia with and without a background infusion after lower abdominal surgery in children. Br J Anaesth 71: 670–673

Doyle E, Harper I, Morton N S 1993b Patient controlled analgesia with low dose background infusions after lower abdominal surgery in children. Br J Anaesth 71: 818–822

Doyle E, Byers G, McNichol L R, Morton N S 1994a Prevention of postoperative nausea and vomiting with transdermal hyoscine in children using patient controlled analgesia. Br J Anaesth 72: 72–76

Doyle E, Mottart K, Marshall C, Morton N 1994b Comparison of different bolus doses of morphine for patient controlled analgesia in children. Br J Anaesth 72: 160–163

Doyle E, Morton N, McNicol L 1994 Comparison of patient controlled analgesia in children by the IV and subcutaneous routes of administration. Br J Anaesth 72: 533–536

Fell D 1993 Postoperative analgesia in children. Br J Anaesth 70: 4–5

Flandin-Blety C, Barrier G 1995 Accidents following extradural analgesia in children: the results of a retrospective study. Paediatr Anaesth 5: 41–46

Gaudreault P, Guay J, Nicol O, Dupuis C 1988 Pharmacokinetics and clinical efficacy of intra-rectal solutions of acetaminophen. Can J Anaesth 35: 149–152

Gianna-Koulopoulos X, Sepulveda W, Kourtis P, Glover V, Fisk N M 1994 Fetal plasma cortisol and B-endorphin response to intrauterine needling. Lancet 344: 77–81

Grunau R V E, Craig K D 1987 Pain expression in neonates: facial action and cry. Pain 28: 395–410

Guinard J P, Borboen M 1993 Probable venous air embolism during caudal anaesthesia in a child. Anesth Analg 76: 1134–1135

Holthusen H, Eichwede F, Stevens M, Willnow U, Lipfert P 1994 Pre-emptive analgesia: comparison of preoperative with postoperative caudal block on postoperative pain in children. Br J Anaesth 73: 440–442

Houck C S, Troshynski T, Berde C B 1994 Treatment of pain in children. In: Wall T D, Malzack R (eds) Textbook of pain. Churchill Livingstone, Edinburg, pp 1419–1434

Johnson M R 1987 Pain response in pre-term infants. Infant Behav Dev 67: A532

Kauffman R E, Nelson M V 1992 Effect of age on ibuprofen pharmacokinetics and anti-pyretic response. J Pediatr 121: 969–973

Kehlet H 1989 Surgical stress: the role of pain and analgesia. Br J Anaesth 63: 189–195

Kehlet H 1994 Postoperative pain relief: what is the issue? Br J Anaesth 72: 375–378

Koren G, Butt W, Chinyonga H, Soldis S, Tan Y K, Pape K 1985 Post-operative morphine infusion in newborn infants: assessment of disposition characteristics and safety. J Pediatr 107: 963–967

Krane E J, Jacobson L E, Lynn A M, Parrot C, Tyler D C 1987 Caudal morphine for postoperative analgesia in children: a comparison with caudal bupivacaine and intrave-nous morphine. Anesth Analg 66: 647–653

Lee J, Rubin A 1994 Comparison of a bupivacaine-clonadine mixture with plain bupivacaine for caudal analgesia in children. Br J Anaesth 72: 258–262

Lejus C, Roussiere G, Testa S, Ganansia F, Meignier M, Souron R 1994 Postoperative extradural analgesia in children: comparison of morphine and fentanyl. Br J Anaesth 72: 156–159

Leslie F M, Tso S, Harlbutt D E 1982 Differential appearance of opiate receptor subtypes in neonatal rat brain. Life Sci 31: 1393–1396

Lloyd-Thomas A R 1990 Pain management in paediatric patients. Br J Anaesth 64: 85–104

Lloyd-Thomas A R 1993 An acute pain service for children. Anaesth Loco Regionale 1993; 2: 71–77

Lloyd-Thomas A R, Howard R F 1992 Postoperative pain control in children. Br Med J 304: 1174–1175

Lloyd-Thomas A R, Howard R F 1994 A pain service for children. Paediatr Anaesth 4: 3–15

Lynn A M, Slattery J T 1987 Morphine phamacokinetics in early infancy. Anesthesiology 66: 136–139

Mather L E, Mackie J 1983 The incidence of post-operative pain in children. Pain 15: 271–282

Maunuksela E-L, Ryhanen P, Janhunen L 1992a Efficacy of rectal ibuprofen in controlling postoperative pain in children. Can J Anaesth 39: 226–230

Maunuksela E-L, Kokki H, Bullingham R E S 1992b Comparison of intravenous ketorolac with morphine for postoperative pain in children. Clin Parmacol Ther 52: 436–443

Maxwell L, Martin L, Yaster M 1994 Bupivacaine induced cardiac toxicity in neonates: successful treatment with intravenous phenytoin. Anaesthesiology 80: 682–686

McCloskey H, Haun S, Deshbande J 1992 Bupivacaine toxicity secondary to continuous caudal epidural infusion in children. Anesth Analg 75: 287–290

McGrath P F, Johnson G, Goodmen J T, Schillinger J, Dunn J, Chapman J 1985 The CHEOPS: a behavioural scale to measure post-operative pain in children. In: Fields H L, Dubner R, Cervero F (eds) Advances in pain research and therapy. Raven Press, New York, pp 395–402

McNicol L R 1993 Postoperative analgesia in children using continuous SC morphine. Br J Anaesth 71: 752–756

McRorie T, Lynn A, Nespeca N, Opheim K, Slattery J 1992 The maturation of morphine clearance and metabolism. Am J Dis Child 146: 972–976

Meignier M, Souronss R, Leneel J 1983 Postoperative dorsal epidural analgesia in the child with respiratory disabilities. Anaesthesiology 59: 473–475

Morselli P L, Franco-Morselli R, Borsi 1980 Clinical pharmacokinetics in newborns and infants: age related differences and therapeutic implications. Clin Pharmacokinet 5: 485–527

Morton N S 1993 Development of a monitoring protocol for the safe use of opioids in children. Paediatr Anaesth 3: 179–184

Murat I, Delleur M M, Esteve C M, Egu J F, Raynaud P, Saint-Maurice P 1987 Continuous extradural anaesthesia in children, clinical and haemodynamic implications. Br J Anaesth 59: 1441–1450

Murrell D, Gibson P, Cohen R 1993 Continous epidural analgesia in newborn infants undergoing major surgery. J Paediatr Surg 28: 548–553

Osborne R, Joel S, Trew D, Slevin M 1988 Analgesic activity of morphine-6–glucuronide. Lancet i: 828–830

Pain after Surgery 1990 Commission on the Provision of Surgical Services. Royal College of Surgeons of England and the College of Anaesthetists, London

Perillo M, Sethna N, Berde C 1993 Intravenous isoprotenerol as a marker for epidural test dosing in children. Anesth Analg 76: 176–181

Peutrell J M, Hughes D G 1993 Epidural analgesia through caudal catheters for inguinal herniotomies in awake ex-premature babies. Anaesthesia 48: 128–131

Porter F 1993 Pain assessment in children: infants. In: Schechter N L, Berde C B, Yaster M (eds) Pain in infants, children and adolescents. Williams & Wilkins, Baltimore pp 87–96

Porter F L, Porges S W, Marshall R E 1988 Newborn pain cries and vagal tone: parallel changes in response to circumcision. Child Dev 59: 495–505

Purcell-Jones G, Dorman F, Sumner E 1987 The use of opioids in neonates: a retrospective study of 933 cases. Anaesthesia 42: 1316–1320

Purcell-Jones G, Dormon F, Sumner E 1988 Pain on the postal survey of members of Paediatric Anaesthetists Pain Association: paediatric anaesthetists' perception of neonatal and infant pain. Pain 32: 181–187

Ready B, Oden R, Chadwick H et al 1988 Development of an anaesthesiology-based postoperative pain management service. Anesthesiology 68: 100–106

Rodgers B M, Webb C J, Stergios D, Newman B M 1988 Patient controlled analgesia in paediatric surgery. J Paediatr Surg 33: 259–262

Schwartz N, Eisenkraft J 1993 Probable venous air embolism during epidural placement in an infant. Anesth Analg 76: 1136–1138

Sethna N, Berde C 1993 Venous air embolism during identification of the epidural space in children. Anesth Analg 76: 925–927

Southern D, Reed M 1994 Over dosage of opiate from patient controlled analgesia devices. Br Med J 309: 102

Taddio A, Goldbach M, Ipp M, Stevens B, Koren G 1995 Effect of neonatal circumcision on pain responses during vaccination in boys. Lancet 344: 291–292

Tyler D C, Crane E J 1990 Paediatric pain: advances in pain research and therapy, Vol 15. Raven Press, New York

Tyler D C, Tu A, Douthit J, Chapman C R 1993 Toward validation of pain measurement tools for children: a pilot study. Pain 52: 301–309

Watcha M F, Jones M B, Lagueruela R G, Schweiger C, White P F 1992 Comparison of ketorolac and morphine as adjuvants during paediatric surgery. Anaesthesiology 76: 368–372

Watcha M, Bras P, Cieslak G, Pennent J 1995 The dose response relationship of ondansetron in preventing postoperative emesis in paediatric patients undergoing ambulatory surgery. Anaesthesiology 82: 47–52

Webster A, McKishnie J, Reid W 1993 Lumbar epidural anaesthesia for inguinal hernia repair in low birth weight infants. Can J Anaesth 40: 670–675

Wilson P T J, Lloyd-Thomas A R 1993 An audit of extradural infusion analgesia in children using bupivacaine and diamorphine. Anaesthesia 48: 718–723

Wolf A R 1994 Treat the babies not their stress responses. Lancet 344: 77–81

Wolf A, Hughes D 1993 Pain relief for infants undergoing abdominal surgery: comparison of infusions of IV morphine and extradural bupivacaine. Br J Anaesth 70: 10–16

Wolf A, Hughes D, Wade A, Mather S, Prys-Roberts C 1990 Postoperative analgesia after orchidopexy: evaluation of a bupivacaine morphine mixture. Br J Anaesth 64: 430–435

Wolf A R, Eyres R L, Laussen P C et al 1993 Effect of extradural analgesia on stress responses to abdominal surgery in infants. Br J Anaesth 70: 654–660

Wood C, Goresky G, Classen K, Niel S 1994 Complications of continuous epidural infusions for postoperative analgesia in children. Can J Anaesth 14: 613–620

Wright J 1993 Controlled trial of wound infiltration with bupivacaine for postoperative pain relief after appendicectomy in children. Br J Surg 80: 110–111

Yaster M, Deshpande J K 1988 Management of pediatric pain with opioid analgesia. J Pediatr 113: 421–429

Yaster M, Maxwell K G 1989 Pediatric regional anaesthesia. Anesthesiology 70: 324–338

Yaster M, Maxwell L G 1993 Opioid agonists and antagonists. In: Schechter N L, Berde C B, Yaster M (eds) Pain in infants, children and adolescents. Williams & Wilkins, Baltimore, pp 145–171

9

Recent advances in oxidant-mediated tissue injury

D. N. Tew   J. G. Jones

The biological significance of oxidants has been debated for at least 30 years in the scientific press (Halliwell & Gutteridge 1989) and is increasingly the subject of public attention (Anon 1994). Oxidants are relevant to the practice of anaesthesia and intensive care since some acute or chronic underlying diseases and perioperative events can involve oxidant mediators. Anaesthetists already use drugs which enhance oxidant production (e.g. high inspired oxygen concentrations and halothane (Knecht et al 1992)) or possess antioxidant properties (e.g. mannitol (Rickels et al 1993) and propofol (Murphy et al 1992, Nelson et al 1993)). As knowledge of the oxidant/antioxidant axis increases so current anaesthetic and intensive care practice may alter, particularly with the introduction of more focused oxidant and antioxidant manipulations.

Oxidants are produced under normal conditions (Table 9.1) both accidentally by leakage from the respiratory chain and deliberately to serve useful biological roles. Under pathological conditions (Table 9.1) oxidant production contributes to many disease states and in some cases may be the

Table 9.1 Oxidant production under normal and pathological conditions

Normal conditions	Pathological conditions
'Leak' from mitochondrial respiratory chain	Increased leak from respiratory chain
Neutrophils	Pathologically activated neutrophils
Catecholamine auto-oxidation	Increased catecholamine auto-oxidation during stress response or inotrope therapy

Background radiation	Exposure to high levels of radiation
	Transition metal ion-catalysed reactions (iron and copper)
	Xanthine oxidase
	Prostaglandin metabolism
	Drugs (bleomycin, xenobiotics)
	Nitric oxide interaction with superoxide
	Inhaled oxidants
	   Ozone
	   Exhaust fumes
	   High inspired oxygen concentrations
	Calcium-mediated

Table 9.2   Endogenous antioxidant defences

Plasma/blood	Cellular	
	Cytosolic	Membranous
Vitamin C	Superoxide dismutase (SOD)	Vitamin E
Urate	Catalase	Phospholipid hydroperoxide glutathione peroxidase (PHGPX)
Haemoglobin	Glutathione peroxidase (GPX)	
Vitamin A	Glutathione-*S*-transferase (GST)	
Glutathione	Glutathione	

Table 9.3   Consequences of oxidant stress

Biological target	Damage
Proteins	Dysfunctional enzymes
	Ultrastructural disruption
Lipids	Disruption of cellular membranes and organelles
	Chain reactions producing further oxidants (lipid peroxidation products)
	Damage to circulating lipids
DNA	Dysfunctional genes
	Mutations, possibly carcinogenic
Connective tissue	Direct: through oxidation of collagen and lipopolysaccharides
	Indirect: through elastase and collagenase released from activated neutrophils

underlying cause. Endogenous antioxidant defences (Table 9.2) have evolved partly to quench the 'leak' of oxidants from normal physiological production and partly to defend against tissue injury in disease. When oxidant activity exceeds antioxidant capacity the resulting 'oxidant stress' can damage lipids, proteins DNA and connective tissue (Table 9.3). The resulting tissue injury may at least amplify if not cause disease processes (reviewed in Halliwell et al 1992, Webster & Nunn 1988, Royston 1988).

This review describes how such exciting biochemical concepts have apparently failed to provide widespread routine therapeutic benefit and how this may be addressed in the future. We also describe recent findings in the contribution of oxidants to normal physiology and the mechanisms of tissue injury in specific pathological conditions listed below.

1. Reperfusion injury
   – Brain
   – Myocardium
   – Gut
   – Kidney
   – Transplanted organs
2. Sepsis/inflammation
3. Shock/trauma
4. Pulmonary toxicity
5. Halothane hepatitis

WHERE IS THE THERAPEUTIC BENEFIT?

Of 40 trials examining the ability of antioxidants to reduce myocardial reperfusion injury, half did find a protective effect and half did not (Kukreja & Hess 1992). Of the many explanations for this discrepancy, one may be that oxidant stress serves no significant part in myocardial reperfusion injury. A more likely alternative is that attempts to manipulate pathophysiological processes before they are fully understood is doomed to produce contradictory results. Thus the simplistic idea that some disease processes involve a torrent of 'oxidants' which can be antagonized by a single general-purpose antioxidant is largely discredited.

The complexion of oxidant type and mechanism of production will vary with specific disease processes, as will the precise anatomical location and biological nature of targets to be attacked. The time course over which damage occurs, and the nature and performance of endogenous defences, will also vary, while it should not be forgotten that oxidants may serve useful functions (Table 9.4) even under conditions of pathological activation. A knowledge of these factors in any disease will allow appropriate selection of an antioxidant strategy, pharmacological agents and timing of administration, to prevent or reverse tissue damage in experimental or clinical settings.

INVESTIGATING THE ROLE OF OXIDANTS

Investigators have been hampered in their attempts to set up or test pathophysiological hypotheses because the tools to measure oxidant production (nature and amount), endogenous antioxidant defences, damage to specific biological targets, action of exogenous antioxidants and clinical outcome are difficult to apply.

Nature and amount of oxidant

Oxidants are by nature extremely reactive, thus short lived and difficult to detect in biological systems (hydroxyl radicals are believed to have a half life of around 10^{-6} s). The only technique able to demonstrate free radicals directly is electron paramagnetic resonance spectroscopy (EPR), and although chemists have been using EPR for 40 years it is only recently that EPR has been applied to animal studies (Bolli et al 1988) and only very recently

Table 9.4 Useful biological roles of oxidants

Controlled release of energy within the respiratory chain
Microbial killing
Tumour surveillance
Intracellular signal transduction
DNA biosynthesis

that it has been applied in vivo to man (Grech et al 1993). Spin traps (typically nitrone molecules such as PBN) are increasingly used to aid detection since they combine with free radicals both in vivo and ex vivo to form more stable and thus longer-lived radicals which can be used to assess the nature and amount of original free radical. However, this technique may underestimate oxidant production by failing to react with all the free radical(s) produced. Spin-traps also 'mop up' free radicals, thereby acting as scavengers and thus they alter the disease process themselves; indeed this is a highly effective therapeutic intervention in an animal model of shock (Novelli 1992). Recently, naturally occurring spin-traps such as vitamin C have been considered as quantitative measures of oxidant production (Buettner & Jurkiewicz 1993, Tew et al 1994a). The mechanisms for oxidant production are referenced above but of particular recent note is the role of nitric oxide in producing hydroxyl radicals through a peroxynitrate reaction with superoxide (Beckman et al 1990).

Some studies make statements about antioxidant activity without being able to show that specific oxidants were produced within a biological system and antagonized by the antioxidant under test. Such studies lack authority since many antioxidants possess other therapeutic properties (e.g. N-acetylcysteine is an antioxidant through possession of sulphydryl groups but also an anticoagulant (Jepsen et al 1992)).

Anatomical location of oxidant activity

The sites of oxidant activity at macroscopic, ultrastructural and molecular levels have only recently been investigated and this information is likely to be crucial when deciding on delivery strategies for antioxidant therapies. Thus magnetic resonance imaging (MRI) can delineate macroscopic oxidant activity in acute lung injury by showing high-intensity spots where lung damage has occurred (Taylor et al 1990).

Techniques have been developed to demonstrate the ultrastructural location of oxidant production related to underlying tissue injury. NADPH oxidase (Murphy & Jones 1991) and cerium chloride (Murphy et al 1991) stains suggest that in acute lung injury oxidant production occurs at the site of epithelial injury (Fig. 9.1) A combination of perfusion with cerium chloride and adminstration of the tracer horseradish peroxidase allows the demonstration of hydrogen peroxide generation and sites of increased vascular leakage (Fig. 9.2).

Site-specific oxidation is now recognized, at the molecular level, whereby oxidants can produce specific genetic or protein modification. This knowledge may be used in treatment, thus oxidative inactivation of α_1-antiproteinase can be virtually abolished by a single amino acid substitution (valine for methionine in position 358) to produce oxidant resistance while retaining antagonism to human neutrophil elastase. The possibility that genetic engineering will permit the development of modified proteins resistant to

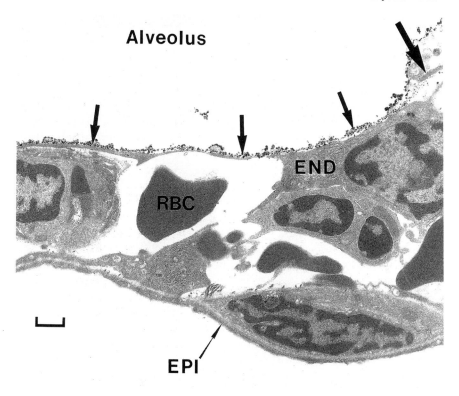

Fig. 9.1   Electron micrograph of the alveolar capillary barrier in experimental acute lung injury. Increase in permeability to ^{99m}Tc-DTPA is associated in one airspace with extensive destructionof the alveolar epithelium (the limit of the epithelium is shown by the large arrow), although the epithelial lining of the adjacent alveolus is intact. The tissue in this preparation has been stained for NADPH oxidase; the resulting electron-dense deposits (small arrows) at the site of epithelial loss suggest that oxygen-derived free radicals are produced at the site of such injury. Marker equals 1 μm; RBC, red blood cell; END, endothelium. EPI (alveolar epithelium). (Reprinted with permission from Murphy & Jones 1991.)

oxidant attack, while retaining their biological function is a promising field (Kalsheker 1989).

Biological targets

Oxidants are very reactive and in achieving a more inert state interact with a wide variety of biological substrates, including proteins, lipids and DNA. The resulting damage leads to *direct effects*; these include denaturing proteins which may lead to structural disruption or reduced activity of enzymes. Lipid peroxidation disrupts cell and organelle membranes leading to cell death and release of previously compartmentalized noxious substances, e.g. free iron or proteolytic enzymes. Oxidation of DNA leads to disordered genetic

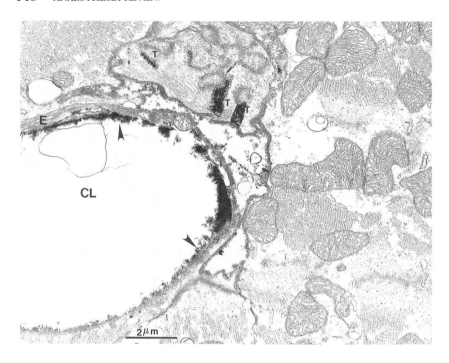

Fig. 9.2 Transmission electron micrograph of porcine myocardium following 20 min ischaemia and 15 min reperfusion with pig blood. Cerium perhydroxide is precipitated (arrows) on the luminal surface of a capillary endothelial cell (E), indicating an anatomical site of oxidant production. Immediately under the damaged capillary, tetramethyl benzadine crystals (T) are present in cardiac myocytes. These are the histochemical reaction products from with horseradish peroxidase which has passed from the capillary lumen (CL) through the leaky endothelium and entered a damaged myocyte. This suggests an association between sites of oxidant production and tissue damage. Reproduced from Tew et al 1994a (by kind permission of J Skepper).

expression of proteins and is believed to be involved in carcinogenesis (Cerruti 1994). *Indirect damage* is expressed in numerous ways, many of which are yet to be fully elucidated. Examples include unopposed proteolytic destruction of lung following oxidative inactivation of α_1-antiproteinase in acute lung injury (Weiss 1989) and the atherosclerotic consequences of low-density lipoprotein (LDL) oxidation (Witztum 1994).

Markers of oxidant damage

The problems in measuring oxidants directly have led to the development of damage markers for oxidant-induced tissue damage, e.g. lipid peroxidation products and modified DNA bases. Many trials have used reductions in these markers as evidence for protection against oxidant attack. Almost all tissue injury, regardless of cause, can produce oxidants and changes in these markers do not necessarily support the role of oxidants as a sole cause of tissue injury. Similarly the changes in damage markers may be statistically significant when clinical significance is in question. Thus without knowledge of the processes concerned it would be unwise to recommend clinical interventions on the basis of their ability to reduce damage markers.

Endogenous antioxidant defences

Table 9.2 outlines how a variety of antioxidants reside at different anatomical locations. These defences can be assessed either as the total radical antioxidant potential (TRAP) (Miller et al in press) of plasma, plasma levels of antioxidant scavengers (Buettner 1993) or as activity of defensive enzymes.

The endogenous defences in Table 9.2 are well characterized (Halliwell & Gutteridge 1989) but a new membranous selenoperoxidase enzyme (phospholipid hydroperoxide glutathione peroxidase, PHGPX) has recently been described. PHGPX is lipophilic and prevents lipid peroxidation by acting on phospholipid hydroperoxide substrates, with the additional advantage of preventing phospholipase A2 activation (Ursini & Bindoli 1987, Thomas et al 1990).

It is now apparent that in addition to specific antioxidants other defensive mechanisms exist to repair damaged DNA (endonuclease enzymes) and restore protein homeostasis (heat shock proteins). Heat shock proteins in particular are attracting considerable attention since they are known to assist in folding nascent proteins to their tertiary structures as they emerge from the ribosomal apparatus under normal conditions [Nature ref 1994]. As cells are subject to thermal or oxidant stress, rapid upregulation of heat shock proteins occurs with suppression of normal protein synthesis and subsequent protection against further stress (Jolliet et al 1994). Ischaemic preconditioning of the myocardium is also attracting attention (Murray et al 1986). A short period of ischaemia offers protection against subsequent ischaemic insults and this appears to be biphasic, with short-term protection (1–2 h) probably mediated through adenosine, and longer protection (24 h or more) mediated through heat shock proteins.

Exogenous antioxidants

Strategies for antagonizing oxidant stress include preventing initial oxidant production and stopping oxidants begetting further oxidants through chain reactions, notably in the lipid phase; for example, scavenging free oxidant with the exogenous application of natural or artificial antioxidants and upregulating naturally occurring defences in vivo through diet or pharmacological manipulation.

Clinical outcome

If the eventual goal of basic scientific and clinical research is to translate concepts into useful therapeutic strategies, then it is particularly important to establish the antioxidant effect on clinical outcome. Endpoints such as mortality and morbidity for antioxidant therapy are still being evaluated but in chronic disease and cancer the early promise of observational studies has been disappointing when subjected to prospective randomized controlled trials. Vitamin E or A supplementation compared with placebo over 6 years in 29 000 Finnish smokers showed no protection against cancer or heart disease, while new lung cancer, haemorrhagic stroke and total mortality increased in the treatment groups (Alpha-Tocopherol BCCpSG 1994). Antioxidant supplements in 800 Americans had no effect on bowel cancer. Vitamins E and A with selenium prevented 1–16% of cancers in 30 000 Chinese subjects (Blot et al 1993). Some of these trials have been criticized in terms of inadequate dose to produce meaningful increases in blood levels and short time span in which a treatment effect is sought (Hennekens et al 1994), emphasizing how difficult it is to apply current knowledge in clinical settings. It is becoming apparent that oxidized low-density lipoprotein (Ox-LDL) may be a major contributor to atherosclerotic disease (Witztum 1994) and although investigation has shown that some antioxidants can reduce Ox-LDL the clinical significance remains to be demonstrated (Steinberg 1993). With acute disease, timing of antioxidant intervention is important, particularly with reperfusion injury. Many animal models of acute oxidant injury show therapeutic benefit with prospective treatment which cannot be matched using retrospective therapy.

Well-designed trials investigating oxidant-mediated processes are difficult and expensive to organize, particularly in man. It is hoped that basic science will continue to furnish the data necessary to focus antioxidant manipulations in experimental settings, particularly in vivo in man.

WIDER ROLES OF OXIDANTS

Life requires energy which is released from biochemical stores in a controlled, efficient manner through single electron transfers. Single electron transfer will thus produce free radicals which are largely controlled within the respiratory chain proteins of the mitochondria. Normal life depends on a controlled production of free radicals and any 'leakage' usually dealt with by endogenous defences.

Neutrophils can produce oxidants through three pathways which in turn they use to kill ingested microbes. This killing role may be extended to abnormal or mutant cells during immune surveillance which may be particularly important in the prevention of cancer.

Stable and transient amino acid radicals and nucleic acid radicals are known to be important in DNA biosynthesis (Stubbe 1994).

Oxidants are recognized as intracellular signals both in upregulating defences during oxidant stress (increased expression of defensive enzymes and other defences such as heat shock proteins) and under normal physiological conditions. Oxidants are involved in protein synthesis through their interaction with redox-sensitive recognition sites (Abate et al 1990). Exogenous antioxidants may interfere with this process in two ways. Firstly, by altering the intracellular level of available oxidant they may indirectly reduce protein synthesis coupled to oxidant stress. Since these proteins would have served a protective role then exogenous antioxidants may, paradoxically, increase the effects of oxidant stress. Secondly, an antioxidant responsive element (ARE) (Rushmore et al 1991) has been identified, which on exposure to redox antioxidants increases the genetic expression of antioxidant enzymes, e.g. glutathione-S-transferase and NADPH reductase (Daniel 1993). Exogenous antioxidants may not act on the ARE to upregulate defensive enzymes in this way.

From this it can be seen that oxidants regulate expression of endogenous defences (Figs. 9.3 and 9.4). Pretreatment of bacteria with low-dose hydrogen peroxide allows their adaptation to previously lethal levels on subsequent exposure. It has been shown that hydrogen peroxide and superoxide, respectively, induce the expression of different antioxidant enzymes through different genes. Of the 30 or so bacterial proteins induced by oxidant stress many are maximally expressed in just 10 min after exposure. The situation

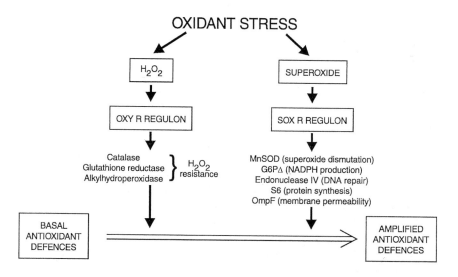

Fig. 9.3   Genetic regulation of bacterial antioxidant defences. As oxidant stress increases, hydrogen peroxide and superoxide induce different amplifications of basal antioxidant defences through different genetic regulons. This upregulation of defence is specific for the stimulating oxidant and leads to the increased expression of appropriately targeted defensive enzymes. (Adapted from Harris 1992.)

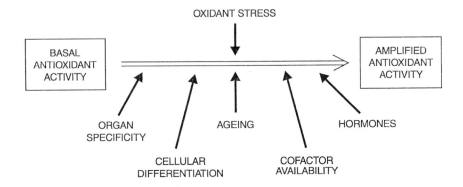

Fig. 9.4 Genetic modulation of antioxidant defences in higher organisms. In higher organisms upregulation of antioxidant defences, although triggered by oxidant stress, is modified by genetic and environmental influences. (Adapted from Harris 1992.)

is more complicated in higher organisms since basal levels of antioxidant enzyme activity are influenced by oxidant stress, cellular differentiation, cofactor availability and hormone activity (Harris 1992).

Endogenous antioxidants may also work synergistically, for example, superoxide dismutase (SOD) promotes the conversion of superoxide to hydrogen peroxide. This is potentially damaging since hydrogen peroxide is a potent source of highly toxic hydroxyl radicals. Catalase and glutathione peroxidase promote the conversion of hydrogen peroxide to water, removing this threat and completing a cascade of antioxidant defence. Trials in which SOD alone has been given may fail to show an effect because of ungoverned conversion of relatively innocuous superoxide to the far more noxious hydroxyl radical through hydrogen peroxide, which overwhelms endogenous clearance mechanisms (Yim et al 1990). Similarly vitamins E and C are believed to act synergistically, with free radical bearing vitamin E in cell membranes being regenerated by aqueous-phase vitamin C (Packer et al 1979). To increase membranous vitamin E without regulating vitamin C levels may not produce the treatment effect anticipated. It has also been suggested that, in some circumstances, excess antioxidant activity could, paradoxically, protect mutagenic DNA from natural destruction, leading to tumour promotion (Cerruti 1994).

Endogenous antioxidant defence is internally regulated and in many cases orchestrated by a number of complementary biologically active molecules. To apply exogenous antioxidants during oxidant stress may improve outcome but equally may produce indifferent or even damaging effects. The mechanisms for deleterious effects include suppressing upregulation of more appropriate endogenous defences, conversion of low-toxity oxidant to higher toxicity oxidant (e.g. superoxide to hydrogen peroxide when using SOD alone) and pro-oxidant activity of vitamin C in the presence of free iron (Halliwell & Gutteridge 1984).

Basic science research will provide more information about the nature of these interactions and permit the development of more sophisticated antioxidant therapies, perhaps using well-timed cocktails of antioxidants for specific clinical circumstances.

EVIDENCE FOR FREE RADICAL INVOLVEMENT IN DISEASE

Reperfusion injury

Enhanced tissue damage by oxidants occurs when reperfusion takes place after temporary vascular occlusion. These oxidants may be derived from the organ in question, from blood elements or from the vascular endothelium of the blood vessels supplying it. Animal studies have provided the majority of evidence for free radical involvement in reperfusion injury. Human studies have provided some evidence for free radical generation and contribution to disease but little data on the efficacy of therapy.

The principal sources of free radicals in reperfusion injury are xanthine oxidase (XO), activated neutrophils, arachadonic acid metabolites, free transition metal ions (iron and copper) and nitric oxide interaction with superoxide. During ischaemia, vascular endothelial xanthine dehydrogenase is converted to XO, which in the presence of molecular oxygen after reperfusion acts on hypoxanthine to produce superoxide radicals (McCord 1985). Activated neutrophils provide superoxide and singlet oxygen through their respiratory burst (Klebanoff 1980, Rosen & Klebanoff 1977). Transitional metal ions catalyse the formation of hydroxyl radicals from hydrogen peroxide (Halliwell & Gutteridge 1989).

XO and iron-mediated radical production occurs rapidly on reperfusion, whereas neutrophil-mediated free radicals may appear over a longer time course particularly associated with prolonged ischaemia and necrosis (Lucchesi & Mullane 1986). The vascular endothelium is now emerging as a highly active metabolic site producing many mediators of acute inflammation, elements promoting free radical production and leucocyte adhesion. It may also be central to ischaemia preconditioning, which thus may apply not only to the myocardium but to any location containing vascular endothelium (Parratt 1994).

Brain

Intracerebral free radical production has been described as a consequence of brain ischaemia/reperfusion (Sakamoto et al 1991, Carney & Floyd 1991, Hall et al 1993) and has been proposed as a causal agent in reperfusion brain injury (Sakamoto & Ogawa 1992) and vasospasm following subarachnoid haemorrhage (MacDonald & Weir 1994).

Several mechanisms have been proposed for free radical generation, including the arachadonic acid cascade, transition metal-catalysed reactions (Gutteridge 1992), ascorbate/haemoglobin interactions (Sadrzadeh & Eaton

1988, Prat & Turrens 1990) and leucocyte activation. XO may not be involved in producing cerebral free radicals since no conversion of XO from xanthine dehydrogenase could be detected during cerebral ischaemia in animals (Betz et al 1991) and no protective effect of allopurinol could be ascribed to XO antagonism (Lindsay et al 1991).

Nitric oxide (itself a free radical) may contribute to ischaemia/reperfusion injury (Oury et al 1992) through cyclic guanosine monophosphate production and/or an interaction with SOD, forming hydroxyl radicals via peroxynitrate (Garthwaite 1991). Interestingly, nitric oxide synthase inhibitors reduce infarct size in rats (Oury et al 1992) and mice (Nowicki et al 1991).

Free iron is a potent source of cerebral radicals, and traumatic release of free iron from injured brain (Halliwell & Gutteridge 1985) cannot be contained by the limited transferrin concentrations in cerebrospinal fluid (Halliwell 1992). An aminosteroid which blocks iron-based radical reactions decreases post-traumatic neurological damage after head injury (Hall & Braughler 1989).

The spin-trap PBN, used in the detection of free radicals through EPR, has been shown to protect against oxidative damage (Carney & Floyd 1991, Cheng et al 1993).

Although allopurinol is predicted to offer poor protection against cerebral reperfusion injury, other antioxidants which are of benefit in animal models should lead to clinically useful applications of these compounds. Most notable of these is Tirilizad, a 21 amino steroid (also termed lazaroid) which offers exceptional protection against lipid peroxidation (without corticosteroid side effects) following both pre- and post-insult administration (Perkins et al 1991, Hall & Yonkers 1988). The ability of Tirilizad to influence neurological outcome when given within 6 h of head injury is currently the subject of a multi-centre clinical trial.

Myocardium

Regional and global myocardial ischaemia/reperfusion are seen following coronary insufficiency, myocardial infarction (particularly after thrombolysis) and cardiac surgery with cardiopulmonary bypass. Reperfusion produces dysrhythmias, temporary reduction in cardiac performance (stunning) and increased infarct size. Free radicals are associated with these changes but a causal relationship is, at present, only suggested (Kukreja & Hess 1992).

Global myocardial ischaemia/reperfusion in intact dogs produces lipid peroxidation products indicative of oxygen free radical-mediated injury (Romaschin et al 1987). Isolated perfused rat hearts are protected from a post-reperfusion increase in radical-generated phosphocreatine kinase by perfusion with SOD, catalase and XO inhibitors (Grisham et al 1986). Some 40 studies have looked at the effect of antioxidants on reperfusion injury and half found no protective effect (Kukreja & Hess 1992). Possible reasons for these discrepancies include inadequate dose and an inappropriate range of antioxidant activity. This may mean that prolonged antioxidant activity and cocktails of agents with activity against a wider spectrum of oxidants will produce more consistent results. The half-life of native SOD is less than 10 min and it has been shown that conjugating SOD to polyethylene glycol (PEGSOD) increases its half-life to 30 h, allowing it to reduce infarct size at 6 h and 4 days in a canine model (Tamura et al 1988). Histidine, which antagonizes singlet oxygen, has been shown to protect against reperfusion injury (Loesser et al 1992) and may be a useful component of future antioxidant cocktails. Increasing endogenous antioxidant defences (enzyme activity) has been shown to protect rat hearts against reperfusion injury (Kirshenbaum & Singal 1993).

Free radical species have now been directly identified using EPR in isolated hearts (Garlick et al 1987, Zweier et al 1988), intact animals (Bolli et al 1988, Bolli & McCay 1990, Zweier et al 1988) and man (Grech et al 1993). It has been suggested that the intensity of free radical generation is related to the severity of ischaemia and contributes to myocardial stunning (Bolli et al 1988).

Lipid radicals have been detected in a patient undergoing coronary angioplasty $2^{1}/_{2}$ h after the onset of chest pain from myocardial infarction. Two peaks of radical intensity were detected at 20 min and at 9 h after angioplasty. These were interpreted as demonstrating early XO and iron-mediated radicals followed by late, neutrophil-derived free radicals (Grech et al 1993).

As might be expected, other mediators are implicated including activated neutrophils, free calcium and complement (Kilgore et al 1994). Our understanding of how these factors combine is improving and it is believed that free radicals cause lipid membrane disruption, which in turn releases excessive free cytosolic calcium and arachadonic acid metabolites (Kuzuya et al 1993), leading to chemotaxis and neutrophil activation. Complement is activated by free radicals and itself generates further oxidants and chemotactic agents as well as producing direct cell damage through membrane attack complexes, which again releases arachadonic acid substrate. By these mechanisms lipid barriers and contractile proteins are disrupted, leading to the clinical consequences of reperfusion. Cellular energy depletion is also increasingly recognized as an important consideration, particularly with the emergence of adenosine as the leading contender for the mediator of early ischaemia preconditioning. This area is already producing therapeutic possibilities since akadesine protects against reperfusion injury through 'pharmacological preconditioning' (Mullane 1993).

The routine use of antioxidants is currently confined to antioxidant cardioplegia in some centres, and antioxidant preservative is used in most heart transplantation programmes. It is anticipated that the administration of a well-timed cocktail of antioxidants, neutrophil adhesion molecule inhibitors, complement inhibitors, adenosine analogues and heat shock protein stimulants will offer very significant myocardial protection particularly with 'elective' reperfusion, e.g. after cardiac surgery and thrombolysis.

Gut

Oxidants almost certainly mediate intestinal reperfusion injury, and anti-oxidant therapy in man has been shown to be effective. Intestinal mucosa is very sensitive to ischaemia/reperfusion injury and quantitative assessment of free radicals using EPR has suggested a causal link between free radical production and histological damage in a feline model (Nilson et al 1993). Calcium-mediated phospholipase A2 activation is also implicated in both mucosal injury and neutrophil recruitment since inhibitors of this enzyme reduce its activity and moderate tissue injury in the rat (Otamiri 1989). Oxidants are the molecular trigger and phosholipase A2 the enzymatic trigger for post-reperfusion gut injury (Schoenberg & Beger 1993). The small intestine is disproportionately susceptible to ischaemia during circulatory shock and endothelial cell XO probably triggers this mucosal reperfusion injury (Schiller et al 1993). Intravenous SOD almost completely abolishes the increases in intestinal permeability following a 1 h period of partial ischaemia in cat intestine (Granger et al 1981). Pretreatment with SOD has been shown to attenuate intestinal epithelial necrosis in models of regional intestinal hypotension and haemorrhagic shock (Schoenberg et al 1983). Pretreatment with the xanthine oxidase inhibitor allopurinol prevents intestinal reperfusion injury (Parks et al 1983, Holgado et al 1989). Agents interfering with leucocyte adherence also protect against reperfusion injury (Arndt et al 1991). The spin-trap PBN acting as an antioxidant has been shown to improve survival in a rat superior mesenteric artery occlusion model of shock from 0/10 (controls) to 8/10 (PBN treated) (Novelli 1992). It seems very likely that free radicals play a pivotal role in gut reperfusion injury and that clinical trials will show which antioxidant strategies are most appropriate. Recent studies in man have shown that allopurinol and desferioxamine improve cure and relapse rates in acute colitis (Salim 1992a) and peptic ulceration (Salim 1992b). In critically ill patients with stress ulceration, free radical-mediated damage secondary to mucosal ischaemia and reperfusion is now recognized as a major contributory factor (Tryba 1992). In a recent clinical trial, 177 patients with haemorrhagic shock received placebo or antioxidant therapy (allopurinol or dimethyl sulphoxide) for stress ulcer prophylaxis. The incidence of endoscopically proven gastric ulceration within 3 days of admission in each treatment group was 22% (placebo), 3% (allopurinol) and 4% (dimethyl sulphoxide), demonstrating the efficacy of antioxidant therapy in this group of critically ill patients (Salim 1991). The link between partial ischaemia an reperfusion injury has interesting clinical correlates since the use of gut mucosal pH as an indicator of intestinal perfusion appears to show a link between inadequate intestinal perfusion and outcome (Gys et al 1988, Maynard et al 1993). It is probable that mucosal villous degradation allows translocation of proteolytic enzymes, bacteria and endotoxin, with adverse cardiopulmonary effects. This villous damage can occur even in the presence of apparently adequate intestinal blood flow, through extravascular short-circuiting of oxygen at the base of villi

(Schoenberg & Beger 1993). Thus therapy targeted to prevent intestinal reperfusion injury would be predicted to offer systemic protection as well.

Organ transplantation

The ischaemic interval between harvest and grafting of transplanted organs has prompted research into the influence of free radicals on performance and survival of these organs.

This ischaemic interval is known to be associated with free radical production, which has been suggested as a mechanism for graft failure (Connor et al 1992). Antioxidants protect lung function after heart-lung transplantation in dogs (Takeuchi et al 1992) and prolong graft survival after liver transplantation in rats (Connor et al 1992). Donor pretreatment with allopurinol improves graft survival and performance in canine renal transplants (Owens et al 1974).

The potential therapeutic strategies for enhancing graft survival in man include donor pretreatment to antagonize XO (allopurinol) or induce antioxidant enzymes in the graft (diet) and recipient perioperative treatment with antioxidants.

Shock/trauma

Shock and trauma produce ischaemia/reperfusion and tissue damage leading to neutrophil activation, cytokine release, transition metal release, free myoglobin and haemoglobin, changes in acute-phase proteins and redistribution of antioxidants. This may increase free radical activity, amplifying the damage sustained during shock/trauma. These free radicals may produce direct tissue damage or indirect damage mediated through inactivation of protective proteins or elevation of intracellular calcium. Allopurinol has been shown to improve survival in canine haemorrhagic shock (Crowell et al 1969) and more recently spin-trapping nitrones (radical scavengers) have been shown to dramatically reduce mortality in three different models of shock in the rat (Novelli 1992).

Sepsis/inflammation

The inflammatory response with or without microbial initiation generates cytokines, interleukins and interferon. This in turn activates complement and neutrophils which, in addition to releasing prostaglandins, leukotrines and proteolytic enzymes, also generate free radicals (Table 9.1). As inflammation progresses the resulting tissue damage will provide further generation of free radicals (Table 9.1).

These appear to be important processes since oxidant production and antioxidant depletion have been reported in septic patients, while septic models have found protective effects of trace elements (zinc, copper and selenium), vitamins E and C, N-acetylcysteine, other glutathione donors, superoxide dismutase and catalase (Goode & Webster 1993). Antioxidants appear to be protective in rat endotoxaemia (Schneider et al 1989) and *Escherichia coli* septicaemia (Broner et al 1989), while in the clinical arena combining selenium, vitamins E and C and N-acetylcysteine reduced mortality in septic ARDS patients (Sawyer et al 1989). Further clinical trials will undoubtedly be necessary since excessive antagonism may reduce endogenous microbial killing and inappropriate antagonism may paradoxically increase oxidant stress (Hoffman et al 1987, Traber et al 1985). Nutritional status may also prove to be significant in survivors and one of the ways in which nutritional therapy may provide immune benefits is through improving antioxidant status.

Pulmonary toxicity

The lung is exposed to higher concentrations of oxygen than other body organs, particularly when higher inspired oxygen concentrations are administered during anaesthesia or intensive care. Lung injury may be produced if hyperoxia increases free radical generation (through semiquinones) and antioxidant defences are reduced, e.g. steroid-mediated reduction in SOD and catalase (Royston 1988). Relative increases in SOD and catalase reduce mortality from oxygen toxicity in the rat (Turrens et al 1984).

Acute lung injury may be mediated by some of the mechanisms in Table 9.1 since many of the predisposing factors to lung injury will produce free radicals through activated neutrophils, free transition metals and prostaglandin synthesis and endothelial nitric oxide. Neutrophils are particularly implicated since large numbers of neutrophils are observed in the lung vasculature in adult respiratory distress syndrome (ARDS), while neutrophil depletion is protective. Free radicals may produce direct damage but they have such a short half-life that alternative mechanisms have been proposed. It may be that the protective screen of antiproteolytic enzymes are inactivated by free radicals, allowing the unopposed action of human neutrophil elastase (Weiss 1989).

Serum antioxidants have been used to predict ARDS in patients (Leff et al 1993), while combination therapy reduced ARDS mortality (Sawyer et al 1989) and heat shock protein induction reduced mortality in an animal model of acute lung injury (Villar et al 1993). Thus application of oxidant biochemistry in acute lung injury offers predictive and therapeutic potential.

Halothane hepatitis

The aetiology of halothane hepatitis is complex since at least two syndromes exist with five possible theoretical explanations (Ray & Drummond 1991). It appears that the biotransformation of halothane through reductive pathways produces free radicals as reactive intermediates which damage the liver. This may cause the less serious but more common form of hepatic damage reflected in elevated serum aminotransferases seen in up to 20% of patients exposed to halothane (Neuberger & Williams 1984). It has been shown that these reactive intermediate molecules, formed through the cytochrome P450 system, initiate lipid peroxidation which may be responsible for hepatocellular damage (de Groot & Noll 1983). Free radical generation has been shown during halothane exposure to intact rats (Knecht et al 1992, Hughes et al 1991) isolated perfused rat liver (Hughes et al 1991) and rat liver microsomes (Janzen et al 1990). Vitamin E given intravenously and by inhalation has been shown to suppress halothane-induced liver damage in the guinea-pig by inhibiting lipid peroxidation (Sato et al 1992).

SUMMARY

The evidence for the role of free radicals in conditions frequently encountered by anaesthetists, as well as the successful use of antioxidants to reduce their effects in numerous experimental models and some clinical trials, begs the question 'Why are antioxidants not more widely used in anaesthetic practice?' The simplest answer is that there are too few prospective clinical trials of antioxidants in humans supporting a role for their routine clinical use.

Why are there so few trials supporting a role for their routine clinical use? Firstly, there are numerous mediators involved in many of the diseases in which free radicals have also been implicated. These variables would be difficult to standardize in prospective trials and may have prevented trial development. Secondly, techniques to measure free radicals and the damage they induce are still being refined and are biochemically complex.

Good trials would need to demonstrate direct evidence of free radical generation in the trial subjects and a causal link between these free radicals and the disease process (with measurements of the induced damage). It should also be shown that reduction of free radical activity with an antioxidant is significantly related to improvement in a clinically important outcome measure. These difficulties should serve to focus research (Halliwell et al 1992, Halliwell & Gutteridge 1985) so that effective therapies can be developed.

Viewing the oxidant system in isolation has contributed to current confusion about the clinical role of antioxidant therapy in practice but it is hoped that a better understanding and application of pathophysiological knowledge will provide routine clinical uses for oxidant manipulation. Timing is perhaps one of the largest obstacles to overcome since the same antioxidant intervention compared before or after oxidant stress gives different results, usually favouring prospective intervention. This suggests that the earliest therapeutic benefits are likely to appear in situations where ischaemia/reperfusion or other triggers can be predicted, for example vascular occlusion and release during aortic aneurysm repair, reconstruction of ischaemic circulations, the use of tourniquets and neurosurgery. Patients at increased risk of acute lung injury or septicaemia may also justify prospective intervention. In clinical scenarios where oxidant production has already occurred the future role of antioxidant manipulation is less easy to predict since oxidant stimulation may have triggered different pathways for tissue injury which, of course, will no longer be prevented by antioxidants.

If oxidants merely amplify tissue damage then antioxidant therapy will have limited ability to treat disease but if, as seems increasingly likely, they are causally involved, then well-targeted antioxidant manipulation offers tremendous potential benefit. However, antioxidants are not benign; therefore such benefit can only be determined through clinical trials.

REFERENCES

Abate C, Patel L, Rauscher III F, CurranT 1990 Redox regulation of Fos and Jun DNA-binding activity in vitro. Science 249: 1157–1161

Alpha-Tocopherol Beta Carotene Cancer Prevention Study Group 1994 The effects of vitamin E and beta carotene on the incidence of lung cancer and other cancers in male smokers. N Engl J Med 330: 1029–1035

Anon 1994 Heroic doses. Economist August 27: 76

Arndt H, Kubes P, Granger D N 1991 Involvement of neutrophils in ischemia-reperfusion injury in the small intestine. Klin Wochenschr 69: 1056–1060

Beckman J, Beckman T, Chen J, Marshall P, Freeman B 1990 Apparent hydroxyl radical production by peroxy nitrate: implications for endothelial injury from nitric oxide and superoxide. Proc Natl Acad Sci USA 87: 1620-1624

Betz A L, Randall J, Martz D 1991 Xanthine oxidase is not a major source of free radicals in focal cerebral ischemia. Am J Physiol 260: H563–H568

Blot W, Li J–Y, Taylor et al 1993 Nutrition intervention trials in Linxian China: supplementation with specific vitamin/mineral combination, cancer incidence and disease-specific mortality in the general population. J Natl Cancer Inst 85: 1483–1492

Bolli R, McCay P B 1990 Use of spin traps in intact animals undergoing myocardial ischemia/reperfusion: a new approach to assessing the role of oxygen radicals in myocardial 'stunning'. Free Radical Res Commun 9: 169–180

Bolli R, Patel B, Jeroudi M, Lai E, McCay P 1988 Demonstration of free radical generation in 'stunned' myocardium of intact dogs with the use of the spin trap alpha-phenyl N-tert-butyl nitrone. J Clin Invest 82: 476–477

Broner C, Cherep J, Stidham G 1989 Effect of antioxidants in experimental Escherichia coli septicaemia. Circ Shock 29: 77–92

Buettner G R 1993 The pecking order of free radicals and antioxidants: lipid peroxidation, alpha-tocopherol, and ascorbate. Arch Biochem Biophys 300: 535–543

Buettner G R, Jurkiewicz B A 1993 Ascorbate free radical as a marker of oxidative stress: an EPR study. Free Radical Biol Med 14: 49–55

Carney J M, Floyd R A 1991 Protection against oxidative damage to CNS by alpha-phenyl-tert-butyl nitrone (PBN) and other spin-trapping agents: a novel series of nonlipid free radical scavengers. J Mol Neurosci 3: 47–57

Cerruti P 1994 Oxy-radicals and cancer. Lancet 344: 862–863

Cheng H Y, Liu T, Feuerstein G, Barone F C 1993 Distribution of spin-trapping compounds in rat blood and brain: in vivo microdialysis determination. Free Radical Biol Med 14: 243–250

Connor H D, Gao W, Nukina S, Lemasters J J, Mason R P, Thurman R G 1992 Evidence that free radicals are involved in graft failure following orthotopic liver transplantation in the rat: an electron paramagnetic resonance spin trapping study.

Transplantation 54: 199–204

Crowell J, Jones C, Smith E 1969 Effect of allopurinol on hemorrhagic shock. Am J Physiol 216: 744–748

Daniel V 1993 Glutathione S-transferase: gene structure and regulation of expression. Crit Rev Biochem Mol Biol 28: 173–207

de Groot N, Noll T 1983 Halothane hepatotoxicity: relation between metabolic activation, hypoxia, covalent binding, lipid peroxidation and liver cell damage. Hepatology 3: 601–660

Garlick P, Davies M, Hearse D, Slater T 1987 Direct detection of free radicals in the reperfused rat heart using electron spin resonance spectroscopy. Cir Res 61: 757–760

Garthwaite J 1991 Glutamate, nitric oxide and cell signalling in the nervous system. Trends Neurosci 14: 60-67

Goode H, Webster N 1993 Free radicals and antioxidants in sepsis. Crit Care Med 21: 1770-1776

Granger D, Rutuli G, McCord J 1981 Superoxide radicals in feline intestinal ischaemia. Gastroenterology 81: 22–29

Grech E, Dodd N, Bellamy C, Perry R, Morrison W, Ramsdale D 1993 Free radical generation during angioplasty reperfusion for acute myocardial infarction. Lancet 341: 990–991

Grisham M, Russell W, Roy R 1986 Reoxygenation injury in the isolated perfused working rat heart: roles of xanthine oxidase and transferrin. In: Rotillo G (ed) Superoxide and superoxide dismutase in chemistry, biology and medicine. Elsevier Science, Amsterdam, p 571

Gutteridge J M 1992 Iron and oxygen radicals in brain. Ann Neurol 32: S16–21

Gys T, Hubens A, Neels H et al 1988 Prognostic value of gastric intramural pH in surgical intensive care patients. Crit Care Med 16: 1222–1224

Hall E, Braughler J 1989 Central nervous system trauma and stroke. Free Radicals Biol Med 6: 303–313

Hall E, Yonkers P 1988 Attenuation of post-ischaemic cerebral hypoperfusion by the 21–aminosteroid U74006F after cardiopulmonary arrest in dogs. Stroke 19: 340-344

Hall E D, Andrus P K, Yonkers P A 1993 Brain hydroxyl radical generation in acute experimental head injury. J Neurochem 60: 588–594

Halliwell B 1992 Oxygen radicals as key mediators in neurological disease: fact or fiction. Ann Neurol 32: S10–15

Halliwell B, Gutteridge J 1984 Oxygen toxicity, oxygen radicals, transition metals and disease. Biochem J 219: 1–14

Halliwell B, Gutteridge J 1985 Oxygen radicals and the nervous system. Trends Neurosci 8: 22–26

Halliwell B, Gutteridge J 1989 Free radicals in biology and medicine. Clarendon Press, Oxford

Halliwell B, Gutteridge J, Cross J 1992 Free radicals, antioxidants and human disease: where are we now? J Lab Clin Med 6: 598–620

Harris E 1992 Regulation of antioxidant enzymes. FASEB J 6: 2675–2683

Hennekens C, Buring J, Peto R et al 1994 Antioxidant vitamins: benefits not yet proven. N Engl J Med 330: 1080-1108

Hoffman H, Siebeck M, Welter H 1987 High dose superoxide dismutase potentiates respiratory failure in septicaemia. (Abstract) Am Rev Respir Dis 135: A78

Holgado M M, Refoyo E A, Marino H E, Martin R C, Garcia G J, Macias N J 1989 Effect of xanthine oxidase inhibitors on the prognosis of acute intestinal ischemia [Spanish.] An Med Intern 6: 177–182

Hughes H M, George I M, Evans J C, Rowlands C C, Powell G M, Curtis C G 1991 The role of the liver in the production of free radicals during halothane anaesthesia in the rat: quantification of N-tert-butyl-alpha-(4-nitrophenyl)nitrone (PBN)-trapped adducts in bile from halothane as compared with carbon tetrachloride. Biochem J 277: 795–800

Janzen E G, Towner R A, Krygsman P H, Haire D L, Poyer J L 1990 Structure identification of free radicals by ESR and GC/MS of PBN spin adducts from the in vitro and in vivo rat liver metabolism of halothane. Free Radical Res Commun 9: 343–351

Jepsen S, Herlevsen P, Knudsen P et al 1992 Antioxidant treatment with N acetyl cysteine during adult respiratory distress syndrome: a prospective randomized placebo controlled study. Crit Care Med 20: 918–923

Jolliet P, Slosman D, Polla B 1994 Heat shock proteins in critical illness: markers of cellular stress or more? In: Vincent J-L (ed) Year book of intensive care medicine. Springer-Verlag, Berlin pp 24–34

Kalsheker N 1989 Alpha-1-antitrypsin: structure, function and molecular biology of the gene. Biosci Rep 9: 129–138

Kilgore K, Friedrichs G, Homeister J, Lucchesi B 1994 The complement system in myocardial ischaemia/reperfusion injury. Cardiovasc Res 28: 437–444

Kirshenbaum L A, Singal P K 1993 Increase in endogenous antioxidant enzymes protects hearts against reperfusion injury. Am J Physiol 265: H484–H493

Klebanoff S 1980 Oxygen metabolism and the toxic properties of phagocytes. Ann Intern Med 93: 480–489

Knecht K T, DeGray J A, Mason R P 1992 Free radical metabolism of halothane in vivo: radical adducts detected in bile. Mol Pharmacol 41: 943–949

Kukreja R, Hess M 1992 The oxygen free radical system: from equations through membrane-protein interactions to cardiovascular injury and protection. Cardiovasc Res 26: 641–655

Kuzuya T, Hoshida S, Kim Y et al 1993 Free radical generation coupled with arachidonate lipoxygenase reaction relates to reoxygenation induced myocardial cell injury. Cardiovasc Res 27: 1056–1060

Leff J, Parsons P, Day C 1993 Serum antioxidants as predictors of adult respiratory distress syndrome in patients with sepsis. Lancet 341: 777–780

Lindsay S, Liu T H, Xu J A et al 1991 Role of xanthine dehydrogenase and oxidase in focal cerebral ischemic injury to rat. Am J Physiol 261: H2051–2057

Loesser K, Qian Y, Wei E et al 1992 In vivo protection of ischaemia/reperfusion injury by histidine, a singlet oxygen scavenger. FASEB J 6: A1342

Lucchesi B, Mullane K 1986 Leukocytes and ischaemia induced myocardial injury. Annu Rev Pharmacol Toxicol 26: 201

MacDoald R, Weir B 1994 Cerebral vasospasm and free radicals. Free Radical Biol Med 16: 633–643

Maynard N, Bihari D, Beale R 1993 Assessment of splanchnic oxygenation by gastric tonometry in patients with acute circulatory failure. JAMA 270: 1203–1210

McCord J 1985 Oxygen-derived free radicals in postischaemia tissue injury. N Engl J Med 312: 159–163

Mergner G W, Weglicki W B, Kramer J H 1991 Postischemic free radical production in the venous blood of the regionally ischemic swine heart: effect of deferoxamine. Circulation 84: 2079–2090

Mullane K 1993 Akadesine: the prototype adenosine regulating agent for reducing myocardial ischaemic injury. Cardiovasc Res 27: 43–47

Murphy P, Jones J. 1991 Acute lung injury: the quantitative evaluation of acute lung injury. Br J Intensive Care 1: 110–117

Murphy P, Myers D, Green M, Jones J 1991 Ultrastructural evidence for free radical production during experimentally induced lung injury. Br J Anaesth 66: 398P

Murphy P G, Myers D S, Davies M J, Webster N R, Jones J G 1992 The antioxidant potential of propofol (2,6–diisopropylphenol). Br J Anaesth 68: 613–618

Murray C, Jennings R, Reimer K 1986 Preconditioning with ischemia: a delay of lethal cell injury in ischaemic myocardium. Circulation 74: 1124–1136

Nelson V, Bennett S, Green T 1993 The nature of free radicals with which 2,6-diisopropylphenol interacts. Br J Anaesth 71(2): 313P

Neuberger J, Williams R 1984 Halothane anaesthesia and liver damage. BMJ 289: 1136–1139

Nilsson U A, Aberg J, Aneman A, Lundgren O 1993 Feline intestinal ischaemia and reperfusion: relation between radical formation and tissue damage. BMJ Eur Surg Res 25: 20–29

Novelli G 1992 Oxygen radicals in experimental shock: effects of spin trapping nitrones in ameliorating shock pathophysiology. Crit Care Med 20: 499–507

Nowicki J, Duval D, Poignet H, Scatton B 1991 Nitric oxide mediates neuronal death after focal cerebral ischaemia in the mouse. Eur J Pharmacol 204: 339–340

Otamiri T 1989 Oxygen radials, lipid peroxidation and neutrophil infiltration after small-intestine ischaemia and reperfusion. Surgery 105: 593–597

Oury T D, Ho Y S, Piantadosi C A, Crapo J D 1992 Extracellular superoxide dismutase, nitric oxide, and central nervous system O2 toxicity. Proc Nat Acad Sci USA 89: 9715–9719

Owens M, Lazarus H, Wolcott M, Maxwell J, Taylor B 1974 Allopurinol and hypoxanthine pre-treatment of canine kidney donors. Transplantation 17: 424–427

Packer J, Slater T, Wilson R 1979 Direct observation of a free radical interaction between vitamin E and vitamin C. Nature 278: 737–738

Parks D, Bulkley G, Granger D 1983 Role of oxygen derived free radicals in digestive tract diseases. Surgery 94: 415–422

Parratt J 1994 Ischaemic preconditioning: a pronounced and endogenous form of protection against tissue injury. In: year book of intensive care medicine. Springer-Verlag. Berlin, pp 279–289

Perkins W, Milde L, Milde J, Michenfelder J 1991 Pretreatment with U74006F improves neurologic outcome following complete cerebral ischaemia in dogs. Stroke 22: 902–909

Prat A G, Turrens J F 1990 Ascorbate- and hemoglobin-dependent brain chemiluminescence. Free Radical Biol Med 8: 319–325

Ray D, Drummond G 1991 Halothane hepatitis. 67: 84–99

Rice-Evans C, Miller NJ 1994 Total status in plasma and body fluids. Methods Enzymol 234: 279–293

Rickels E, Gaab M R, Heissler H, Dietz H 1993 The effect of mannitol and nimodipine treatment in a rat model of temporary focal ischaemia. Zentralbl Neurochir 54: 3–12

Romaschin A, Rebekia I, Wilson G, Mickle D 1987 Conjugated dienes in ischaemic and reperfused myocardium: an in vivo chemical signature of oxygen free radical mediated injury. J Mol Cell Cardiol 19: 289–302

Rosen H, Klebanoff S 1977 Formation of singlet oxygen by the myeloperoxidase mediated antimicrobial system. J Biol Chem 252: 4803–4806

Royston D 1988 Free radicals. Anaesthesia 43: 315–320

Rushmore T, Morton M, Pickett C 1991 The antioxidant resposive element: activation by oxidative stress and identification of the DNA consensus sequence required for functional activity. J Biol Chem 266: 11632–11639

Sadrzadeh, Eaton 1988 Hemoglobin mediated oxidant damage to the central nervous system requires endogenous ascorbate. J Clin Invest 82: 1510–1515

Sakamoto A, Ogawa R 1992 ESR study of free radical formation during ischaemia-reperfusion injury in the rat brain and the protective effect of a new antioxidant. [Japanese.] Masui Jpn J Anesthesiol 41: 595–602

Sakamoto A, Ohnishi S, Ohnishi T, Ogawa R 1991 Relationship between free radical production and lipid peroxidation during ischaemia/reperfusion injury in the rat brain. Brain Res 554: 186–192

Salim A 1991 Protection against stress-induced acute gastric mucosal injury by free radical scavengers. Intensive Care Med 17: 455–460

Salim A 1992a Role of oxygen-derived free radical scavengers in the management of acute attacks of ulcerative colitis: a new approach. J Lab Clin Med 119: 710-717

Salim A 1992b Allopurinol and dimethyl sulphoxide improve treatment outcomes in smokers with peptic ulcer disease. J Lab Clin Med 119: 702–709

Sato N, Fujii K, Yuge O, Tanaka A, Morio M 1992 Suppressive effect of vitamin E on lipid peroxidation in halothane administered guinea pig liver. In-vivo 6: 503–550

Sawyer M, Mike J, Chavin K 1989 Antioxidant therapy and ARDS. (Abstract.) Crit Care Med 17: S153

Schiller H J, Reilly P M, Bulkley G B 1993 Tissue perfusion in critical illnesses: antioxidant therapy. Crit Care Med 21: S92–102

Schneider J, Friderichs E, Giertz J 1989 Protection by recombinant human SOD in lethal rat endotoxaemia. Prog Clin Biol Res 308: 913–917

Schoenberg M H, Beger H G 1993 Reperfusion injury after intestinal ischemia. [Review.] Crit Care Med 21: 1376–1386

Schoenberg M, Younes M, Muhl E, Selin D, Fredholm B, Schildberg F 1983 Free radical involvement in ischaemic damage of the small intestine. In: Greenwald R, Cohen G (eds) Oxy-radicals and their scavenger systems: cellular and molecular aspects. Elsevier Science, New York, pp 154–157

Steinberg D 1993 Antioxidant vitamins and coronary heart disease. N Engl J Med 328: 1587–1589

Stubbe J 1994 Controlling radical reactions. Nature 370: 502

Takeuchi K, Suzuki S, Kako N et al 1992 A prostacyclin analogue reduces free radical generation in heart–lung transplantation. Ann Thoracic Surg 54: 327–332

Tamura Y, Chi L, Driscoll E et al 1988 Superoxide dismutase conjugated to polyethylene glycol provides sustained protection against myocardial ischaemia/reperfusion injury in the canine heart. Circ Res 63: 944–959

Taylor C, Towner R, Janzen E, Bray T 1990 MRI detection of hyperoxia-induced lung edema in Zn deficient rats. Free Radical Biol Med 9: 229–233

Tew D, Bacon P, Pierson R, Menon D, Jones J 1994a Ascorbate as an endogenous spin trap to detect free radicals during ischaemia and reperfusion of isolated working hearts. Br J Anaesth 73: 267P

Tew D, Bacon P, Pierson R, Skepper J, Menon D, Jones J 1994b Oxidant stress, antioxidant defences and ultrastructural damage during myocardial ischaemia and reperfusion. Association of Cardiothoracic Anaesthetists, 10th Anniversary Meeting, Cambridge

Thomas J P, Maiorino M, Ursii F, Girotti A W 1990 Protective action of phospholipid hydroperoxide glutathione peroxidase against membrane-damaging lipid peroxidation: in situ reduction of phospholipid and cholesterol hydroperoxides. J Biol Chem 265: 454–461

Traber D, Adams T, Sziebert L, Stein M, Traber L 1985 Potentiation of lung vascular responses to endotoxin by superoxide dismutase. J Appl Physiol 58: 1005–1009

Tryba M 1992 Stress ulcer prophylaxis and gastric alkalinization: death of a myth? [Editorial comment] Intenstive Care Med 18: 1–3

Turrens J, Crapo J, Freeman B 1984 Protection against oxygen toxicity by intravenous injection of liposome-entrapped catalase and superoxide dismutase. J Clin Invest 73: 87–95

Ursini F, Bindoli A 1987 The role of selenium peroxidases in the protection against oxidative damage of membranes. Chem Physics Lipids 44: 255–276

Villar J, Edelson J, Post M, Mullen J, Slutsky A 1993 Induction of heat stress proteins is associated with decreased mortality in an animal model of acute lung injury. Am Rev Respir Dis 147: 172–181

Webster N, Nunn J 1988 Molecular structure of free radicals and their importance in biological reactions. Br J Anaesth 60: 98–108

Weiss S 1989 Tissue destruction by neutrophils. N Engl J Med 320: 356–376

Witztum J 1994 The oxidation hypothesis of atherosclerosis. Lancet 344: 793–795

Yim M, Chock P, Stadtman E 1990 Copper-zinc superoxide dismutase catalyses hydroxyl radical production from hydrogen peroxide. Proc Natl Acad Sci USA 87: 5006–5010

Zweier J, Flaherty J, Weisfelt M 1988 Direct detection of free radical generation following reperfusion of ischaemia myocardium dysfunction (stunned myocardium). J Am Coll Cardiol 12: 239–249

10

The metabolic fate of newer anaesthetic drugs

T. Durcan   G. Philpott

In this review we examine some of the newer drugs which are currently or may soon be used by anaesthetists with regard to what is known about their metabolic fate.

The safe use of the many potent drugs available today requires a sound knowledge of basic pharmacokinetics and pharmacodynamics. Anaesthetic drugs may be required for short day case procedures, prolonged major surgery, patients in the intensive care situation and for those requiring alleviation of acute and chronic pain. Patients requiring anaesthesia may present with hepatic or renal impairment; therefore, in the interests of safety, anaesthetists must know and understand the drugs they use. Metabolism is one aspect of the pharmacokinetic profile of a drug which may be important in determining its duration of action, pharmacological effect and toxicity.

Generally, metabolism makes drugs more water soluble and facilitates excretion, although occasionally active and/or toxic metabolites are produced. Biotransformation can be a double-edged sword; with the development of more potent and specific drugs and drugs 'designed' to undergo rapid metabolic degradation, it is important to know their metabolic fate. Many drugs used in anaesthesia are lipid soluble and undergo biotransformation before excretion by renal, biliary or other routes.

Metabolic reactions can be classified as functionalization (phase I) or conjugation (phase II) reactions.

Phase I reactions are mainly oxidative, reductive or hydrolytic, oxidative pathways playing the major role and are catabolized by the cytochrome P450 family of pigments. These enzymes are characterized by a maximum absorption wavelength of 450 nm in their reduced state in the presence of carbon monoxide and reside in the microsomal fraction of cells in the liver, the zone III (periportal) hepatocytes undertaking the bulk of drug biotransformation. Families of cytochrome P450 enzymes have an amino acid sequence homology of 40–50%, subfamilies have homology of >55%. Individual cytochrome P450 enzymes differ from each other with respect to their ability to metabolize different substrates, their induction or inhibition by different substances, by the presence or absence of genetically determined polymorphism and by their variability of distribution and concentration.

The metabolites generated may be pharmacologically active, as in the case of codeine, which is metabolized to morphine (i.e. it is a prodrug), inactive (as is more usual) or, under certain conditions, toxic, e.g. paracetamol overdose or norpethidine accumulation resulting in seizures.

Phase II reactions involve conjugation of the parent drug or its phase I metabolites with an endogenous substrate, usually rendering the compound inactive and hydrophilic, so enhancing renal excretion, or allowing excretion in bile if more lipid soluble. Morphine-6-glucuronide (M-6-G) is an example of an active phase II metabolite which, by virtue of molecular folding, is more lipophilic than expected and is thus able to cross the blood-brain barrier. Toxic effects have been ascribed to accumulation of M-6-G (Osbourne 1986). The liver is the major site of metabolism by virtue of the large amount of cytochrome present; however, other sites, including the gastrointestinal tract, kidneys, lungs, skin and brain, have all been identified as potential sites of drug metabolism (Devarakonda et al 1994).

Non-specific esterases are widely distributed in different tissues including blood, liver and gastrointestinal tract. These enzymes metabolize many different drugs, including procaine, diamorphine, methylprednisolone and esmolol. Of particular interest to anaesthetists is plasma cholinesterase. Plasma cholinesterase is a tetrameric glycoprotein consisting of four identical subunits, each having a catalytic site. It has a molecular weight of 342 000, is synthesized by the liver and is involved in the metabolism of several drugs, including suxamethonium, mivacurium, cocaine, procaine and heroin. The recognition and study of suxamethonium apnoea led to the realization of its genetic determination and the birth of pharmacogenetics.

Several new facts have emerged about plasma cholinesterase over the last few years. The enzyme is encoded on chromosome 3 and all variants are determined by mutations of one gene. Both quantitative and qualitative variants exist; for example, increased activity with the 'cynthiana' variant is due to a three-fold increase in enzyme levels, whilst the 'Johannesburg' variant demonstrates twice the normal activity at each active site.

Conversely, three variants of plasma cholinesterase have been identified having normal catalytic activity, but because of altered bioproduction or stability have reduced plasma concentrations – 'K' variant has 33% less activity, 'J' 66% and 'H' 90%.

Modern techniques of molecular genetics have already begun and will continue to identify other variants in plasma cholinesterase. The traditional tests used over the last 30 years (measurement of esterase activity with a variety of substrates; dibucaine inhibition; fluoride inhibition and RO2–0683 inhibition) cannot identify or explain all variants or prolonged responses to succinylcholine. Interested readers are referred to the articles by La Du (1993) and Pantuck (1993).

Proteases and peptidases in plasma, erythrocytes and many other tissues are involved in the biotransformation of polypeptide drugs. These enzymatic reactions will probably assume greater importance in the future.

PROPOFOL

Propofol (2,6–diisopropylphenol) is an intravenous induction and anaesthetic maintenance agent that, due to its water insolubility, is presented as a 1% aqueous emulsion containing 10% soya bean oil, 1.2% egg phosphatide and 2.25% glycerol. It has a short duration of action due to rapid metabolism and elimination from the body, with rapid recovery characteristics and a low incidence of nausea and vomiting due to possible antiemetic properties. These features make it an ideal agent for outpatient anaesthesia as well as being a useful sedative agent for ventilated patients on the intensive care unit. Following bolus doses, propofol has a metabolic clearance eight times that of thiopentone and an elimination half-life of 50%. Recovery following intravenous infusion is more rapid with propofol in comparison to thiopentone, benzodiazepine or opioid infusions.

Servin et al (1990) studied the pharmacokinetics of propofol infusion in patients with cirrhosis, who all exhibited moderate liver dysfunction. They discovered that total body clearance was not significantly reduced, although mean time to recovery was longer in the cirrhotic group. They concluded that the pharmacokinetics of propofol given by infusion were not affected markedly by moderate cirrhosis.

The metabolic clearance of propofol exceeds the hepatic blood flow, suggesting that extra hepatic sites are also involved in its metabolism. Veroli et al (1992) demonstrated the occurrence of extrahepatic metabolism with the appearance of urinary metabolites of propofol occurring during the an hepatic phase of orthotopic liver transplantation. Gray et al (1992) found there was no difference in metabolite levels between arterial and central venous samples, indicating that metabolism of propofol may not occur in the lungs as was originally thought. Although the exact site of extrahepatic metabolism is not known, it is thought to occur in the gastrointestinal tract and may account for up to 10% of propofol's metabolic fate. Following a dose of propofol, 0.3% of the drug is excreted unchanged and 88% is eliminated as metabolites in the urine. The principal metabolite is propofol glucuronide (50%), together with 2,6-diisopropyl-1,4-quinol, which is further conjugated with glucuronide and sulphate (Simons et al 1985). The quinol metabolite is responsible for the green coloration of urine and breast milk in some patients, but none of the metabolites are thought to be active in man. This has been confirmed by a study of endstage renal failure patients (Nathan et al 1993), where conjugated metabolites of propofol accumulated in the blood, but there was no difference in time to eye opening compared with healthy controls following discontinuation of the propofol infusion.

There are problems associated with propofol's presentation as an emulsion that is identical to the intralipid component of parenteral nutrition. Fat overload syndrome can result following prolonged infusions leading to fever, jaundice, cerebral irritability and hyperlipidaemia, with fatty infiltration of the heart, lungs, liver and kidneys. Fat is cleared principally by the liver.

Recommendations to reduce the risk of fat overload include the omission of fat from TPN regimes during propofol infusions for sedation and the regular screening of patients' serum for lipaemia and elevated triglyceride levels which necessitates discontinuation of the infusion.

Propofol is no longer recommended as a sedative agent for children following the deaths of five children under the age of 6 years who received prolonged propofol infusions whilst being ventilated for upper respiratory tract infections (Park et al 1992). They subsequently developed lipaemic serum, metabolic acidosis and myocardial failure and, although the exact cause of death remains unknown, fatty infiltration of the liver was discovereed in the three children who underwent post-mortem examination.

VOLATILE ANAESTHETIC AGENTS

Background

The continuing search for new volatile agents attempts to meet the requirements of the ideal agent as outlined by Heijke & Smith (1990).

The compound should be easily and cheaply manufactured and remain stable over a range of climatic conditions, with a long shelf life. It should be pleasant to inhale, with a high potency and low blood gas solubility, allowing smooth and rapid induction and recovery from anaesthesia. It should have minimal side effects on the cardiovascular, respiratory and central nervous systems and should be devoid of organotoxic potential.

Metabolism of the fluorinated volatile anaesthetic agents is important historically because of the resultant nephro- and hepatotoxicity that has occurred with methoxyflurane and halothane respectively. As a result, the two new fluorinated ether volatile agents sevoflurane and desflurane have undergone extensive animal and human research to investigate their metabolic fate and potential organotoxicity.

The potential of the volatile anaesthetic agents to cause nephrotoxicity or hepatotoxicity is consequent on the extent of their metabolism by the hepatic cytochrome P450 isoenzymes and subsequent liberation of toxic metabolites (Table 10.1).

Their nephrotoxic potential is due to the release of free fluoride ions which result in renal impairment when their concentration exceeds 50 μM and in polyuric nephropathy with concentrations above 90 μM (Cousins & Mazze 1973).

Methoxyflurane, a fluorinated ether now withdrawn from clinical use, is metabolized in the liver mainly by cytochrome P450 2E1 (Kharasch & Thummel 1993), although multiple isoforms of the enzyme are thought to be involved as well, which may explain its extensive biotransformation. Plasma concentrations of fluoride ions exceed 50 μM in patients anaesthetized with methoxyflurane for 2.5–3.00 MAC hours, and although enflurane, isoflurane, sevoflurane and desflurane are similar in structure to

Table 10.1 Percentage metabolism of volatile anaesthetic agents

Agents	%
Methoxyflurane	50
Halothane	20
Sevoflurane	4.6
Enflurane	2.4
Isoflurane	0.2
Desflurane	0.02

methoxyflurane, they appear less susceptible to cytochrome P450–mediated oxidative defluorination. Plasma fluoride ion concentrations greater than 50 μM may be encountered with sevoflurane, enflurane and isoflurane under certain risk conditions, but are usually short lived and unlikely to result in nephrotoxicity. These factors include prolonged anaesthesia, obesity and cytochrome P450 isoenzyme 2E1–inducing drugs such as ethanol and isoniazid.

Nephrotoxicity related to methoxyflurane has not been encountered in infants and children, possibly because of reduced activity of hepatic microsomal enzymes, reduced fat stores and increased elimination of the compound.

Halothane, a halogenated hydrocarbon, is also metabolized by the cytochrome P450 system, with the P450 2E1 isoenzyme being predominantly responsible under oxidative and possibly reductive conditions, although its metabolism does not result in the liberation of free fluoride ions and hence nephrotoxicity. However, biotransformation of halothane leads to two distinct types of hepatic damage.

Type I occurs in up to 20% of patients and is a mild form of damage characterized by minor elevations of serum aminotransferase levels occurring up to 2 weeks after exposure to halothane. Type II is characterized by severe disturbance of liver function and is associated with fulminant hepatic failure. The incidence of massive liver necrosis (National Halothane Study 1966) is approximately 1 in 35 000 patients exposed to halothane, increasing to 1 in 3700 patients receiving halothane on multiple occasions within a one–month period.

Evidence suggests that type II damage occurs as a result of an oxidative metabolite of halothane, possibly trifluoracetyl halide, binding covalently with hepatocyte macromolecules to form a hapten, thus altering its structure and inducing an autoimmune reaction against the liver cell (Gut et al 1993).

Sevoflurane

Sevoflurane, a polyfluorinated methyl isopropyl ether, has been in clinical use in Japan since 1990 and is undergoing trials in Europe and the USA. Its low blood gas partition coefficient of 0.62 places it between isoflurane and desflurane for speed of induction and emergence. Its lack of respiratory tract irritability may make it a suitable induction agent for children. Sevoflurane is metabolized by the cytochrome P450 isoenzymes, with the major metabolic products being free fluoride ions and hexafluorisopropanol, which is rapidly glucoronidated. Frink et al (1992) measured plasma fluoride ion levels in 50 ASA I and II adult surgical patients following between 1–5 h anaesthesia with sevoflurane and found peak plasma concentrations of $29.3 \pm 1.8\ \mu M$, 2 h after anaesthesia. Standard renal function tests showed no deterioration in these patients.

Evidence suggests that sevoflurane can produce plasma fluoride levels greater than 50 μM in animals (Cork et al 1978). Unpublished human data from volunteers exposed to 9 MAC hours of sevoflurane have shown plasma levels to exceed 50 μM (Frink et al 1992). These subjects, however, did not display any urinary concentrating problems in response to desmopressin or any alteration in standard renal function tests of plasma sodium, osmolality or creatinine clearance. Hepatoxicity is also less likely to occur than with halothane, due to the significantly reduced level of biotransformation of sevoflurane. Its organic metabolite, hexafluorisopropanol, appears less reactive than trifluoracetyl halide due to rapid glucuronidation by the fast phase II reaction in the liver, thus preventing hapten formation.

Animal experiments aimed at producing hepatotoxicity have failed to demonstrate any significant hepatic impairment and there have been no case reports of hepatic toxicity following the use of sevoflurane in Japan. One potential problem attributed to sevoflurane, with the increasing use of low-flow anaesthetic breathing systems, is its breakdown by soda lime to vinyl derivatives. Frink et al (1992) studied a group of surgical patients exposed to 3 h of low-flow sevoflurane anaesthesia and subsequently were unable to demonstrate any postoperative problems or any alteration in hepatic or renal function. Organotoxicity, due to vinyl derivatives, may be more theoretical than practical.

Desflurane

Desflurane is a polyfluorinated methyl ethyl ether, which differs from isoflurane only by the substitution of a fluoride ion for a chloride ion at the α-ethyl carbon atom. This confers a high degree of chemical stability on the compound. It has a mild odour with a boiling point of 23.5°C, necessitating a temperature-controlled pressurized vaporizer. It is stable in soda lime and has a very low blood gas partition coefficient of 0.42, potentially allowing a rapid induction, although in children it has proven irritant to the upper airway, causing coughing, laryngospasm and breath holding.

Jones et al (1990) were unable to demonstrate any increase in serum or urinary inorganic fluoride levels nor any change in renal or hepatic function in 10 healthy volunteers exposed to an average inspired concentration of 3.6% desflurane in oxygen for $1\frac{1}{2}$ h. Hence its stability and minimal biotransformation, together with low tissue solubility, ensure rapid elimination from the body and low organotoxic potential.

MUSCLE RELAXANTS

Background

Several new muscle relaxants have recently been developed. These include the long-acting drugs (greater than 30–40 min) pipecuronium and doxacurium, the intermediate-acting drug (approximately 20–30 min) rocuronium and the short-acting mivacurium (less than 20 min). More recently clinical reports about ORG9487 have appeared. This drug could be classified as ultra-short acting, after one bolus dose, if reversal agents are given.

The introduction of vecuronium and atracurium in the 1980s allowed anaesthetists much greater flexibility, but the non-depolarizing fast-onset ultra-short-acting replacement for suxamethonium is still awaited. The use of these shorter-acting drugs reduced the incidence of drug interactions and residual neuromuscular blockade. Older long-acting agents such as gallamine, tubocurare and pancuronium had other disadvantages such as slow onset time, cardiovascular side effects, obligatory renal elimination and the potential for inadequate reversal.

The independence of vecuronium and atracurium from renal elimination stems from the increased contribution of distribution and/or of metabolism to their plasma clearance (Table 10.2). In the case of vecuronium 19–30% of a dose has been estimated to be eliminated in human bile (Sohn et al 1982). This may be an underestimate of biliary excretion, or may be due to extensive uptake of vecuronium in special organelles. Hepatic uptake is responsible for the rapid clearance of vecuronium, with metabolism

Table 10.2 Percentage elimination of muscle relaxants via kidney and liver and proportion metabolized (figures are estimates)

	Kidney	Liver	Metabolism
Allcuronium	80–85	15–20	0
Atracurium	6–10	0	90
Doxacurium	25–50		?6
Gallamine	95–98	<0.5	0
Mivacurium	5–10		95
ORG 9478*	?12–20	30–80	30–80
Pancuronium	45–65	5–10	35
Pipecuronium	30–40	5	35
Rocuronium	30–35		
Tubocurarine	45–65	10–15	0
Vecuronium	15–30	30–40	35

* Values are putative: insufficient human data available.
Adapted with permission from Booij (1994).

and biliary excretion being of secondary importance. Liver failure can therefore prolong the action of vecuronium (Lebrault et al 1985). The 3–hydroxy metabolite of vecuronium does have activity and may contribute to persistent paralysis in patients with renal failure who receive prolonged infusions (Segredo et al 1992).

Atracurium is a mixture of 10 stereoisomers (Amaki et al 1985) having varying pharmacokinetic parameters. All isomers are unique in that they are metabolized throughout the body by carboxylases and by spontaneously undergoing pH and temperature-dependent Hofmann elimination (Stenlake and Hughes 1987). One molecule of atracurium ultimately yields two molecules of laudanosine. Also produced as an intermediate is a highly electrophilic acrylate which in vivo is probably rapidly metabolized by hydrolysis or conjugation. Laundanosine was a cause of concern as it is known to produce excitatory EEG changes and seizures in animals and it was felt that accumulation might occur after prolonged infusions in man. Extensive experience with atracurium in critically ill patients has so far failed to support this hypothesis (Coakley 1994), perhaps because serum levels of laudanosine which may be removed by the liver (Nigrovic & Fox 1991) have never been shown to exceed the seizure threshold in humans. Use of a more potent isomer of atracurium (51 W89) in the future may allow a reduction in dose and consequently reduce production of laudanosine (Miller 1995).

Newer muscle relaxants

Pipecuronium

Pipecuronium is a longer-acting 2,16-diaminosteroid which has piperazine rings at positions 2 and 16 (vecuronium and pancuronium having two piperidine groups). It is 20–30% more potent than pancuronium and vecuronium. It has a slow onset time (4–6 min) depending on the dose used. Duration of action varies from 29 min (ED_{95}) to 94 min ($2 \times ED_{95}$) (Wierda et al 1989, Sanfilippo et al 1992).

Pipecuronium is predominantly renally eliminated. Wierda et al (1990), in a study on patients undergoing coronary artery bypass graft, showed that 56% of the original dose was recovered in the urine over the next 24 h; 75% of this was unchanged and 25% was in the form of the 3-desacetyl pipecuronium metabolite. The liver may have a role in pipecuronium clearance (Pittet et al 1990).

Doxacurium

Doxacurium is a bisquaternary benzylisoquinolinium diester. It resembles atracurium, but does not undergo Hofmann degradation. It is the most potent muscle relaxant (ED_{95} 0.03 mg/kg), having a slow onset of action.

Doxacurium is hydrolysed by plasma esterase in vitro, but at 6% of the rate of suxamethonium (Booij 1994). It is excreted in urine and bile.

Rocuronium

Rocuronium was developed from the vecuronium molecule, from which it differs in four positions (notably the 2b-morphalino and the 16-pyrrolidino function attached to a 16-N-allyl group) (Marshall et al 1994). The structural changes render rocuronium 5–10 times less potent than vecuronium. It was developed because of its fast onset time in cats. In humans intubation is possible at 60–90 s (still 40–60 seconds slower than suxamethonium). Rocuronium undergoes hepatobiliary elimination. The putative metabolites, 17-desacetylrocuronium and 16–N-desallylrocuronium, are usually not detectable in plasma. Following a bolus dose of rocuronium only a very small amount was detectable in urine within 6 h (Wierda et al 1991). Although biotransformation occurs in the liver, there is no evidence that decreased metabolism in hepatic disease prolongs its duration of action (Bevan 1994). The effect of rocuronium appears to be prolonged in the elderly because of decreased liver extraction, most likely secondary to reduced hepatic cell mass (Matteo et al 1993). In hepatic failure, Magorian et al (1991) showed an increased clinical duration with rocuronium.

ORG 9487

In the last year clinical reports on ORG 9487 have appeared in the literature. It is a 16-N-allyl 17b-propionate analogue of vecuronium. It is claimed to have an ED_{90} of 1.15 mg/kg and a dose of 1.5 mg/kg is said to provide good to excellent intubating conditions at 1 min (Wierda et al 1993, 1994). The duration of action of this dose was 26.6 min (70% recovery of train of four response): neostigmine given 2 min after the bolus dose led to recovery in 11.6 min.

ORG 9487 has a urinary excretion fraction of about 12%. Like other steroidal relaxants it undergoes redistribution and is metabolized in the liver by hydrolysis at the 3 and 17 positions (Bowman et al 1988). The main metabolite is the active 3-desacetyl metabolite, in the cat the potency ratio is 1 : 0.5 (parent : metabolite).

Van den Broek et al (1994) estimated that, assuming the same potency ratio in man, after an infusion of about 1 h, the percentage contribution of the 3-OH metabolite to the neuromuscular block was about 6%. They also estimated that at clinically adequate recovery the contribution of the metabolite to residual block was about 27%. It remains to be seen if there are conditions in humans where the rate of formation of this metabolite could exceed its elimination with clinical consequences. In their paper Van den Broek et al (1994) found that renal excretion was of minor importance; only 17% of parent and metabolite were renally excreted in the first 8 h, with only a further 5% in the next 16 h.

Mivacurium

This bis-benzylisoquinolinium diester compound was 'designed' to undergo hydrolysis by plasma cholinesterase. It was hoped that a molecule which underwent rapid hydrolysis and had increased neuromuscular blocking potency would lack cumulation and have reduced histamine release. The recovery rate would thus be constant over a wide range of dosages and infusion rates. Mivacurium has a duration of action about half that of atracurium and vecuronium, but a similar onset time. It is hydrolysed by plasma cholinesterase at a rate some 70–88% of suxamethonium (Saverese et al 1988). The disproportionately small increase in length of action as dosage is increased suggests that plasma concentrations of substrate may not approach V_{max} for plasma cholinesterase within the clinical dose range.

Hydrolysis of mivacurium results in the production of a quaternary amino alcohol (15–50%), a quaternary mono ester (30–80%) and a dicarboxylic acid. None of these metabolites are active and are excreted in urine and bile. Like suxamethonium, mivacurium will be subject to unpredictable prolongation of action in patients with qualitative or quantitative deficiencies in cholinesterase. These can occur in patients with liver disease, renal disease and patients with genetic variants of cholinesterase (Hilmi & Ginsburg 1994). Unlike suxamethonium, evidence suggests that early reversal with anticholinesterases is possible, especially where there is some spontaneous recovery of neuromuscular function (Goudsouzian et al 1993).

REMIFENTANIL

Background

Remifentanil, like fentanyl, alfentanil and sufentanil, is a phenylpiperidine derivative having potent opioid actions. Unlike fentanyl, alfentanil and sufentanil, it is structurally unique by virtue of its ester linkage. Remifentanil's ester structure renders it susceptible to hydrolysis by non-specific esterases and rapid degradation (Egan et al 1993). The rate of metabolic breakdown of remifentanil contrasts sharply with that of its older congeners fentanyl, alfentanil and sufentanil, whose primary route of elimination is via hepatic metabolism (Bovil 1991).

The main metabolic pathway for all three compounds is *N*-dealkylation by phase I cytochrome P450 isoenzymes. Oxidative *O*-demethylation is a minor pathway which, in the case of sufentanil, produces the active metabolite desmethyl-sufentanil (Weldon et al 1985). Desmethyl-sufentanil has about one-tenth the potency of the parent compound (equivalent to that of fentanyl). Neither fentanyl nor alfentanil has active metabolites. Whilst fentanyl and sufentanil have high hepatic extraction ratios, that of alfentanil is lower (0.3–0.5) (Chauvin et al 1986). Alfentanil metabolism is therefore more susceptible to changes in liver blood flow and/or enzyme capacity.

Bartkowski & McDonnell (1990) showed that treatment with erythromycin could delay recovery and prolong respiratory depression after surgery due to reduced clearance of alfentanil. The development of these opioids focused on increasing potency, reducing cardiac toxicity and developing more readily titratable pharmacokinetics. Despite its short elimination half-life, an infusion of alfentanil does not necessarily lead to more predictable recovery. Rate of recovery is also determined by the duration of the infusion, as well as the rate of distribution and elimination (Glass et al 1993).

Remifentanil (which is currently undergoing phase II and III trials) may fulfil the requirements for an ultra short-acting opioid with a rapid onset of action and a short duration. This would effectively be a more titratable opioid for use by infusion.

Metabolism

Remifentanil is the hydrochloride salt of 3-(4-methoxycarbonyl-4-[(1-oxopropyl)phenylamino]-1-piperidine]propanioc acid methyl ester. By virtue of its ester linkage, it is susceptible to rapid hydrolysis by circulating and tissue non-specific esterases. The elimination half-time is about 10–20 min, with a clearance of 3–4 litres/min; 88% of the dose of reminfentanil was recovered in the urine as the major carboxylic acid metabolite GI90291. This metabolite has 1/300–1/1000 the potency of the parent compound in animals (Glass et al 1993) but this is not yet confirmed in humans (Fig. 10.1).

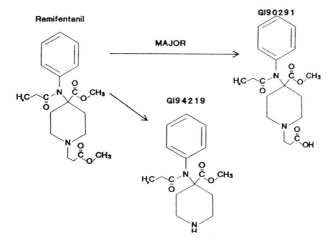

Fig. 10.1   The metabolic pathway of remifentanil is illustrated. Remifentanil is metabolized by ester hydrolysis, primarily to GI90291, of which over 80% is subsequently recovered in urine. GI90291 is approximately 1/300 to 1/1000 the potency of the parent compound. (From Glass et al 1993.)

In vitro studies indicate remifentanil is not a good substrate for serum cholinesterase and that its clearance is not affected by the presence of anticholinesterases such as neostigmine. There are no data on its use in patients with cholinesterase deficiency (Roscow 1993).

Two pharmacokinetic studies, one in volunteers and another in elective surgical inpatients, both using computer simulations, showed that the duration of infusion (Egan et al 1993, Westmoreland et al 1993) of remifentanil should have little influence on the context-sensitive half-life, i.e. time required for a 50% decrease in plasma or effect site concentration in the context of the duration of the infusion (Hughes et al 1992, Shafer & Varvel 1991).

Clearance was unaffected by patient demographics. The context-sensitive half-life for remifentanil by computer simulation was calculated to be 3.65 min, compared with sufentanil 33.9, alfentanil 58.5 and fentanyl at 262.5 min. Westmoreland et al (1993) showed that at steady state the concentration of the active metabolite was about 12 times that of the steady-state levels of remifentanil. The elimination of the metabolite will be prolonged in renal failure and may accumulate after long infusions.

Remifentanil may allow rapid titration of drug effect intraoperatively, with possible reduced incidence of postoperative side effects and lack of drug accumulation. It may also be relatively unaffected by hepatorenal disease. Further clinical trial data are awaited with interest.

TRAMADOL

Background

Tramadol, introduced in Germany in 1970s, was recently introduced in the UK as Zydol. It is a weak opioid with an atypical profile, in that it is claimed to have little or no respiratory depression, smooth muscle effects and a low abuse potential.

Tramadol appears to cause weak activation of the opioid as well as the descending monoaminergic system, resulting in a synergistic effect of analgesia. Its use in acute pain appears to show that it is a weak opioid with an analgesic potency roughly equalling that of pethidine (Vickers et al 1992). It also appears to spare morphine requirements after orthopaedic surgery. The unique mode of action of tramadol appears to be beneficial in chronic pain, extending its therapeutic range. A survey of chronic pain studies suggests tramadol causes less constipation than morphine (Beeson & Vickers 1994).

Metabolism

Tramadol is a synthetic 4-phenyl-piperidine analogue of codeine. It can be administered orally or parenterally and is formulated as a racemic mixture with each enantiomer displaying differing opioid receptor-binding properties, and monoaminergic reuptake inhibition.

Tramadol is metabolized in the liver by the two main metabolic pathways forming N- and O-demethylated compounds (phase I), while the O-demethylated compounds are further conjugated (phase II). There are 11 metabolites, of which only the O-demethylated or 'M1' metabolite is active. It has between 4 and 200 times greater affinity for the mu opioid receptor than tramadol. Of an oral dose of tramadol, some 85% is metabolized. The cumulative renal excretion of M1 in young volunteers was approximately 7.5% (Lintz et al 1981, 1986).

The elimination half-life of tramadol was 5–6 h and that of M1 6.7 h (Lintz et al 1986, Liao et al 1992) or up to 9 h. Within 48 h of commencing a regime of tramadol 100 mg four times daily the parent drug and its metabolite M1 had accumulated in plasma approximately two-fold.

Tramadol metabolism by O-demethylation was inhibited by quinidine, a selective inhibitor of the polymorphic CYP2D6 cytochrome P450 isoenzyme, and M1 production is influenced by debrisoquine-type polymorphism.

Collart et al (1993) studied the effects of quinidine and naloxone on tramadol action in 12 healthy subjects after a single 100 mg dose. The main decrease in peak tramadol analgesia by naloxone was 31% whereas quinidine had no effect on tramadol analgesia. This suggests that M1 does not contribute to the analgesic effect of tramadol in man. This study looked at single-dose and multiple-dose situations, such as in chronic pain, where accumulation of tramadol and M1 may have potential clinical significance.

The effect of liver disease has been studied in 12 patients with advanced cirrhosis. It was found that tramadol elimination was prolonged and it was recommended that in severe impairment the dosage interval should be increased to 12 h (Grünenthal report FOPK 228). In a study of volunteers with varying degrees of renal insufficiency, after a single dose of tramadol elimination half-lives of both tramadol and M1 were increased. Consequently, it was concluded that for patients with creatinine clearance <30 ml/min the dosage interval should be increased to 12 h. Where creatinine clearance is <10 ml/min tramadol is not recommended (Grünenthal report FOPK 218).

The metabolism of tramadol can also be influenced by other drugs. Carbamazepine, as a result of enzyme induction, caused a reduction in plasma concentration and elimination half-life of tramadol of 50%. The maximum plasma concentration of the active metabolite M1 was also reduced by 9% and the elimination half-life by 33%, suggesting that carbamazepine induces metabolism of M1 as well as tramadol.

Concomitant use of cimetidine increased the elimination half-lives of both tramadol and M1 by 19% and 25% respectively. The cumulative renal excretion of tramadol was increased by 29% and that of M1 decreased by 27%. These are probably not clinically significant (Lee et al 1993). In conclusion, tramadol is a central analgesic, having synergistic actions on the opioid and monoaminergic systems. It is of intermediate potency, being a step II drug in the World Health Organization analgesic ladder for the management of chronic pain. It appears effective and safe in a variety of pain situations. Its dual mode of action may help in its efficacy in certain chronic pain conditions such as neuropathic pain. The clinical significance of its active metabolite is unclear; it may accumulate with chronic use, especially where renal insufficiency supervenes.

Possible drug interactions due to enzyme induction and/or inhibition may render certain individuals liable to adverse drug interactions or changes in dose requirements. Such problems do not currently appear to be of clinical significance. Further comparative multiple dose studies are awaited.

Tramadol may well represent a useful analgesic with an increased safety margin; it remains to be seen if clinical experience with this drug will clarify these issues.

REFERENCES

Amaki Y, Waud B E, Waud D R 1985 Atracurium receptor kinetics: sample behaviour from a mixture. Anaesth Analg 64: 777–780
Bailie G R, Cockshott I D, Douglas E J et al 1992 Pharmacokinetics of propofol during and after long term continuous infusion for maintenance of sedation in ICU patients. Br J Anaesth 68: 486–491
Bartkowski R R, McDonnell T E 1990 Prolonged alfentanil effect following erythromycin administration. Anesthesiology 73: 566–568
Beeson J M, Vickers M D (eds) 1994 Tramadol analgesia: synergy in research and therapy. Drugs 47 (Suppl 1): 1–46
Bevan D R 1994 Rocuronium bromide and organ function. Eur J Anaesthesiol 11 (Suppl 9): 87–91
Booij L 1994 Pharmacokinetics of muscle relaxants. In: Goldhill D R, Flynn P J (eds) Ballière's clinical anaesthesiology, Vol 8(2), London: Baillière Tindall: pp 349–367
Bovil J G 1991 Opioids. In: Dundee J W, Clarke R S J, McCaughey W (eds) Clinical anaesthetic pharmacology. Churchill Livingston, Edinburgh, pp 231–238
Bowman W C, Rodger I W, Houston J et al 1988 Structure – action relationships among some desacetoxy analogues of pancuronium and vecronium in the anaesthetised cat. Anesthesiology 69: 57–62
Chauvin M, Bonnet F, Montembault C et al 1986 The influence of hepatic plasma flow on alfentanil concentration plateaus achieved with an infusion model in humans: measurement of alfentanil extraction coefficient. Anaesth Analg 62: 966–974
Coakley J 1994 Muscle relaxants and neuromuscular disorders in the intensive care unit. Ballière's clinical anaesthesiology, Vol 8 (2), pp 349–367
Collart L, Luthy C, Dyaer P 1993 Multimodal analgesic effect of Tramadol. Annual Meeting of the American Society of Clinical Pharmacology and Therapeutics, Honolulu, March 1993. Clin Pharmacol Ther 54: 339–344
Cork T L, Beppu W J, Hitt B A et al 1978 Renal effects and metabolism of sevoflurane in Fischer 344 rats. Anesthesiology 43: 70–77
Cousins M J, Mazze RI 1973 Methoxyflurane nephrotoxicity: a study of close response in man. J Am Med Assoc 225: 1611–1616
Devarakonda R, Klotz K, Klotz U 1994 Extrahepatic metabolism of drugs in humans. Clin Pharmacokinet 26(2): 144–160
Egan T D, Lemmens H J M, Fiset P et al 1993 The pharmacokinetics of the new short-acting opioid reminfentanil (GI 87084B) in healthy adult male volunteers. Anesthesiology 79: 881–892
Frink E J, Ghantous H, Malam T P et al 1992 Plasma inorganic fluoride with

sevoflurane anaesthesia: correlation with indices of hepatic and renal function. Anaesth Analg 74: 231–235

Glass S A, Hardman D, Kamhama Y et al 1993 Preliminary pharmacokinetics and pharmacodynamics of an ultra-short-acting opioid: remifentanil (GI87084B). Anaesth Analg 77: 1031–1040

Goudsouzian N G, d'Hollander A A, Viby-Mogensen J 1993 Prolonged neuromuscular block from mivacurium in two patients with cholinesterase deficiency. Anaesth Analg 77: 183–185

Gray P, Park G R, Cockshott I D et al 1992 Propofol metabolism in man during the anhepatic and reperfusion phases of liver transplantation. Xenobiotica 22: 105–114

Grünenthal. Data on file. Report Nos FOPK 228 and FOPK 218 (courtesy of Searle)

Gut J, Christen V, Huwyler J 1993 Mechanisms of halothane toxicity: novel insights. Pharmacol Ther 58: 133–155

Heijke S, Smith G 1990 Quest for the ideal anaesthetic agent. Br J Anaesth 64: 3–6

Hilmi I, Ginsburg R 1994 Mivacurium. In: Kaulman L, Ginsbury R (eds) Anaesthesia review, Vol 11. Churchill Livingstone, Edinburgh, pp 109–120

Hughes M A, Glass P S A, Jacobs J R 1992 Context sensitive half-time in multi-compartment pharmacokinetic models for intravenous anaesthetic drugs. Anaesthesiology 76: 334–341

Jones R M, Cashman J N, Eger I I E I et al 1990 Kinetic and potency of desflurane (I-653) in volunteers. Anaesth Analg 70: 3–7

Kharasch E D, Thummel K E 1993 Identification of cytochrome P450 2EI as the predominant enzyme catalysing human liver microsomal defluorination of sevoflurane, isoflurane and methoxyflurane. Anaesthesiology 79: 795–807

La Du B N 1993. Human serum butyrylcholinesterase and the hydrolysis of succinylcholine. Anaesth Pharmacol Rev 1: 354–361

Lebrault C, Berger J L, d'Hollander A A et al 1985 Pharmacokinetics and pharmacodynamics of vecuronium in patients with cirrhosis. Anaesthesiology 62: 601–605

Lee C R, McTavish D, Sorgin E 1993. Tramadol: a preliminary review of its pharmacodynamic and pharmacokinetic properties and therapeutic potential in acute and chronic pain states. Drugs 46(2): 313–340

Liao S, Hill J F, Nayak R K 1992. Pharmacokinet4ics of tramadol following single and multiple oral doses in man. Abstract No PPDM 8206. Pharm Res 9 (Suppl) : 308

Lintz W, Erlacin S, Frankus E et al 1981 Biotransformation of tramadol in man and animal. Drug Res 31: 1932–1943

Lintz W, Barth H, Osterloh G et al 1986 Bioavailability of enteral tramadol formulations. Drug Res 36: 1278–1283

Magorian T, Wood P, Caldwell J E et al 1991 Pharmacokinetics onset and duration of action of rocuronium in humans: normal vs hepatic dysfunction. Anaesthesiology 75: A 1069

Marshall R J, Muir A W, Sleigh T et al 1994 An overview of the pharmacology of rocuronium bromide in experimental animals. Eur J Anaesthesiol 11 (Suppl 9): 9–15

Matteo R S, Ornstein E, Schwartz E et al 1993 Pharmacokinetics and pharmacodynamics of rocuronium (ORG 9426) in elderly surgical patients. Anaesth Analg 77: 1193–1197

Miller R D 1995 Is 51 W89 an improvement compared with atracurium? (Editorial.) Br J Anaesth 74: 1–2

Nathan N, Debord J, Narcisse F et al 1993 Pharmacokinetics of propofol and its conjugates after continuous infusion in normal and in renal failure patients: a preliminary study. Acta Anaesthesiol Belg 44: 77–85

National Halothane Study 1966 Summary of the national halothane study. JAMA 197: 775–788

Nigrovic V, Fox J 1991 Atracurium decay and the formation of laudanosine in humans. Anaesthesiology 74: 446–454

Osborne R J, Simon J P, Slevin M L 1986 Morphine intoxication in renal failure: the role of morphine-6-glucuronide. BMJ 292: 1548–1549

Pantuck E J 1993 Plasma cholinesterase: gene and variations. Anaesth Analg 77: 380–386

Park T J, Stevens J E, Rice A S C et al 1992 Metabolic acidosis and fatal myocardial failure after propofol infusion in children: five case reports. Br Med J 305: 613–616

Pittet J F, Tassonyi E, Schopfer C et al 1990 Dose requirements and plasma concentrations of pipecuronium during bilateral renal exclusion and orthopic liver transplantations in pigs. Br J Anaesth 65: 779–785

Roscow C 1993 Reminfentanil: a unique opioid analgesic. Anaesthesiology 79: 875–876

Sanfilippo M, Fierrog G, Villardi V et al 1992 Clinical evaluation of different doses of pipecuronium bromide during nitrous oxide–fentanyl anaesthesia in adult surgical patients. Eur J Anaesthesiol 9: 49–53

Savarese J J, Ali H H, Basta S J et al 1988 The clinical neuromuscular pharmacology of mivacurium chloride. Anaesthesiology 68: 723–732

Segredo V, Caldwell J E, Matthay M A et al 1992 Persistent paralysis in critically ill patients after long-term administration of vecuronium. N Engl J Med 327: 524–528

Servin F, Cockshott D, Farihott R et al 1990 Pharmacokinetics of propofol infusions in patients with cirrhosis. Br J Anaesth 65: 177–183

Shafer S L, Varvel J R 1991 Pharmacokinetics, pharmacodynamics and rational opioid selection. Anaesthesiology 74: 53–63

Simons P J, Cockshott I D, Douglas E J et al 1985 Blood concentrations, metabolism and elimination after sub anaesthetic intravenous dose of 14C-propofol to male volunteers. Postgrad Med J 61 (Suppl 3): 64

Sohn Y J, Bencini A, Scaf A J H et al 1982 Pharmacokinetics of vecuronium in man. Anaesthesiology 57: A256

Stenlake J B, Hughes R 1987. In vitro degradation of atracurium in human plasma. Br J Anaesth 59: 806–807

Van den Broek L, Wierda J M K H, Smeulers N J et al 1994 Pharmacodynamics and pharmacokinetics of an infusion of ORG 9487, a new short-acting steroidal neuromuscular blocking agent. Br J Anaesth 73: 331–335

Veroli P, O'Kelly B, Bertrand F et al 1992 Extrahepatic metabolism of propofol in man during the anhepatic phase of orthotopic liver transplantation. Br J Anaesth 68: 183–186

Vickers M D, O'Flaherty D, Szekely S M et al 1992 Tramadol: pain relief by an opioid without depression of respiration. Anaesthesia 47: 291–296

Weldon S T, Perry D F, Cork R C et al 1985 Detection of picogram levels of sufentanil by capillary gas chromatography. Anaesthesiology 65: 684–687

Westmoreland C L, Hoke J F, Sebeld P S et al 1993 Pharmacokinetics of remifentanil (GI87084B) and its major metabolite (GI90291) in patients undergoing elective inpatient surgery. Anaesthesiology 79: 893–903

Wierda J M K H, Richardson F J, Agostons S 1989. Dose response relation and time course of action of pipecuronium bromide in humans anaesthetised with nitrous oxide and isoflurane, halothane or droperidol and fentanyl. Anaesth Analg 68: 208–213

Wierda J M K H, Karliczek G F, Vandenbrom R H G et al 1990 Pharmacokinetics and cardiovascular dynamics of pipecuronium bromide during coronary artery surgery. Can J Anaesth 37: 183–191

Wierda J M K H, Kleef U W, Lambalk L M et al 1991 The pharmacokinetics or ORG 9426, a new non-depolarising neuromuscular blocking agent in patients anaesthetised with nitrous oxide, halothane and fentanyl. Can J Anaesth 38: 430–435

Wierda J M K H, Van Den Broek L, Proost J H et al 1993 Time course of action and endotracheal intubating conditions of ORG 9487, a new short-acting steroidal muscle relaxant: a comparison with succinylcholine. Anaesth Analg 77: 579–584

Wierda J M K H, Beaufort A M, Kleef U W et al 1994 Preliminary investigations of the clinical pharmacology of three short-acting non-depolarising neuromuscular blocking agents, ORG 9453, ORG 9489 and ORG 9487. Can J Anaesth 41: 213–220

11

Epidural anaesthesia

P. I. E. Jones   G. O'Sullivan

The epidural space has, for most of this century, been used mainly for the delivery of local anaesthetic agents. It is now being studied with renewed enthusiasm, however, as a route for the administration of an increasing variety of pain-modifying drugs, in the pursuit of improved analgesia in labour, during and after surgery and in chronic pain states. It would be impossible to cover, in this chapter, all the available ground. Thus, we have selected and concentrated upon some of the topics which have generated most interest in the recent literature.

THE EPIDURAL SPACE AND ITS ANATOMY

Our understanding of epidural anatomy has been enhanced by the work of Gaynor (1990) in cadavers, and Blomberg (1993) using the epiduroscope. These studies have confirmed (1) that the epidural space is at its deepest at the 2nd lumbar interspace (4–8 mm from the posteromedial border of the ligamentum flavum to the dura), (2) that it is deeper posteromedially than in the midline, and (3) that there is a definite gap between the ligamenta flava, which will provide little resistance to an epidural needle inserted precisely in the midline. Gaynor's studies have also shown that an epidural catheter, when passed via the paramedian route, usually takes up a midline position and travels a straight cephalad path, and, because of the oblique angulation, tends not to tent the dura. Patchy or unilateral blocks have been ascribed to the prevention, by a dural fold, of the passage of injected local anaesthetics across the midline. Anatomical and magnetic resonance imaging (MRI) studies, however, have failed to confirm the presence of this 'plica medialis durae matris', possibly because previous methods of identifying it have involved insertion of dye, resin or an epiduroscope into the epidural space, with resulting distortion. Okutomi et al (1993) have recently investigated one of the traditional methods for identifying the epidural space – the demonstration of negative pressure after passage of the needle through the ligamentum flavum. They confirmed that there is indeed a negative pressure on insertion of the needle, but that it reverts to a positive pressure within 30 s. This suggests that the negative pressure is an artefact generated by the technique, possibly 'tenting' of the dura. This has been confirmed by Shah (1994).

Clinical studies, supported by data from computed tomography (CT), have shown the average distance from the surface of the skin to the epidural space to be 4–5 cm, with a range of 2–9 cm, and that the distance does not always correlate with height or weight. However, Upton et al (1992), from measurements made during epidural insertion in 400 obstetric patients, determined that the depth, from the skin, to which the needle could be safely passed before testing for loss of resistance, correlated well with body weight (formula: 'safe' depth (cm) = body weight (kg)/25). A skin-to-dura distance of >6 cm is associated with an increased likelihood of poor-quality analgesia, and, if the depth is <4 cm, there is a three-fold increase, in obstetric patients, in the rate of dural puncture (Sutton & Linter 1991).

DRUGS USED VIA THE EPIDURAL ROUTE

The agents most commonly administered into the epidural space are local anaesthetics, opioids and, more recently, α-adrenergic agonists. Studies of neuraxially administered benzodiazepines have been mainly confined to animals.

Local anaesthetic agents

Ropivacaine is a new amide-linked local anaesthetic which has similar characteristics when used clinically to those of bupivacaine but with a shorter duration of motor block and lower cardiotoxicity. Epidural administration of ropivacaine 1% was as effective and safe as bupivacaine 0.75% (Wood & Rubin 1993).

Opioids

The mechanisms of action and clinical use of spinal opioids have been extensively reviewed in a recent edition in this series (Green 1992). The main controversies surrounding their use remain: are opioids more effective when given intraspinally than by other routes and, if they are, do the benefits outweigh the risks of side effects and complications?

α-adrenergic agonists

Alquist classified adrenergic receptors as α and β. α Receptors have since been subdivided into α_1 and α_2 and, more recently, the α_2 group has been further split into A, B, C and D subclasses, α_{2A} being predominant in the human spinal cord (Lawhead et al 1992). The involvement of the adrenergic system in nociception was suggested by Weber's observation (Weber 1904) that intrathecally administered adrenaline reduced reflex response to thermally induced pain in the rabbit. Furthermore, Priddle & Andros (1950) demonstrated, in labouring women, that adrenaline in relatively high doses (up to 1 mg intrathecally!) produced analgesia by itself, prolonged the action of added local anaesthetic and generated no neurological sequelae. Yaksh (1984) was the first to demonstrate an adrenergic pain-modulating system at the spinal level. In animals, experimentally induced bulbospinal activity has induced the release of noradrenaline in the spinal cord, accompanied by impairment of response to painful stimuli. The ability of adrenaline to enhance the analgesic effects of epidurally administered drugs may be due to its local actions as a vasoconstrictor (α_1) in preventing vascular absorption of local anaesthetics or opioids. It also has weak α_2 agonist properties and may therefore produce analgesia by its effect on the dorsal horn, where it is known to inhibit the release of substance P. α_2 adrenoceptor agonist and their role in clinical anaesthesia have been extensively reviewed by Maze & Tranquilli (1991). Clonidine, the most investigated of the α_2 agonists, has been shown experimentally to act as an inhibitor pre- and postsynaptically at α_2 adrenoceptors in the spinal cord. Analgesia is superior when clonidine is given epidurally compared with similar doses given intravenously (De Kock et al 1993). The high lipid solubility of clonidine and its rapid absorption and elimination from cerebrospinal fluid (CSF) provide rapid onset of analgesia and thus limited possibilities for rostral spread. In humans, epidural clonidine produces postoperative analgesia, prolonged in doses >600 µg (Eisenach et al 1989). Large doses (700–900 µg) provide longer-lasting analgesia but more pronounced hypotension, as do thoracic placement of the epidural catheter and pre-existing hypovolaemia. Eisenach et al (1993), based on measurements of CSF and plasma levels, have suggested of epidural clonidine that analgesia is predominantly a spinal action, whereas hypotension, bradycardia and sedation are more likely to be central effects resulting from systemic absorption. Rauck et al (1993) produced sustained pain relief in 19 of 26 patients with chronic sympathetic dystrophy by epidurally administered clonidine, initially by bolus and subsequently by infusion. The catheter was placed at C7–T1 if the symptoms were in the upper limb, or L2–3 if in the lower. The effects on blood pressure and pulse rate were the same whether the epidural injection was lumbar or cervical. Eisenach & Tong (1991) showed greater falls in blood pressure in sheep, when intrathecal clonidine was injected at thoracic as opposed to cervical levels. These observations suggest that rostral spread of clonidine in the CSF does not play a prominent role in the production of haemodynamic changes. Liu et al (1993), in a study of 30 patients undergoing orthopaedic surgery, demonstrated that the α_2 adrenoceptor antagonist yohimbine given orally did not reverse the haemodynamic effects (hypotension and bradycardia) produced by extradural clonidine, suggesting that these effects are not mediated by a supraspinal action of clonidine. Epidural clonidine enhances the analgesic effects of opioids (Vercauteren et al 1990) and local anaesthetics (Carabine et al 1992a). Carabine et al (1992a) compared an extradural bupivacaine-clonidine mixture with bupivacaine and clonidine alone, administered at the end of surgery in 95 patients undergoing total hip replacement under general anaesthesia. They found that clonidine produced superior analgesia to bupivacaine and that the combination significantly prolonged analgesia without causing respiratory depression. The same group (Carabine et al 1992b) also noted enhanced analgesia when epidural clonidine was given postoperatively by continuous infusion. Jamali et al (1994) showed a similar benefit following caudal block in children with the addition of clonidine 1 μg/kg to bupivacaine.

Mogensen et al (1992) added low-dose clonidine (75 μg bolus followed by 18.75 μg/h) to a postoperative epidural infusion regimen of bupivacaine-morphine. They noted enhanced analgesia, particularly during coughing or movement, but significant hypotension. Carroll et al (1993) compared intravenous with epidural clonidine in 10 patients with chronic back pain and found a high incidence of troublesome side effects in both groups. They discerned no analgesic benefit in the use of the epidural route. O'Meara & Gin (1993) added a small dose of clonidine (120 μg) to the bolus injection of 8 ml 0.125% bupivacaine for initiation of epidural analgesia in labour. Compared with the same dose of bupivacaine alone, there was better analgesia at 15 min but this was accompanied by sedation. Huntoon et al (1992) found in women who had undergone Caesarean section that either 400 μg or 800 μg epidural clonidine followed by an infusion of 40 μg/h provided adequate analgesia when bupivacaine, but not chlorprocaine, had been used to establish the initial block.

TEST DOSE

There is still no universal agreeement on the constituents of the perfect epidural test dose. Ideally, it should enable precise identification of intrathecal or intravascular placement of an epidural catheter. Inadvertant position of the catheter in an epidural vein may complicate up to 5% of epidurals in the general population, with two or three times that incidence in parturients. The use of adrenaline in the test dose was described by Moore & Batra (1981), in whose original study intravenous placement was reliably identified if a 3 ml injection containing 15 μg of adrenaline caused a mean increase in heart rate of 30 beats/min occurring within 20–40 s. Several other methods for avoiding intravascular catheterization and its consequences have been suggested. Aspiration of the catheter prior to injection and fractionation of the total dose are used routinely by the majority of anaesthetists but these often fail. Lignocaine 100 mg or 2-chlorprocaine 150 mg as an intravenous bolus rapidly produces tinnitus and perioral numbness. Morris et al (1994) found that fentanyl 100 μg via an epidural catheter in labour produced symptoms of sedation and dizziness which was >90% predictive in identifying intravascular injection.

All the above methods were utilized in an obstetric patient during preparation for Caesarean section but failed to prevent her from having a grand mal seizure (McClean et al 1992). Concerns have been expressed (Chestnut et al 1988a) that variations in maternal heart rate during labour, and possible adverse effects on uteroplacental blood flow, make the intrapartum use of adrenaline in the test dose questionable. Leighton et al (1987) showed a maternal heart rate variability in labour greater than 30 beats/min and pointed out the limited predictive value of adrenaline as an intravenous marker in this context. Precordial Doppler detection, after injection of 1 ml of air via an intravascular epidural catheter, is highly sensitive (Leighton et al 1990). Thiopentone can be used to distinguish CSF from local anaesthetic solution in the aspirate from an epidural catheter; if the aspirate is added to thiopentone, the mixture will become turbid with the less alkaline bupivacaine (pH 5) but not with CSF (pH 7).

EPIDURAL ANALGESIA IN OBSTETRICS

The use of regional blockade for operative delivery has burgeoned in recent years. General anaesthesia is now viewed as second best by mothers, who wish increasingly to be awake during childbirth whatever the circumstances, and by anaesthetists, who are attracted by the improved neonatal outcome and postoperative analgesia, as well as a reduction in maternal mortality associated with general anaesthesia. It is the use of epidural analgesia for pain relief in labour which has been, and remains, controversial. Although this chapter is concerned with epidural, not spinal, anaesthesia, the traditional distinction between the two methods has become unclear, no more so than in the field of obstetrics, with the introduction and increasing popularity of combined spinal/epidural techniques.

Combined spinal/epidural (CSE)

This technique was originally described, for management of anaesthesia for Caesarean section, by Brownridge (1981), who used lignocaine, and then by Carrie & O'Sullivan (1984), who used bupivacaine for the intrathecal injection. It involves the intrathecal injection of local anaesthetic, with or without additional opiate, as well as the insertion of an epidural catheter, allowing the possibility of subsequent epidural drug administration. It is the method of choice in many maternity units and has recently been adapted for use in labour (Collis et al 1994) – the 'walking epidural'.

Epidural analgesia in labour has been criticized for, among other things, altering adversely the course of labour and increasing the incidence of instrumental and operative intervention. Attempts at solving these problems have been directed towards the reduction of motor block, either by reducing the concentration of local anaesthetic employed or by the use of an opioid, or both. Although epidural opioids alone have not been associated with satisfactory analgesia in labour, local anaesthetic/opioid combinations have been more successful (Chestnut et al 1988b) while simultaneously allowing a reduction in the quantity of local anaesthetic used. The method of CSE described by Collis and colleagues (1994), using a needle-through-needle-technique with a 27G pencil-point spinal needle, refines this in several ways. First of all, the onset of analgesia is hastened and the motor block generated by the first injection is minimized by an initial subarachnoid injection of bupivacaine 2.5 mg and fentanyl 25 µg. Secondly, rather than an infusion, intermittent epidural top-ups of 10–15 ml of a solution containing 0.1% bupivacaine and 0.002% fentanyl are employed. This, combined with intermittent connection to the intravenous infusion, allows considerable mobility during labour. In spite of an incidence of failed subarachnoid block (10.7%), pruritus (17.3%), postdural puncture headache (2.3%) and blood patching (2%), 95% of mothers reported complete satisfaction both with mobility and analgesia. Enthusiasm for the potential benefits of this technique, especially the mobility of the parturient, should be tempered by other considerations. A recent report from Buggy et al (1994) recorded impairment of proprioception in association with top-ups of 15 ml 0.1% bupivacaine containing fentanyl 2 µg/ml. Another, from Cohen et al (1992), showed that ambulation was impaired even during ultra low-dose (0.03%) patient-controlled bupivacaine infusion. Furthermore, Harding et al (1994) have reported two cases of meningitis following the use of CSE in labour (see below).

Most authors, emphasizing the simplicity of the method, favour a single-space, needle-through-needle technique. Some advocate rotation of the epidural needle through 180° after the intrathecal injection and before the insertion of the epidural catheter, as a way of avoiding the passage of the catheter through the dural hole. The objection to this manoeuvre is that it is itself associated with inadvertant dural puncture (Meiklejohn 1987).

Epidural analgesia in labour

Concern persists that, by availing herself of an epidural for pain relief in labour, a woman is compromising her birth experience and increasing the likelihood of operative intervention and peripartum morbidity.

Attempts at improving maternal satisfaction have centred around the use of local anaesthetic/opioid epidural infusions to provide adequate analgesia while minimizing motor blockade. The lipophilic opioids fentanyl and sufentanil are the most widely used in this context. Sufficiently dilute epidural infusions may allow mobility comparable with the CSE method above. Breen et al (1993) compared fentanyl-low-dose bupivacaine-adrenaline with fentanyl alone in an effort to provide adequate analgesia combined with the ability to ambulate in labour. A similar number in each group (68% and 70% respectively) successfully ambulated. There were no fetal or neonatal problems in either group. They stressed that under these conditions a parturient should only be allowed to ambulate if (1) she is accompanied at all times, (2) there is no tendency to orthostatic hypotension, (3) motor testing reveals normal leg strength and (4) she can perform a partial knee bend while standing on one leg. The use of patient-controlled epidural analgesia (PCEA), a further step towards increased control by the parturient over her labour, may be associated with yet further dose reductions, as was shown by Ferrante et al (1994). Using PCEA bupivacaine–fentanyl with a background epidural infusion, they found that, by delivering 33% of the maximum hourly demand dose by infusion, the incidence of top-up doses was minimized and there was a 35% dose-sparing effect when compared with continuous infusion alone. A loading dose of opioids is frequently added to the initial blocking dose of local anaesthetic, but Russell et al (1993a) found no benefit in the addition of sufentanil to a bolus dose of bupivacaine prior to a bupivacaine–sufentanil infusion. The same group (Russell & Reynolds 1993), in a study of nulliparae in labour, showed that 0.0625% bupivacaine containing 0.25 µg/ml sufentanil or 2.5 µg/ml fentanyl at 12 ml/h were equally effective in labour, that there was a low incidence of motor block (15%) and that only 10–15% required more than one top-up.

Despite increasing interest in the use of drug combinations, by bolus, infusion, PCEA or a combination, some workers are continuing to examine the effects of epidural analgesia using local anaesthetic alone. Chestnut et al (1987), in a double-blind randomized study, compared two groups of nulliparae in labour, both receiving an epidural infusion of 0.125% bupivacaine and intravenous syntocinon. In one group, at 8 cm dilatation, saline was substituted for bupivacaine and, in the other, bupivacaine was continued into the second stage. In the latter group, there was denser perineal analgesia in the second stage of labour, a longer second stage and a higher incidence of forceps delivery, but no increase in abnormal rotation of the head or in the rate of Caesarean delivery (13% in each group). There were no differences in neonatal outcome. The influence of timing of epidural analgesia with bupivacaine in labour has been subsequently examined by the same group (Chestnut et al 1994a, 1994b). Their results indicated that, in women in spontaneous labour or in those already receiving syntocinon, whether the epidural was sited at <5 cm or >5 cm cervical dilatation, there were no differences in the Caesarean section or instrumental delivery rates. However, in the group already receiving syntocinon, the Caesarean section rate was higher (18–19%) than in those in spontaneous labour (8–10%). These results are in stark contrast to those produced by Thorp et al (1993), who found, in 90 randomized nulliparae, that those who received epidural analgesia with bupivacaine in labour had a 25% chance of a Caesarean delivery, mainly as a result of failure to progress, whereas in those having parenteral pethidine–chlorpromazine it was only 2.2%! The lack of standardization of management of labour may help to explain these startling figures.

SIDE EFFECTS AND COMPLICATIONS

Scott & Hibbard (1990) used a retrospective postal study of UK obstetric units to determine the incidence of serious non-fatal complications of extradural block. These included significant hypotension, unexpected widespread nerve block, acute toxicity with convulsions, dural puncture and subsequent headache, extradural abscess, extradural haematoma, damage to a single spinal nerve, paraplegia, backache and urinary problems. Some of these feature in the recent literature.

Neurological

Although very uncommon, neurological damage may follow epidural analgesia. The damage may be the result of local pressure caused by haematoma, air or an abscess, by the inadvertent injection of toxic substances or by a toxic reaction to a drug which is normally given by this route, or by trauma and ischaemia.

Infective

The incidence of extradural abscess in the general hospital population is estimated to be 0.2–1.2 per 10 000 admissions. Scott & Hibbard (1990) quoted an incidence of extradural abscess as 1 in 505 000 obstetric extradural blocks. Despite its rarity, it is a feared complication which appears to be occurring with increasing frequency. The majority of the epidural catheter-related cases (1) have been reported since the mid-1980s, (2) have not been associated with prolonged catheterization, (3) have often had other risk factors increasing susceptibility to infection and (4) have mainly involved thoracic placement. It should be emphasized, however, that most epidural abscesses occur in the absence of anaesthetic intervention, as in the case reported by Kitching & Rice (1993). They described an extradural abscess presenting in a woman 8 weeks after delivery with mid-thoracic back pain, difficulty with micturition and leg weakness. She had not had epidural analgesia during labour and delivery had been uneventful. *Staphylococcus aureus* was grown from the abscess but no focus was found. Typically, there is back pain followed by root pain, lower limb weakness, paralysis and pyrexia. Pain is the most reliable feature; pyrexia and neurological deficit less so. When there are suggestive neurological signs in the absence of pain, MRI is the most reliable diagnostic tool.

Transmission of infection from members of staff, from contaminated injectate, for example from multi-dose vials, or from an adjacent area on the patient have all been implicated. The presence of blood and the potential for lapses in aseptic technique associated with a difficult epidural insertion may have contributed to the development of an epidural abscess in the case reported by Ngan Kee et al (1992). They described a woman who developed pyrexia, rigors and backache 5 days after Caesarean section, quickly followed by neurological deficit involving the bladder and lower limbs. Laminectomy and decompression resulted in complete recovery within 2 months. Cultures from the abscess and from blood grew *Staph. aureus*, as did that from a pustule on her back. Steroids have been implicated by Bromage (1993), who reported a case of cervical epidural abscess following several thoracic extradural injections of methylprednisolone, and by Sowter et al (1992) following the delayed development of a thoracic extradural abscess in a patient taking prednisolone for rheumatoid arthritis. Mamourian et al (1993) reported three cases of epidural abscess. All presented with back pain and fever between 3 and 14 days after epidural injection, all abscesses were confirmed by MRI and all grew *Staph. aureus*. One patient received intraoperative urokinase and postoperative heparin, another was given an epidural injection of steroid, and the third had preoperative systemic steroids, perioperative heparin and postoperative coumarin.

Two cases of meningitis were reported by Harding et al (1994), following combined spinal/epidural analgesia for labour. In the first, signs of meningitis developed within 24 h and cleared within 5 days. CSF specimens taken before and after the administration of antibiotics failed to grow any organisms. This was therefore thought to be a chemical meningitis, possibly related to contamination of the equipment by the solution used for skin preparation, in this case chlorhexidine. In the other case, a second spinal injection was required to provide adequate conditions for Caesarean section. On the third day after delivery, postdural puncture headache (PDPH) was diagnosed and blood patch was performed. Twelve hours later, there were signs of meningitis and pyrexia. Lumbar puncture revealed turbid CSF from which *Staph. epidermis* was cultured. Carp & Bailey (1992), in a study in rats with *Escherichia coli* bacteraemia, reported that, of 40 undergoing cisternal puncture with a 26G needle, 12 developed meningitis, which did not develop in another group pretreated with gentamicin. There were also no instances of meningitis in those rats which were not subjected to dural puncture. If the results of this study were applied to clinical practice, dural puncture might be avoided altogether when there is a high risk of bacteraemia, for example at delivery, or at least covered with antibiotics.

It is clear that, although central nervous system infection is only rarely associated with epidural or intrathecal instrumentation, it may be occurring more often. Increasing use of these routes for various types of pain management may be part of the explanation. The use of strict asepsis must be maintained when performing these procedures. Bromage (1994) insists that the anaesthetist should wear a mask as part of a 'full' aseptic technique, since in at least one reported case the phage type of the *Staph. aureus* grown from the extradural abscess was the same as that grown from the anaesthetist's nose. The use of steroids, in particular epidural steroids, should now be re-examined.

Non-infective

In a parturient (Ben-David et al 1994), the features of anterior spinal artery syndrome appeared after delivery, following the uneventful use of epidural bupivacaine via a catheter for the preceding 5 h. This rapidly responded to removal of the catheter, suggesting transient impairment of blood flow in anterior spinal or segmental radicular vessels caused by the local irritant effect of the epidural catheter.

Air, used to identify the epidural space, may create its own problems and has been associated with unblocked segments, incomplete analgesia and even air embolus (Schwarz & Eisenkraft 1993). Four attempts at identification of the epidural space under general anaesthesia in a 52-year-old woman were followed by persistent leg weakness and numbness 8 h later. CT revealed gas displacing the cauda equina. Complete resolution occurred within 24 h. The use of saline for epidural space identification would avoid these problems. Theoretically, nitrous oxide might also have contributed to the size of the gas bubble.

Dural tap

In their retrospective of 34 819 obstetric epidurals in Birmingham over 20 years, Stride & Cooper (1993) found an overall incidence of dural tap of 1.3%. Identification of the epidural space using loss of resistance to saline was associated with the lowest incidence of all. They also found that the elective use of forceps following dural tap did not affect the incidence of PDPH. Blood patching was attended by a much lower success rate (complete success with the first attempt in only 68%) than in most other studies.

In order to avoid the uncertainty involved in the use of continuous epidural analgesia in labour in the presence of a large hole in the dura, it has been suggested by Cohen et al (1989) that the epidural catheter should be placed intrathecally and used for labour analgesia.

BLOOD PATCH

Since its original description over 30 years ago (Gormley 1960), epidural blood patching has become the standard method of management of PDPH. Beards et al (1993) used MRI to examine five patients following blood patching. They noted that the spread of the injected blood extended over only three to five spinal segments and more cephalad than caudad, giving rise to the recommendation that the point of injection should be at the level of the previous dural puncture or below. The initial haematoma was seen to compress the thecal sac and nerve roots and subsequently to form a clot adherent to the dura. These findings might explain the backache sometimes associated with blood patching (Carrie 1993, Westbrook et al 1993). Headache and transient bradycardia have been shown to occur

(Andrews et al 1992), but less markedly if the blood is injected slowly. The ECG should be monitored. The maintenance of the lateral decubitus position for 1–2 h after blood patching may improve its efficacy (Martin et al 1994). Even if blood patching is performed correctly under aseptic conditions, there may still be danger in the use of early blood patching after childbirth (Harding et al 1994). Infecting organisms entering the maternal bloodstream at delivery may be transferred into the epidural space. Reassuringly, Tom et al (1992) were unable to identify any morbidity attributable to blood patching during the subsequent 2 years in 6 HIV-seropositive patients. Kanumilli et al (1993) described an interesting modification of the blood patch in a Jehovah's Witness. They established a continuous circuit, containing a three-way tap and linking an arm vein with the previously placed epidural needle, before transferring blood from the arm to the epidural space using the tap and a syringe.

ASPIRIN AND ANTICOAGULANTS

Anaesthetists have traditionally been extremely cautious in their use of intraspinal techniques in patients with potential bleeding problems, especially in pregnant women in whom there may be an incidence of 15% or more of vessel puncture during epidural cannulation. The puncture of an epidural vessel or the tearing of an intracranial vessel following inadvertent dural tap may lead to uncontrolled bleeding. Thus, a bleeding diathesis or full therapeutic anticoagulation have been viewed as absolute contraindications to the use of spinal or epidural block. It seems, however, that resistance among practitioners to the use of epidural or spinal analgesia in those receiving or about to receive anticoagulant therapy has weakened. It is now accepted (Letsky 1991) that the use of perioperative prophylaxis against venous thrombosis with low doses of heparin does not interfere with normal haemostasis. Aspirin, even in low doses (60 mg per day), permanently impairs platelet function by irreversible inhibition of cyclooxygenase and may therefore prolong the bleeding time. However, the randomized, multi-centre Collaborative Low-dose Aspirin Study in Pregnancy (CLASP 1994) showed that the concern over the concurrent use of aspirin and epidural anaesthesia was not substantiated. Of 9364 women recruited to the study, 2783 had epidural anaesthesia (1422 in the aspirin group against 1361 who had placebo). There were 79 adverse experiences in relation to the epidural (46 vs. 23); haemorrhage occurred on three occasions (1 vs. 2) and this was described as blood-stained fluid in the cannula. Also, Williams et al (1993), in a study of the use of aspirin in pregnancy, showed no difference between aspirin and placebo in bleeding times, none of which were longer than 10 min. Horlocker et al (1994) reported no spinal haematoma in 188 patients with an indwelling epidural catheter who were given low-dose warfarin postoperatively following knee-joint replacement surgery.

However, Onischchuk & Carlsson (1992) reported a painless epidural haematoma, visualized by MRI and extending T10–L2, in a patient who received an epidural, perioperative thrombolytic therapy and subsequent postoperative heparin infusion. A delayed diagnosis of severe neurological deficit was made but spinal decompression failed to produce a recovery.

The association between epidural block and epidural haematoma may not necessarily be one of cause and effect, as shown in the case reported by Lao et al (1993). They described a subdural haematoma in a pre-eclamptic parturient. There had been an episode of severe back pain the previous day and a generalized seizure after two small doses of epidural lignocaine with adrenaline. The day after delivery, loss of sphincter control and leg weakness were noted. Laminectomy and decompression were followed by a full recovery.

BACKACHE

There has been renewed interest in the possibility of an association between the use of epidural analgesia, particularly during labour, and long-term back pain. MacArthur et al (1990), from the results of a retrospective postal survey covering 11 701 deliveries over a 9–year period, concluded that the use of epidural analgesia was the main predisposing factor in the development of 'new' long-term backache (onset within 3 months of delivery and lasting at least 6 weeks). They found an incidence of 19% in those who had received an epidural for vaginal delivery and 10% in those who had not. The response rate, however, was only 39% in contrast to Russell et al (1993b), who achieved a 68% response rate from 1015 primiparae but, nevertheless, obtained similar results (18% in those who had an epidural, 12% in those who had not). Another retrospective postal survey of postnatal women, however, revealed no association between insertion of an epidural, whether difficult or not, and subsequent backache (Clark & McQueen 1993). Furthermore, in a prospective study of 1185 parturients of whom they succeeded in following up 88%, Breen et al (1994) found that new-onset backache was related to weight, inversely related to height and not related to the use of epidural analgesia. Their use of relatively dilute solutions of bupivacaine in labour (0.04–0.125), compared with 0.25%–0.5% quoted by MacArthur et al, might support the concept that the problem arises from a sensory and possibly motor block sufficiently profound that the mother may adopt positions during labour that would otherwise be uncomfortable. This might generate the injury which manifests itself as back pain. If this analysis is correct, then the increasing use of progressively more dilute local anaesthetic solutions in labour should see a reduction in the incidence of this problem.

PAEDIATRIC APPLICATIONS

This has been recently reviewed by Dalens (1989). Attitudes to the delivery of analgesia to children have, until recently, been very conservative.

Indeed, because of the inability of young children, and particularly neonates, to articulate their pain and of the difficulties in making objective measurements, analgesia has been used sparingly or even withheld. The growing realization that, like adults, children need adequate relief from pain has generated much recent interest in the use of the epidural route for delivery of analgesia in this age group (Berde 1994).

Single-injection caudal administration of local anaesthetics has proved both popular and safe for peri- and post-operative analgesia. Simple dosage regimens for bupivacaine, such as that of Armitage (1979) utilizing concentrations of 0.19–0.25%, allow for adequate spread up to the mid-thoracic dermatomes, and are suitable for minor procedures below the umbilicus, even in day surgery. Caudal morphine 30 µg/kg is also effective and for a longer period. Using caudal epidural infusions of bupivacaine at 1.25–2.5 mg/kg per hour for postoperative analgesia, McCloskey et al (1992) reported systemic toxicity in three children. Serum levels of bupi-vacaine in each case exceeded the 4 µg/ml (2–10 µg/ml) toxic threshold for adults. They thus modified their infusion regimen to 0.2–0.4 mg/kg per hour in infants and 0.2–0.75 mg/kg per hour in children. Berde (1992) has subsequently recommended that doses of this order should be strictly   adhered to and should be reduced in patients who have risk factors for seizures. He also emphasized that caudal infusions of local anaesthetics should not be expected to supply adequate analgesia for thoracic or upper abdominal surgery. The addition of fentanyl 1 µg/kg to caudal bupivacaine 0.125% 1 ml/kg was not found to be of additional benefit when compared with bupivacaine alone in children undergoing urological surgery (Campbell et al 1992).

The lumbar (Murat et al 1987) and thoracic (Meignier et al 1983) routes are finding wider acceptance especially when infusions of local anaesthetics or opioids or both are used. Experience from Britain and from Canada has been recently reported. Wilson & Lloyd-Thomas (1993) audited 150 children, ranging from neonates to 16 years, who were scheduled for major surgery and who received intraoperative epidural analgesia (lumbar 125, thoracic 25) with bupivacaine 0.25% 0.5–0.75 ml/kg together with, in some cases, diamorphine 25–50 µg/kg. They used a 19G needle/23G catheter or an 18G needle/21G catheter. Post-operatively, analgesia was provided by epidural infusion of bupivacaine 0.125% 0.1–0.5 ml/kg per h, each 60 ml of solution containing 3, 6 or 10 mg diamorphine, and the patients were looked after by specially trained nurses supervised by a pain team. Previously, in the same unit, the use of postoperative epidural infusions, using local anaesthetic alone, had been associated with inadequate sedation. The addition of diamorphine, either because of the sedative effects resulting from systemic absorption or because of the improved analgesia, increased the acceptability of the technique in the ward setting. Pruritus (10%) and nausea (<5%) were minor difficulties compared with technical catheter-related problems. 16.7% of infusions were terminated prematurely due to catheter occlusion, blockage, leakage or disconnection, occupying much nursing time in the process. Two cases of respiratory depression were easily treated with naloxone; one was an 8-week-old infant (born at 31 weeks' gestation) and the other a child of 9 kg. Since both received diamorphine in the higher dose ranges, these workers now recommend the 3 mg/60 ml dilution. Subsequently, Wood et al (1994) reviewed 2 years' experience with postoperative epidural analgesia in 190 children who were thought likely to have moderate to severe postoperative pain in the thoracic, lumbar or sacral dermatomes. Using infusions containing 0.1–0.25% bupivacaine, with or without adrenaline, and fentanyl 1 μg/ml, they noted only a 5.2% incidence of pruritus but more nausea and vomiting (23%) than Wilson & Lloyd-Thomas. Again, 17% of infusions were stopped due to technical problems with the catheters. There was one instance each of respiratory depression, seizure and insertion site infection. None of these was associated with short- or long-term disability.

In both of these series, although the patients were nursed on general wards, it was clear that this form of analgesic management was very labour intensive and that special nurse training was required, so that side-effects and technical complications would be recognized and dealt with swiftly.

CONCLUSION

Despite considerable improvements in the use of epidural anaesthesia, controversy still surrounds the practical application of the newer methods and there is still a price to be paid in terms of side effects and complications.

REFERENCES

Andrews P J D, Ackerman W E, Juneja M et al 1992 Transient bradycardia associated with extradural blood patch after inadvertent dural puncture in parturients Br J Anaesth 69: 401–403
Armitage E N 1979 Caudal block in children. Anaesthesia 34: 396
Beards S C, Jackson A, Griffiths A G et al 1993 Magnetic resonance imaging of extradural bloodpatches: appearances from 30 minutes to 18 hours. Br J Anaesth 71: 182–188
Ben-David B, Vaida S, Collins G et al 1994 Transient paraplegia secondary to an epidural catheter. Anesth Analg 79: 598–600
Berde C B 1992 Convulsions associated with pediatric regional anesthesia. Anesth Analg 75: 164–166
Berde C 1994 Epidural analgesia in children. (Editorial) Can J Anaesth 41: 555–560
Blomberg R G 1993 Recent insights in the anatomy and physiology of the epidural space and some clinical consequences, In: Aken H V (ed) Clinical anaesthesiology, Vol 7. Ballière Tindall, London, pp 535–556
Breen T W, Shapiro T, Glass B et al 1993 Epidural anesthesia for labor in an ambulatory patient. Anesth Analg 77: 919–924
Breen T W, Ransil B J, Groves P A et al 1994 Factors associated with back pain after childbirth. Anesthesiology 81: 29–34
Bromage P R 1993 Spinal extradural abscess: pursuit of vigilance. Br J Anaesth 70: 471–473
Bromage P R 1994 (Letter.) Anaesthesia 49: 260

Brownridge P 1981 Epidural and subarachnoid analgesia for elective caesarean section. Anaesthesia 36: 70

Buggy D, Hughes N, Gardiner J 1994 Posterior column sensory impairment during ambulatory extradural analgesia in labour. Br J Anaesth 73: 540–542

Campbell F A, Yentis S M, Fear D W et al 1992 Analgesic efficacy and safety of a caudal bupivacaine-fentanyl mixture in children. Can J Anaesth 39: 661–664

Carabine U A, Milligan K R, Moore J 1992a Extradural clonidine and bupivacaine for postoperative analgesia. Br J Anaesth 68: 132–135

Carabine U A, Milligan K R, Mulholland et al 1992b Extradural clonidine infusions for analgesia after total hip replacement. Br J Anaesth 68: 338–343

Carp H, Bailey S 1992 The association between meningitis and dural puncture in bacteremic rats. Anesthesiology 76: 739–742

Carrie L E S 1993 Postdural puncture headache and extradural blood patch. Br J Anasth 71: 179–181

Carrie L E S, O'Sullivan G M 1984 Subarachnoid bupivacaine 0.5% for caesarean section. Eur J Anaesthesiol 1: 275–283

Carroll D, Jadad A, King V et al 1993 Single-dose, randomized, double-blind, double-dummy cross-over comparison of extradural and IV clonidine in chronic pain. Br J Anaesth 71: 665–669

Chestnut D H, Vandewalker G E, Owen C L et al 1987 The influence of continuous epidural bupivacaine analgesia on the second stage of labor and method of delivery in nulliparous women. Anesthesiology 66: 774–780

Chestnut D H, Owen C L, Brown C K et al 1988a Does labor affect the variability of maternal heart rate during induction of epidural anesthesia? Anesthesiology 68: 622–625

Chestnut D H, Owen C L, Bates J N et al 1988b Continuous infusion epidural analgesia during labor: a randomized, double-blind comparison of 0.0625% bupivacaine/0.0002% fentanyl versus 0.125% bupivacaine. Anesthesiology 68: 754–759

Chestnut D H, Vincent R D, McGrath J M et al 1994a Does early administration of epidural analgesia affect obstetric outcome in nulliparous women who are receiving intravenous syntocinon? Anesthesiology 80: 1193–1200

Chestnut D H, McGrath J M, Vincent R D et al 1994b Does early administration of epidural analgesia affect obstetric outcome in nulliparous women who are in spontaneous labour? Anesthesiology 80: 1201–1208

Clark V A, McQueen M A 1993 Factors influencing backache following epidural analgesia in labour. Int J Obstet Anesth 2: 193–196

CLASP 1994 A randomised trial of low-dose aspirin for the prevention and treatment of pre-eclampsia among 9364 pregnant women. Lancet 343: 619–629

Cohen S, Daitch J S, Goldiner P L 1989 An alternative method for management of accidental dural puncture for labour and delivery. Anesthesiology 70: 164–165

Cohen S, Amar D, Pantuck C B et al 192 Adverse effects of epidural 0.03% bupivacaine during analgesia after cesarean section. Anesth Analg 75: 753–756

Collis R E, Baxandall M L, Srikantharajah I D et al 1994 Combined spinal epidural (CSE) analgesia: technique, management and outcome of 300 mothers. Int J Obstet Anesth 3: 75–81

Dalens B 1989 Regional anaesthesia in children. Anesth Analg 68: 654–672

De Kock M, Crochet B, Morimont C et al 1993 Intravenous or epidural clonidine for intra- and postoperative analgesia. Anesthesiology 79: 525–531

Eisenach J C, Tong C 1991 Site of haemodynamic effects of alpha-2 adrenergic agonists. Anethesiology 74: 766–771

Eisenach J, Lysack S, Viscomi C 1989 Epidural clonidine analgesia following surgery: phase 1. Anesthesiology 71: 640–646

Eisenach J, Detweiler D, Hood D 1993 Hemodynamic and analgesic actions of epidurally administered clonidine. Anesthesiology 78: 277–287

Ferrante F M, Rosinia F A, Gordon C et al 1994 The role of continuous background infusions in patient-controlled epidural analgesia for labor and delivery. Anesth Analg 79: 80–84

Gaynor A 1990 The lumbar epidural region: anatomy and approach. In: Reynolds F (ed) Epidural and spinal blockade in obstetrics: epidural and spinal blockade in obstetrics. Ballière Tindall, London, pp 3–18

Gormley J B 1960 Treatment of post-spinal headache. Anesthesiology 21: 565–566

Green D W 1992 The clinical use of spinal opioids. In: Kaufman L (ed) Anaesthesia Review 9. Churchill Livingstone, London, pp 80–111

Harding S A, Collis R E, Morgan B M 1994 Meningitis after combined spinal-epidural anaesthesia in obstetrics. Br J Anaesth 73: 545–547

Horlocker T T, Wedel D J, Schlichting J L 1994 Postoperative epidural analgesia and oral anticoagulant therapy. Anesth Analg 79: 89–93

Huntoon M, Eisenach J C, Boese P 1992 Epidural clonidine after cesarean section: appropriate dose and effect of prior local anaesthetic. Anesthesiology 76: 187–193

Jamali S, Monin S, Begon C et al 1994 Clonidine in paediatric caudal anaesthesia. Anesth Analg 78: 663–666

Kanumilli V, Kaza R, Johnson C et al (Letter) 1993 Epidural blood patch for Jehovah's Witness patient. Anesth Analg 77: 872–873

Kitching A J, Rice A S C 1993 Extradural abscess in the postpartum period (Letter). Br J Anaesthesia 70: 703

Lao T T, Halpern S H, MacDonald D et al 1993 Spinal subdural haematoma in a parturient after attempted epidural anaesthesia. Can J Anaesth 40: 340–345

Lawhead R G, Blaxall H S, Bylund D B 1992 Alpha-2A is the predominant alpha-2 subtype in human spinal cord. Anesthesiology 77: 983–991

Leighton B L, Norris M C, Sosis M et al 1987 Limitations of epinephrine as a marker of intravascular injection in laboring women. Anesthesiology 66: 688–691

Leighton B L, Norris M C, DeSimone C A et al 1990 The air test as a clinically useful indicator of intravenously placed epidural catheters. Anesthesiology 73: 610–613

Letsky E A 1991 Haemostasis and epidural anaesthesia. Int J Obstet Anesth 1: 51–54

Liu N, Bonnet F, Delaunay L et al 1993 Partial reversal of the effects of extradural clonidine by oral yohimbine in postoperative patients. Br J Anaesth 70: 515–518

MacArthur C, Lewis M, Knox E G et al 1990 Epidural anaesthesia and long-term backache after childbirth. Br Med J 301: 9–12

McClean B Y, Rottman R L, Kotelko D M 1992 Failure of multiple test doses and techniques to detect intravascular migration of an epidural catheter. Anesth Analg 74: 454–456

McCloskey J J, Haun S E, Deshpande J K 1992 Bupivacaine toxicity secondary to continuous caudal epidural infusion in children. Anesth Analg 75: 287–290

Mamourian A C, Dickan C A, Drayer B P et al 1993 Spinal epidural abscess: three cases following spinal epidural injection demonstrated with magnetic resonance imaging. Anesthesiology 78: 204–207

Martin R, Jourdain S, Clairoux M et al 1994 Duration of decubitus position after epidural blood patch. Can J Anaesth 41: 23–25

Meignier M, Souron R, Le Neel J C 1983 Postoperative dorsal epidural analgesia in the child with respiratory disabilities. Anesthesiology 59: 473–475

Meiklejohn B H 1987 The effect of rotation of an epidural needle. Anaesthesia 42: 1180–1182

Maze M, Tranquilli W 1991 Alpha-2 adrenoceptor agonists: defining the role in clinical anesthesia. Anesthesiology 74: 581–605

Mogensen T, Eliasen K, Ejlersen E et al 1992 Epidural clonidine enhances postoperative analgesia from a combined low-dose epidural bupivacaine and morphine regimen. Anesth Analg 75: 607–610

Moore D C, Batra M S 1981 The components of an effective test dose prior to an epidural block. Anesthesiology 55: 693–696

Morris G F, Gore-Hickman W, Lang S A et al 1994 Can parturients distinguish between intravenous and epidural fentanyl? Can J Anaesth 41: 667–672

Murat I, Delleur M M, Levy J et al 1987 Continuous epidural anaesthesia for major abdominal surgery in young children. Eur J Anaesthesiol 4: 327–335

Ngan Kee W D, Jones M R, Thomas P et al 1992 Extradural abscess complicating extradural anaesthesia for caesarean section. Br J Anaesth 69: 647–652

Okutomi T, Watanabe S, Goto F 1993 Time course in thoracic epidural pressure measurement. Can J Anaesth 40: 1044–1048

O'Meara M E, Gin T 1993 Comparison of 0.125% bupivacaine with 0.125% bupivacaine and clonidine as extradural analgesia in the first stage of labour. Br J Anaesth 71: 651–656

Onishchuk J L, Carlsson C 1992 Epidural haematoma associated with epidural anaesthesia: complications of anticoagulant therapy. Anesthesiology 77: 1221–1223

Priddle H D, Andros G J 1950 Primary spinal anaesthetic effects of epinephrine. J Curr Anesth Analg 29: 156–162

Rauck R L, Eisenach J C, Jackson K et al 1993 Epidural clonidine treatment for refractory reflex sympathetic dystrophy. Anesthesiology 79: 1163–1169

Russell R, Reynolds F 1993 Epidural infusions for nulliparous women in labour. Anaesthesia 48: 856–861

Russell R, Groves P, Reynolds F 1993a Is opioid loading necessary before opioid/local anaesthetic epidural infusions? A randomized double-blind study in labour. Int J Obstet Anesth 2: 78–84

Russell R, Groves P, Taub N et al 1993b Assessing long-term backache after childbirth. Br Med J 306: 1299–1303

Schwartz N, Eisenkraft J B 1993 Probable venous air embolism during epidural placement in an infant. Anesth Analg 76: 1136–1138

Scott D B, Hibbard B M 1990 Serious non-fatal complications associated with extradural block in obstetric practice. Br J Anaesth 64: 537–541

Shah J L 1994 Positive lumbar extradural space pressure. Br J Anaesth 73: 309–314

Sowter M C, Burgess N A, Woodsford P V et al 1992 Delayed presentation of an extradural abscess complicating thoracic extradural analgesia. Br J Anaesth 68: 103–105

Stride P C, Cooper G M 1993 Dural taps revisited. Anaesthesia 48: 247–255

Sutton D N, Linter S P K 1991 Depth of extradural space and dural puncture. Anaesthesia 46: 97–98

Thorp J A, Hu D H, Albin R M et al 1993 The effect of intrapartum analgesia on nulliparous labour: a randomized, controlled, prospective trial. Am J Obstet Gynaecol 169: 851–858

Tom D J, Gulevich S J, Shapiro H M et al 1992 Epidural blood patch in HIV-positive patient. Anesthesiology 76: 943–947

Upton P M, Carrie L E S, Reynolds K 1992 Epidural insertion: how far should the epidural needle be inserted before testing for loss of resistance? Int J Obstet Anesth 1: 71–73

Vercauteren M P, Lauwers E, Meert T et al 1990 Comparison of epidural sufentanil plus clonidine with sufentanil alone for postoperative analgesia. Anaesthesia 45: 531–534

Weber H U 1994 Anasthesia durch adrenalin. Verh Dtsch Ges Inn Med 21: 616–619

Westbrook J L, Renowden S A, Carrie L E S 1993 Study of the anatomy of the extradural region using magnetic resonance imaging. Br J Anaesth 71: 495–498

Williams H D, Howard R, O'Donnell N et al 1993 The effect of low dose aspirin on bleeding times. Anaesthesia 48: 331–333

Wilson P T J, Lloyd-Thomas A R 1993 An audit of extradural infusion analgesia in children using bupivacaine and diamorphine. Anaesthesia 48: 718–723

Wood C E, Goresky G V, Klassen K A et al 1994 Complications of continuous epidural infusions for postoperative analgesia in children. Can J Anaesth 41: 613–620

Wood M B, Rubin A P 1993 A comparison of epidural 1% ropivacaine and 0.75% bupivacaine for lower abdominal gynecologic surgery. Anesth Analg 76: 1274–1278

Yaksh T L 1984 Pharmacology of spinal adrenergic systems which modulate spinal nociceptive processing. Pharmacol Biochem Behav 22: 845–858

12

Prevention of perioperative venous thrombosis

D. J. Gerrard   J. A. Skinner

Patients admitted to hospital for surgical procedures are at risk of postoperative deep vein thrombosis (DVT) and subsequent pulmonary embolism (PE). Extensive DVT may lead to the development of chronic venous insufficiency characterized by discomfort, oedema, varicose veins, cutaneous pigmentation, induration and ulceration. PE may present an immediate threat to life or result in chronic pulmonary hypertension from recurrent embolism. These sequelae represent a significant proportion of hospital morbidity and mortality and have a considerable impact on the cost of health care.

Effective prophylaxis can significantly reduce the incidence of DVT in hospitalized patients (Kakkar & Adams 1986). In a retrospective study, Sandler & Martin (1989) found that in over 2300 autopsies performed over a 5-year period 10% of in-hospital deaths were directly related to PE. Of those patients, 83% had thrombus in the deep veins of the legs yet only 19% had been symptomatic.

PE is difficult to diagnose because the spectrum of symptoms and clinical signs varies widely. Monreal et al (1992) found that 22% of all patients with DVT has scintigraphic evidence of PE. However, clinicians often fail to diagnose even the most important emboli. In an autopsy study of patients dying after hip fracture surgery, there was great discrepancy between the autopsy report and the clinically recorded cause of death (Fitts et al 1964). Other studies have shown that 38% of patients who die following hip fracture have evidence of PE at postmortem but only 2% of these are detected clinically.

RISK FACTORS FOR VENOUS THROMBOEMBOLISM

Risk of thromboembolic disease increases with age, becoming significant in otherwise low-risk patients after 40 years. Patients with thrombophilia may develop thromboembolic disease at an early age and those with previous episodes of thromboembolic disease have a 50% incidence of further thrombosis following surgery (Kakkar et al 1970). These and other risk factors for venous thromboembolic disease are well recognized and are listed in Table 12.1.

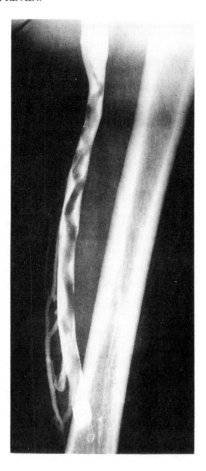

Fig. 12.1 Venogram showing a large 'free-floating', non-occlusive thrombosis in the left femoral vein. Patients with this type of thrombus are often asymptomatic but sudden collapse may occur secondary to embolization.

The clinical problem of identifying patients at greatest risk is by no means straightforward. Mathematical formulae have been developed to predict the risk for individual patients (Breneman 1965). These vary in complexity but often involve measuring coagulation parameters which are not routinely available at most hospitals. While the idea is appealing, these methods are not sufficiently accurate to reliably identify patients in whom thrombo-prophylaxis may be safely withheld.

The most useful clinical method of classifying the degree of risk is that first proposed by Salzman & Hirsh (1987) and later modified by the THRIFT consensus group (1992). This is shown in Table 12.2.

All surgical patients should be assessed for thromboembolic risk factors prior to surgery (Table 12.1). Essentially, the incidence of thromboembolism in patients in the low-risk group undergoing minor surgical procedures is

Table 12.1   Risk factors for thromboembolic disease

Congenital	Acquired
Antithrombin III deficiency	Age over 40 years
Protein S deficiency	Previous thromboembolic disease
Protein C deficiency	Major surgery
Activated protein C resistance	Malignant disease
Dysfibrinoginaemia	Obesity
Antiphospholipid antibody	Trauma
Lupus anticoagulant	Myocardial infarction
Family history	Congestive cardiac failure
Homocystinuria	Cerebrovascular accident (stroke)
Paroxysmal nocturnal	Fracture of hip, pelvis
haemaglobinuria	or lower limb long bone
	Oestrogen therapy (high dose)
	Prolonged immobilization
	Pregnancy and the puerperium
	Varicose veins
	Inflammatory bowel disease
	Respiratory infections
	Behçet's syndrome
	Paralysis

Table 12.2   Incidence of venous thromboembolism in hospital patients according to risk group

	Deep vein thrombosis	Proximal vein thrombosis	Fatal pulmonary embolism
Low-risk groups	<10%	<1%	0.01%
Moderate-risk groups	10–40%	1–10%	0.1–1%
High-risk groups	40–80%	10–30%	1–10%
Low-risk groups	Minor surgery (<30 min); no risk factors other than age Major surgery (>30 min); age < 40, no other risk factors* Minor trauma or medical illness		

Moderate-risk groups	Major general, urological, gynaecological, cardiothoracic,
	    vascular, or neurological surgery; age ≥ 40 years or other risk factor*
	Major medical illness: heart or lung disease, cancer,
	    inflammatory bowel disease
	Major trauma or burns
	Minor surgery, trauma, or illness in patients with previous deep
	vein thrombosis, pulmonary embolism, or thrombophilia		

High-risk groups	Fracture or major orthopaedic surgery of pelvis, hip or lower limb Major pelvic or abdominal surgery for cancer Major surgery, trauma or illness in patients with previous deep vein thrombosis, pulmonary embolism or thrombophilia Lower limb paralysis (e.g. hemiplegic stroke, paraplegia) Major lower limb amputation		

Table: British Medical Journal 1992; 305: 567–574 (with permission)
*Additional risk factors are listed in Table 12.1.

such that the potential complications and expense of prophylaxis may not be warranted. However, patients who may be classified as low risk according to the type of surgery may in fact be at much higher risk of DVT if they have one or more of these risk factors. Similarly, findings on clinical examination such as varicose veins, obesity and heart failure may lead to modification of thromboprophylaxis. Thrombophilia should be excluded in patients who have presented with thrombosis at an early age. Certain other groups of patients should also be screened for thrombophilia and these are shown in Table 12.3.

A large number of screening tests for thrombophilia are now available. However, many of these tests can only be performed in specialized centres. The most frequent causes of thrombophilia can be detected using the tests listed in Table 12.4, which should be readily available in most hospitals or health districts.

Pregnant women and those on hormonal therapy require special consideration. It is important to establish whether women of reproductive age undergoing surgery are taking the oral contraceptive pill (OCP). Vessey et al (1986) retrospectively analysed the data on 5603 women undergoing surgery, 34 of whom subsequently developed DVT and/or PE. The incidence of thromboembolism was found to be approximately 1% (12/1244) for pill users and 0.5% (22/4359) for non-users. However, it does not necessarily follow that all women scheduled to undergo surgery should be advised to stop the OCP. It must be borne in mind that these women may

Table 12.3   Indications for thrombophilia screening

Unexplained venous thrombosis before the age of 40
Family history of venous thrombosis or thrombophilia
Recurrent unexplained venous thrombosis*
Unexplained skin necrosis in patients taking coumarins[†]
Unexplained arterial thrombosis
Unexplained prolongation of the activated partial thromboplastin time
Unexplained recurrent fetal abortion
Idiopathic thrombocytopenia
Systematic lupus erythematosus

* Also exclude underlying malignancy.
[†] Patients with protein C deficiency may develop coumarin-induced skin necrosis.

Table 12.4   Suggested screening tests for thrombophilia. aPPT, activated partial thromboplastin time. PT, prothrombin time. ATIII, antithrombin III. APC resistance, activated protein C resistance.

Full blood count
Activated partial thromboplastin time (a PTT)
Prothrombin time (PT)
Protein C
Protein S
Antithrombin III (AT III)
Reptilase time
Activated protein C (APC) resistance
Plasminogen
Fibrinogen
Lupus anticoagulant
Anti-cardiolipin antibodies

be at risk of an unplanned or unwanted pregnancy, with the subsequent risk to both mother and fetus during surgery. Patients with additional risk factors should, in most circumstances, receive thromboprophylaxis but each case should be assessed individually.

Although even low doses of oestrogen have been shown to have significant effects on coagulation parameters, the risk of thrombosis seems to be directly related to the dose of oestrogen contained in oral contraceptive preparations. The progesterone-only pill does not seem to confer a greater risk of DVT.

Patients receiving hormone replacement therapy (HRT) may also be at greater risk of DVT. However, no randomized studies have been performed to confirm this. Although the HRT preparations currently in use contain much lower doses of oestrogen than the combined OCP, the increased age of this group of patients makes them more likely to have additional risk factors for postoperative DVT. Consequently, although there is no evidence to suggest that withdrawal of HRT prior to surgery is necessary, this group of patients should probably receive thromboprophylaxis.

Pregnancy itself is a risk factor for venous thromboembolism and PE is now one of the leading causes of maternal death in pregnancy and the puerperium. However, routine prophylaxis during an uncomplicated pregnancy is not justified. Obesity, age over 35, parity of three or greater and prolonged bed rest are additional risk factors and thromboprophylaxis should be considered for these women, especially if they are immobilized for any reason, either in the pre- or postpartum period. In most circumstances, thromboprophylaxis should be given to pregnant women undergoing surgery (including Caesarean section). Pregnant women with thrombophilia are at greater risk of developing DVT and if possible should be referred to a specialist who is able to advise on appropriate management throughout their pregnancy.

It has been suggested that there is an increased incidence of pulmonary embolism in patients undergoing laparoscopic surgery due to the fact that increased intra-abdominal pressure for any length of time interferes with the venous return from the legs (Naef & Mitchell 1994).

DIAGNOSIS OF DEEP VIEN THROMBOSIS

The clinical diagnosis of DVT is notoriously unreliable. This is particularly so after surgery to the lower limb, when some degree of swelling is normal. Diagnostic methods available include plethysmography, thermography, ultrasound Doppler techniques and venography. Venography is the most reliable method of diagnosing DVT, although its disadvantages are that it is invasive and expensive. The other diagnostic methods all tend to be highly effective in the diagnosis of occlusive thrombi in the proximal veins which are often symptomatic. The non-invasive tests are less reliable in diagnosing calf vein thrombi and non-occlusive, 'free floating' proximal thrombi, which are often silent (Fig. 12.1). This may be important as there is no evidence to suggest that symptomatic thrombi are more likely to be complicated by embolization; in fact it has been demonstrated that the converse may be true (Sandler & Martin 1989).

Duplex scanning is an attractive alternative to venography and as equipment and scanning techniques improve, it is likely that it will become the diagnostic method of choice in the future. However, at present, it should be remembered that all ultrasound techniques are operator dependent and published studies have shown sensitivities varying from 38% to over 90%.

The radiolabelled fibrinogen uptake test (FUT) is still used in some specialized centres. It is highly sensitive in diagnosing thrombi in the calf, popliteal and distal femoral veins. However, it cannot be reliably used to diagnose proximal femoral and iliac vein thrombi. This is due to high background radiation counts in the pelvic vasculature and viscera. The FUT is a useful screening technique in general, urological, gynaecological and neurosurgical procedures but inappropriate in orthopaedic surgery. Here, extravasated blood in the operative field may mask the popliteal vein following total knee replacement and the femoral vein following total hip replacement. Similar problems arise in screening patients undergoing peripheral vascular reconstruction.

METHODS OF PREVENTING DEEP VEIN THROMBOSIS

Thromboprophylaxis can be directed towards reducing venous stasis, preventing the hypercoaguable state induced by tissue trauma or using a combination of the two methods. Whichever method is used, thromboprophylaxis should probably be initiated prior to induction of anaesthesia, as it has been demonstrated that the thrombotic process commences intraoperatively (Kakkar et al 1969).

The ideal thromboprophylactic agent would prevent all DVTs, be free from side effects, be applicable to all surgical specialities and be simple to apply or administer. No such agent exists. Therefore, the selection of a particular thromboprophylactic method depends on the type of surgery, the overall risk category into which the patient falls and the preference of the responsible clinician. For example, it may not be appropriate to treat a patient undergoing neurosurgical or spinal procedures with anticoagulants, or to use an intermittent pneumatic compression device on a patient who has undergone vascular reconstruction.

Mechanical methods

Graduated compression stockings (GCS)

It is by no means clear how GCS achieve a thromboprophylactic effect. It has been shown that they increase the velocity of venous blood flow

(Meyerowitz & Nelson 1964, Sigel et al 1973, Lawrence & Kakkar 1980) and this may reduce the activation of coagulation systems associated with stasis. It has also been proposed that anaesthesia causes venous dilatation and that in unsupported veins this may cause microtears in the endothelium. GCS may prevent this dilatation and therefore prevent exposure of pro-coagulant subendothelial collagen to circulating coagulation factors (Comerota et al 1989).

GCS are a simple, safe and moderately effective form of thromboprophyl-axis. The only major contraindication is peripheral vascular disease. The majority of studies in patients undergoing general, gynaecological and neuro-surgical procedures have shown a reduction in the incidence of DVT. A comprehensive meta-analysis by Wells et al (1994) concluded that, in studies using sound methods, there was a highly significant risk reduction of 68% in patients at moderate risk of postoperative thromboembolism. Only one methodologically sound study has been performed in orthopaedic surgery (Fredin et al 1989). This showed a strong trend in favour of the treatment arm but no conclusions could be made in this high-risk group of patients. In addition, there is no conclusive evidence that GCS are effective in reducing the incidence of fatal and non-fatal PE (Kakkar 1993). It is not known whether wearing GCS following discharge from hospital is efficacious.

Intermittent pneumatic compression (IPC)

The early IPC devices were uncomfortable and poorly tolerated. How-ever, the devices currently in use are more comfortable to wear, less bulky and have been designed to allow greater knee movement.

IPC influences all three components of Virchow's triad, namely blood flow, factors within the blood itself and the vascular endothelium. Blackshear et al (1987) showed that flow velocity and volume flow rate are improved and Summaria et al (1988) showed that the fibrinolytic response is enhanced by IPC. By inhibiting venous stasis, IPC prevents venous dilatation, thereby preventing endothelial microtears (Comerota et al 1989). Studies compar-ing IPC with control, pharmacological agents and combined methods of prophylaxis have been performed in general, orthopaedic, gynaecological, urological and neurosurgical procedures. In each trial, IPC has been shown to be more or equally as effective in preventing DVT. However, prospec-tive, randomized, double-blind trials have had insufficient power to show that IPC reduces the incidence of postoperative pulmonary embolism. Although the optimal duration of application of IPC has not been firmly established, several studies have shown that commencing IPC prior to surgery and maintaining it during the intraoperative and postoperative periods until the patient is mobile without requiring aid is more effective than commencing IPC only in the postoperative period. Combined use of IPC with graduated compression stockings may also be more effective than either IPC or GCS alone (Nicolaides et al 1983).

There are few contraindications for using IPC. Care should be taken in patients with heart failure and a significant degree of leg oedema. Care should also be taken in using IPC for patients suspected of existing DVT, since compression of the leg may promote embolization of the thrombus. Patients undergoing knee arthroplasty often find IPC uncomfortable, and despite the improvement in the design of the devices they may still limit postoperative mobilization.

Foot pumps

Flattening of the plantar arch on weight bearing has been shown to activate a physiological venous pump mechanism which is capable of ejecting venous blood through an occlusive tourniquet inflated to a pressure of 100 mmHg (Gardner & Fox 1983). Wilson et al (1992) showed a reduction in the incidence of DVT in patients undergoing total knee replacement from 68.7% in untreated controls to 50% in those treated with a foot pump in the postoperative period. Six proximal thrombi were observed in the control group whereas there were no proximal thrombi in the treated group. Fordyce & Ling (1992) investigated the efficacy of the venous foot pump in preventing postoperative DVT in patients undergoing total hip replacement. They demonstrated venographically proven DVT in 40% of untreated controls compared with 5% of the treated group. Whilst these results are promising, the study groups have been small and no trials have been performed in surgical groups other than orthopaedics. In order to assess both the intermittent calf compression and foot pump devices, large randomized trials comparing them with heparin and low molecular weight heparin should be performed.

Pharmacological methods

Dextran

Dextran is a high molecular weight glucose polymer formed by enzymatic degradation of saccharose. The molecular weight of the most commonly used 'dextrans' in clinical practice are 40 000 and 70 000. Dextran is principally excreted renally at a rate proportional to its molecular weight.

Dextrans exert their antithrombotic effects by reducing red cell aggregation, providing a protective coating over the vascular endothelium and erythrocytes, reducing platelet aggregation and by a specific inhibitory effect on Von Willebrand factor. There is also evidence that dextran may facilitate endogenous thrombolysis and reduce venous stasis by expanding plasma volume.

Early trials comparing dextran prophylaxis with untreated controls in orthopaedic patients showed dextran to be of benefit in reducing postoperative DVT. No reliable conclusions can be drawn from these studies because many were poorly designed. However, a meta-analysis performed by Clagett & Reisch

(1988), which included only trials using sound methodology, showed a significant reduction in the incidence of postoperative DVT. Clinicial trials in general, orthopaedic, urological and gynaecological surgery comparing dextran with other anticoagulants have shown it to be less effective than low-dose unfractionated heparin, low molecular weight heparin and warfarin in reducing postoperative DVT. Dextran does, however, seem to be effective in reducing extension of DVT beyond the calf and may reduce the incidence of PE.

The combination of dextran with either aspirin or dihydroergotamine was investigated in a double-blind, randomized trial by Pini et al (1985). The trial was performed on 83 patients undergoing surgery for hip fracture. There was no difference in the incidence of DVT between the two groups but there was significantly more postoperative bleeding in the aspirin group. Dextran used in combination with either GCS (Bergqvist & Lindblad 1984) or intermittent pneumatic compression (Smith et al 1978) has been shown to be more effective than dextran alone.

The use of dextran in the UK is limited and this may be related to its side effects. These include fluid overload, allergic reactions and anaphylaxis. There is a risk of bleeding and wound oozing comparable to that observed with low-dose heparin. Dextran must also be administered by intravenous infusion and the optimal dosage regimen is not established.

Aspirin and other antiplatelet agents

Antiplatelet agents inhibit cyclooxygenase, a key enzyme involved in the formation of thromboxane A_2. Thromboxane A_2 is synthesized and released by platelets in response to various stimuli, such as adenosine diphosphate, thrombin and collagen. By inhibiting the formation of thromboxane A_2, antiplatelet agents are able to reduce platelet aggregation and inhibit interaction with the vascular endothelium.

A large number of clinical trials have investigated the possible thromboprophylactic effect of antiplatelet agents. Many of these have been small or poorly designed studies and the few high-quality studies which have been performed have shown conflicting results. However, there are potential advantages of using aspirin and other antiplatelet agents. The drugs are cheap, active when given orally and are well   tolerated when given at doses which effectively inhibit platelets.

A recent meta-analysis by the Antiplatelet Trialists' Collaboration (1994) recommended that antiplatelet treatment either alone or, for greater effect, in addition to other proven forms of thromboprophylaxis should be considered for patients at high risk of thromboembolism. However, antiplatelet agents resulted in a risk reduction of 25% for DVT, which compares poorly with the result of a similar study with heparin that showed a risk reduction of 58% (Collins et al 1988); the comparison of the results for PE showed similar efficacy. Furthermore, the results of this meta-analysis have been questioned on the grounds that the studies are clinically and statistically heterogeneous and therefore cannot be meaningfully analysed in this way (Cohen et al 1994). A large, multicentre prospective trial, in which aspirin is added to conventional therapy for the prevention of DVT in patients with hip fracture, is currently underway (PEP trial), but other studies are needed to directly compare heparins with antiplatelet agents.

Oral anticoagulants

Oral anticoagulants inhibit the synthesis of vitamin K-dependent coagulant factors (prothrombin, factor VII, factor IX and factor X). However, on commencing treatment with a vitamin K antagonist, there is a latent period before the anticoagulant effects are manifested. The length of this latent period is determined by the rate of disappearance of preformed vitamin K-dependent coagulation factors.

Paiement et al (1987) found that oral anticoagulants, administered at the time of surgery, were effective in reducing the incidence of DVT in orthopaedic patients when the international normalised ratio (INR) was maintained between 2.0 and 2.5. Oral anticoagulants also seem to be effective when commenced 10–14 days preoperatively in small doses, which are able to produce a slight elevation in the INR, followed by an increase in the postoperative dose to maintain the INR at approximately 2.0 (Francis et al 1983). In randomized trials, oral anticoagulants were found to be less effective than low molecular weight heparin following hip surgery (Gerhart et al 1991) and knee surgery (Heit et al 1991). In general and gynaecological surgery, oral anticoagulants have also been shown to be effective in reducing the incidence of DVT and PE.

A major disadvantage of using oral anticoagulants is the high risk of major haemorrhage (between 2% and 7%). Other disadvantages are the need to monitor therapy with laboratory tests and the potential risks of drug interactions. However, randomized trials are underway to assess whether warfarin given in a small dose (1 mg per day) will be effective in preventing thromboembolism without the requirement for laboratory monitoring and without producing an unacceptably high incidence of major bleeding.

Heparin and low molecular weight heparin

Low-dose unfractionated heparin (UFH) has been used as a thromboprophylactic agent for over 20 years. Heparin binds to antithrombin III, inducing a structural change which increases the antithrombin catalytic activity several thousand fold. Heparin also inhibits activated factors IX, X and XII and at higher concentrations is able to inhibit thrombin by activating heparin cofactor II. In addition, heparin inhibits the interactions of coagulant factors on the platelet surface.

Many clinical trials have demonstrated that heparin is effective in reducing the incidence of DVT in surgical patients. In 1975, an international multicentre trial demonstrated conclusively that unfractionated heparin not only reduces the incidence of DVT, but also reduces the incidence of PE (Kakkar et al 1975). In a recent meta-analysis of over 70 randomized, placebo-controlled trials in general surgical, urological and both elective and traumatic orthopaedic procedures, the incidence of DVT was reduced by approximately two-thirds, and fatal PE by 60%. There was no statistical difference in mortality from other causes. Although there was no difference in the incidence of fatal bleeds, there was a 2% increase in the incidence of minor bleeding events. In addition to bleeding, heparin has other side effects. It has to be administered either two or three times daily, starting the day before surgery and continuing usually until the patient is mobile. Pain and bruising may occur at the injection site and heparin can induce a transient thrombocytopenia. Osteoporosis is a rare complication after prolonged administration.

Low molecular weight heparins (LMWHs) are derived by depolymerization of heparin by either chemical or enzymatic degradation. Conventional unfractionated heparin molecules have molecular weights ranging from 5000 to 30 000 Da, whereas LMWH molecules range from 2000 to 8000 Da. All the currently marketed LMWHs have different pharmacological profiles and therefore data from one cannot be extrapolated to another. Several studies in animals have shown that LMWH produces less bleeding than unfractionated heparin while retaining an equivalent antithrombotic effect. This has been explained by the fact that LMWHs have a more specific effect on activated factor X (Xa) than on factor II (thrombin). However, the exact mechanism is far from clear. The animal studies have been reinforced by data from a recent multicentre trial in which patients undergoing major abdominal surgery were randomized to receive one of two doses of LMWH or UFH (Kakkar et al 1993). This trial confirmed that the LMWH had a thromboprophylactic effect equivalent to unfractionated heparin. It also showed that there was a statistically lower incidence of wound haematoma. Although a 23% reduction in the incidence of major bleeding was found, this was not statistically significant.

Several meta-analyses have investigated the relative safety and efficacy of LMWH compared to UFH. The study of Nurmohamed et al (1992) chose rigorous criteria for inclusion of studies in the analysis. This found that in general surgical patients there was no convincing evidence to show that LMWHs had a greater benefit-to-risk ratio than UFH. However, studies using strong methodology in orthopaedic surgery demonstrated a significant risk reduction of 0.75 (CI 0.56−0.99) for DVT. Although not statistically significant, there was a trend in favour of a reduction in PE. There was no significant difference in major bleeding events. Large-scale randomized, double-blind trials comparing LMWHs with UFH are underway.

ANAESTHESIA AND THROMBOEMBOLISM: EFFECTS OF GENERAL AND REGIONAL ANAESTHESIA

Studies have shown that continuous lumbar epidural anaesthesia significantly reduces the incidence of postoperative DVT in patients undergoing total hip replacement (Modig et al 1981, 1983). In 40 patients randomized to receive either general or spinal anaesthesia undergoing 'pin and plate' fixation of fractured neck of femur, 76% of patients in the general anaesthesia group developed venographically proven postoperative DVT, whereas only 40% of patients in the spinal anaesthesia group developed proven DVT. The effect of lumbar epidural anaesthesia on the flow velocity in the femoral vein was measured by Polkolainen & Hendolin (1983). They found the velocity of flow in the femoral veins measured by Doppler ultrasound techniques to be higher in those patients receiving epidural anaesthesia than in those patients receiving general anaesthesia. They also found the incidence of postoperative DVT to be lower in the epidural anaesthesia group. However, studies comparing the incidence of DVT following general anaesthesia or thoracic extradural anaesthesia in abdominal surgery have not shown significant differences (Mellbring et al 1983).

The mechanisms underlying the apparent positive thromboprophylactic effect of epidural and spinal anaesthesia were investigated by Modig (1985). He identified properties of epidural anaesthesia which influence all three of the factors affecting thrombosis initially proposed by Virchow, described earlier. His investigations showed that arterial inflow and venous emptying rate were greater in patients given lumbar epidural anaesthesia than in those given general anaesthesia. In the same study, patients undergoing hip arthroplasty under epidural anaesthesia had significantly lower postoperative factor VIII activity than those patients having hip arthroplasty under general anaesthesia. There was also greater inhibition of natural fibrinolytic activity in patients having general anaesthesia. Release of plasminogen activators from the vascular endothelium and the resting levels of plasminogen activators in the blood were significantly greater during and after epidural anaesthesia than during and after general anaesthesia. The differences in coagulation and fibrinolysis between the two groups of patients cannot easily be explained. It is possible that local anaesthetics have a direct effect, or that the neuroendocrine responses to surgery are altered by afferent and efferent neural block. It is also possible that sympathomimetics given to counter hypotension are responsible for enhancing fibrinolytic activity. In addition, local anaesthetic agents have been shown to have an anti-aggregating effect on platelets in vitro, and may have a stabilizing effect on their interaction with the vascular endothelium. Therefore the lower incidence of DVT in patients undergoing regional anaesthesia may be a result of a combination of factors.

Regional anaesthesia combined with heparin/LMWH

Although regional anaesthesia reduces the incidence of DVT following surgery, it is unlikely that it will provide adequate prophylaxis when used alone in high-risk patients. As yet it is not clear whether this thromboprophylactic effect is potentiated by combining regional anaesthesia with heparin or LMWH.

Spinal haematoma is a recognized complication of epidural and spinal anaesthesia and there are obvious concerns regarding the safety of combining these invasive techniques with anticoagulant thromboprophylactic agents. However, intraspinal haemorrhage may occur spontaneously or in conjunction with coexisting pathology, such as bleeding disorders, spinal neoplasia and vascular abnormalities lying in close proximity to the spinal cord. They are also well documented in association with therapeutic anticoagulation.

The complications of regional anaesthesia have been investigated in three studies with a total of 164 701 patients. There were no reported cases of spinal haematomas. Bergqvist et al (1992) reviewed the clinical trials of patients undergoing surgery using heparin/LMWH as thromboprophylaxis where the type of anaesthesia was defined. No intraspinal haematomas were reported in 9013 patients receiving LMWH in combination with epidural or spinal anaesthesia. There is one case report of a spinal haematoma in a patient receiving prophylactic unfractionated heparin in combination with epidural anaesthesia, and two case reports of spinal bleeding in patients receiving LMWH prophylaxis. However, only one of these patients had epidural catheterization. This data suggest that there is little or no increased risk associated with a combination of regional anaesthesia and heparin thromboprophylaxis.

In patients undergoing major surgery, particularly those at high risk of thromboembolic disease, the risks of DVT and fatal pulmonary embolism far outweigh the risks of spinal haemorrhage. Bergqvist et al (1992) concluded from their review of the literature that the combination of heparin with epidural or spinal anaesthesia is safe, provided normal safety precautions are respected.

THE FUTURE OF THROMBOPROPHYLAXIS

Our understanding of the cellular and molecular biology of thrombosis has advanced considerably over the last few years. This, together with a greater awareness of the magnitude of the problem of thromboembolic disease and the more widespread use of thromboprophylactic agents, should lead to a reduction in the mortality from postoperative PE. There should also be a reduction in the number of patients with the chronic sequelae of DVT and PE. At present, however, all the thromboprophylactic agents currently in use have potential side-effects or limitations in their application. In addition, the incidence of thromboembolic disease remains above 18% for those at highest risk despite thromboprophylactic measures. Further large clinical trials are required to evaluate LMWHs in different types of surgery and to compare them with mechanical methods of prophylaxis and antiplatelet agents. A prospective, multicentre, randomized study of 30 000 patients undergoing major surgery is currently underway with the primary objective of comparing the efficacy of heparin with aspirin in preventing fatal PE. Newer agents, such as ultra low molecular weight heparins and highly specific thrombin inhibitors, are currently being evaluated.

SUMMARY

A range of therapies are available to prevent DVT and PE, which are major causes of morbidity and mortality in patients undergoing surgery. Certain thromboprophylactic agents have been shown to reduce the incidence of DVT and PE and should be used in all patients at moderate or high risk of thromboembolism. The choice of a suitable agent depends upon the type of surgery and other risks factors associated with each patient. So far, the evidence from clinical trials does not demonstrate a clear advantage of any one particular agent in preventing thromboembolism. However, a combination of a pharmacological agent with GCS has been shown to be efficacious and should probably be given to both moderate- and high-risk patients. IPC is an effective alternative, particularly in those patients for whom anticoagulants are contraindicated. Further large clinical trials and evaluation of more specific antithrombotic agents are underway.

REFERENCES

Antiplatelet Trialists' Collaboration 1994 Collaborative overview of randomised trials of antiplatelet therapy III: reduction in venous thrombosis and pulmonary embolism by antiplatelet prophylaxis among surgical and medical patients. Br Med J 308: 235–246
Bergvist D, Lindblad B 1984 The thromboprophylactic effect of graded elastic compression stockings in combination with dextran 70. Arch Surg 119: 1329–1331
Bergvist D, Lindblad B, Matzsch T 1992 Low molecular weight heparin for thromboprophylaxis and epidural/spinal anaesthesia: is there a risk? Acta Anaesthesiol Scand 36: 605–609
Blackshear V W, Precott C, LePain F et al 1987 Influence of sequential pneumatic compression on postoperative venous function. J Vasc Surg 5: 432–436
Breneman J C 1965 Postoperative thromboembolic disease: computer analysis leading to statistical prediction. JAMA 193: 576–580
Clagett G P, Reisch J S 1988 Prevention of venous thromboembolism in general surgical patients. Ann Surg 208: 227–240
Cohen A T, Skinner J A, Kakkar V V 1994 Antiplatelet treatment for thromboprophylaxis: a step forward or backwards. Br Med J 309: 1213–1217
Collins R, Scrimgeour A, Yusuf S et al 1988 Reduction in fatal pulmonary and venous thrombosis by perioperative administration of subcutaneous heparin: overview of randomised trials of general or orthopaedic and urological surgery. N Engl J Med 318: 1162–1173

Comerota A J, Stewart G J, Alburger P D et al 1989 Operative venodilation: a previously unsuspected factor in the cause of postoperative deep vein thrombosis. Surgery 106: 301–309

Fitts W T J, Lehr H B, Bitner R L et al 1964 An analysis of 950 fatal injuries. Surgery 56: 663–668

Fordyce M J F, Ling R S M 1992 A venous foot pump reduces thrombosis after total hip replacement. J Bone Joint Surg 74–B: 45–49

Francis C W, Marder V J, Evarts C M et al 1983 Two-step warfarin therapy: prevention of postoperative venous thrombosis without excessive bleeding. JAMA 249: 374–378

Fredin H, Bergqvist D, Cederholm C et al 1989 Thromboprophylaxis in hip arthroplasty: dextran with graded compression or preoperative dextran compared in 150 patients. Acta Orthop Scand 60: 678–681

Gardner A M N, Fox R H 1983 The venous pump of the foot: preliminary report. Bristol Med Chir J 98: 109–114

Gerhart T N, Yett H S, Robertson L K et al 1991 Low-molecular-weight heparinoid compared with warfarin for prophylaxis of deep-vein thrombosis in patients who are operated on for fracture of the hip. J Bone Joint Surg 73A: 494–502

Heit J, Kessler C, Mammen E et al 1991 Efficacy and safety of R D heparin (a LMWH) and warfarin for prevention of deep-vein thrombosis after hip or knee replacement. Blood 78: 187A

Kakkar V V 1993 Prevention of fatal pulmonary embolism. Haemostasis (Suppl 1): 42–50

Kakkar V V, Adams P C 1986 Preventive and therapeutic approach to venous thromboembolism: can death from pulmonary embolism be prevented? J Am Coll Cardiol 8: 146B–158B

Kakkar V V, Howe C T, Flanc C et al 1969 Natural history of postoperative deep-vein thrombosis. Lancet ii: 230–233

Kakkar V V, Howe C T, Nicolaides A N et al 1970 Deep vein thrombosis of the leg: is there a high risk group? Am J Med 120: 527–530

Kakkar V V, Corrigan T P, Fossard D P 1975 Prevention of fatal postoperative pulmonary embolism by low doses of heparin: an International Trial. Lancet ii: 45–51

Kakkar V V, Cohen A T, Edmondson R A et al 1993 Low molecular weight versus standard heparin for the prevention of venous thrombo-embolism after major abdominal surgery. Lancet 341: 259–265

Lawrence D, Kakkar V V 1980 Graduated, static, external compression of the lower limb: a physiological assessment. Br J Surg 67: 119–121

Mellbring G, Dahlgren S, Reiz S et al 1983 Thromboembolic complications after major abdominal surgery: effect of thoracic epidural anaesthesia. Acta Chir Scand 149: 263–268

Meyerowitz B R, Nelson R 1964 Measurement of the velocity of blood in lower limb veins with and without compression. Surgery 56: 481–486

Modig J 1985 the role of lumbar epidural anaesthesia as antithrombotic prophylaxis in total hip replacement. Acta Chir Scand 151: 589–594

Modig J, Hjelmet A, Sahlstedt B et al 1981 Comparative influences of epidural and general anaesthesia on deep venous thrombosis and pulmonary embolism after total hip replacement. Acta Chir Scand 147: 125–130

Modig J, Borg T, Karlstorm G et al 1983 Thromboembolism after total hip replacement: role of epidural and general anaesthesia. Anaesth Analg 62: 174–180

Monreal M, Ruiz J, Olazabal A et al 1992 Deep venous thrombosis and the risk of pulmonary embolism: a systematic study. Chest 102: 677–681

Naef M M, Mitchell A 1994 Anaesthesia for laparoscopy. In: Kaufman L, Ginsburg R (eds). Anaesthesia Review 11. Churchill Livingston, Edinburgh, pp 39–55

Nicolaides A N, Fernandes e Fernandes J, Pollock A V 1980 Intermittent sequential pneumatic compression of the legs in the prevention of venous stasis and postoperative deep vein thrombosis. Surgery 87: 69–76

Nurmohamed M T, Rosendaal F R, Buller H R et al 1992 Low molecular weight heparin versus standard heparin in general and orthopaedic surgery: a meta-analysis. Lancet 340: 152–156

Paiement G D, Bell D, Wessinger S J et al 1987 New advances in the prevention, diagnosis and cost effectiveness of venous thromboembolic disease in patients with total hip replacement. In: Brand R A (ed) The hip. C V Mosby, St Louis, pp 94–119

Pini M, Spadini E, Carluccio L et al 1985 Dextran/aspirin versus heparin/dihydroergotamine in preventing thrombosis after hip fractures. J Bone Joint Surg 67–B: 305–309

Polkolainen E, Hendolin H 1983 Effects of lumbar epidural analgesia and general anaesthesia on flow velocity in the femoral vein and postoperative deep vein thrombosis. Acta Chir Scand 149: 361–364

Salzman E W, Hirsh J 1987 Prevention of venous thromboembolism. In: Colman R W, Hirsh J, Marder V J, Salzman E W (eds) Haemostasis and thrombosis (2nd end). Lippincott, New York, pp 1252–1265

Sandler D A, Martin J F 1989 Autopsy proven pulmonary embolism in hospital patients: are we detecting enough deep vein thrombosis? J R Soc Med 82: 203–205

Sigel B, Edelstein A L, Felix W R 1973 Compression of the deep venous system of the lower leg during inactive recumbency. Arch Surg 106: 38–43

Smith R C, Elton R A, Orr J D 1978 Dextran and intermittent pneumatic compression in prevention of postoperative deep vein thrombosis: multi-unit trial. Br Med J i: 952–954

Summaria L, Caprini J, McMillan R 1988 Relationship between postsurgical fibrinolytic parameters and deep vein thrombosis in surgical patients treated with compression devices. Am Surg 54: 156–160

THRIFT (Thromboembolic Risk Factors) Consensus Group (1992) Risk of and prophylaxis for venous thromboembolism in hospital patients. Br Med J 305: 567–574

Vessey M P, Mant D, Smith A et al 1986 Oral contraceptives and venous thromboembolism: findings in a large prospective study. Br Med J 292: 526

Wells P S, Lensing A W A, Hirsh J 1994 Graduated compression stockings in the prevention of postoperative venous thromboembolism: a meta-analysis. Arch Intern Med 154: 67–72

Wilson N V, Das S K, Kakkar V V et al 1992 Thrombo-embolic prophylaxis in total knee replacement: evaluation of the A-V impulse system. J Bone Joint Surg 74–B: 50–52

13

Anaesthesia for the thermally injured

L. T. A. Rylah   N. Harper

The anaesthetist is an essential burn team member possessing both the skills and knowledge required at all treatment stages of the thermally injured. More people are surviving major burns than ever before and the percentage of total body surface area (% TBSA) burn that is lethal to half the victims (i.e. the LD_{50}) is now in the region of 70% in the population up to the age of 45 years (Muller & Herndon 1994). Improved survival rates are due to the adoption of early tangential excision of the wound; infection control techniques, up-to-date cardiac, respiratory and renal support in the intensive care unit, and an overall more aggressive approach to the management of this injury by intensivists.

The need for specialist burn anaesthesia is obvious as these patients will undergo many operations, sometimes in a short period of time; they will need large blood transfusions following extensive blood losses; and they will need an integrated approach by the whole burn team to achieve lower morbidity and mortality.

Three phases can be identified after a major burn. First, there is the initial resuscitation phase; this is followed by the hypermetabolic stabilization phase (when skin grafts will be used to cover the defects); and third is the reconstructive phase, where form and function are restored. This chapter will encompass the treatment of the thermally injured after the initial fluid resuscitation has been successfully completed, i.e. the second and third phases.

PATHOPHYSIOLOGY

It is important to understand the early physiological changes that occur with thermal injury as successful ongoing management relies on the response to resuscitation.

A major burn is defined as: 'Any burn of 20% TBSA or more in an adult; any burn of 10% or more in a child under 10 years of age or an adult over the age of 50; any burn of 10% full thickness or more; any burn associated with an inhalation injury or major trauma; any burn affecting the functional areas of the hands, feet, face or perineum.'

Thermal injury produces many of the physiological changes that are seen in major trauma but are yet more profound and longer lasting. The extent of these changes is proportional to the size of the injury. If over 20% TBSA burn is sustained, there is a loss of capillary integrity which will result in a loss of plasma volume into the interstitial space and the burn wound. During this resuscitation phase, lasting some 36–72 h, aggressive fluid replacement is essential to maintain the perfusion of the vital organs. This can be performed by following one of the many available formulae and the reader is referred to a review of resuscitation techniques, as this is beyond the scope of this text (Hunt et al 1992). For a simple fluid resuscitation regimen the reader is referred to Milner et al (1995). Major trauma will complicate the resuscitation as the resultant blood loss must also be replaced. Adequate intravenous analgesia must be administered as pain will alter the vital signs that are so useful during resuscitation.

Inhalation injury may result in airway obstruction, or respiratory exchange may be compromised and necessitate intubation and mechanical ventilation. If an inhalation injury is suspected it is vital that the airway be secured at the earliest possible time. It is wise to avoid performing a tracheostomy on these patients as this procedure is associated with a higher mortality (Eckhauser et al 1974). Intubation is mandatory in a large burn with an inhalation injury as resuscitation may cause massive swelling and jeopardize the patency of the airway.

The burn injury results in a massive catecholamine output. The outcome is the hypermetabolic state that follows such injuries, during which it is not uncommon for an insulin-resistant diabetes reaction to develop. Nutrition becomes a problem as a high caloric intake is necessary to minimize the catabolism of the body mass and may prove difficult to administer by the enteric route alone. Early enteral feeding will attenuate the burn response, limit bacterial translocation from the gut and reduce the incidence of stress ulceration (Deitch, 1990). If enteral feeding is successful, the associated hazards of parenteral nutrition will be avoided.

The loss of skin and the increased metabolic rate impair the thermoregulation of the patient, who responds by increasing his core temperature to 38.5°C. This persistent pyrexia may mask the early signs of sepsis, which is the most common cause of death once the patient has reached a burns unit. A high index of clinical suspicion, supported by haematological and bacteriological surveillance, is essential and aggressive antibiotic therapy must be initiated early. As is the case in major trauma, supportive therapy on the intensive care unit may be essential if not just humane. Similarly, support may be needed postoperatively as surgery can be extensive and blood loss massive.

The above factors must be taken into account on the preoperative visit to a patient that the surgeons wish to operate upon.

PREOPERATIVE VISIT

In the preoperative visit, the anaesthetist must assess whether the patient will benefit from the surgery and whether the risk from the operation is outweighed by the benefit obtained. The normal preoperative parameters must be examined. Haemoglobin concentration, electrolytes, blood urea concentration, chest X-ray and ECG are the baseline requirements. In addition, the anaesthetist should:

1. Look for a near normal intravascular volume.
2. Look for any signs of sepsis.
3. Assess current intravenous access and whether the current site needs changing.
4. Establish whether other sites are available for intravenous access.
5. Assess the airway and predict if a difficult intubation is likely.
6. Ascertain the respiratory status and perform blood gas analysis if necessary.

The previous analgesic requirements should be noted. Fasting should be limited to 2 h preoperatively as gastric motility is not adversely affected (Hu et al 1993). If the patient is already intubated, this time can be limited to 1 h. Surgery should be scheduled as early in the day as possible.

Reassurance is essential and an explanation of the methods of postoperative analgesia (see below) will allay some of the fears. Patience and understanding are vital and continuity of care is important as the patient must have confidence in the anaesthetist and the rest of the burn team during this painful and frightening period. If such care is not taken and confidence is lost, further care and management may become very difficult.

Preoperative medication is to be avoided in order to prevent delayed recovery from the anaesthetic, decrease the likelihood of postoperative nausea and vomiting and limit the starvation time by encouraging early postoperative feeding. Regular analgesia should not be omitted.

OPERATIVE PROCEDURES

There are four main types of operation that these patients will encounter: escharotomy; primary excision and grafting; dressing and debridement procedures; and reconstructive operations.

Escharotomy

A full or sometimes partial circumferential full-thickness burn to the trunk, neck or the limbs may result in the compromise of the respiratory system, the airway patency, or jeopardize the circulation to the limbs. The eschar or burned tissue must be incised down to viable tissue to release the con-striction and improve the circulation or chest compliance. Classically, this is performed without anaesthesia as the eschar is 'dead', but this can be a very painful procedure and general anaesthesia is recommended for hu-manitarian reasons, viable tissue being easily identifiable.

Primary excision and grafting

Excision of the burn wound can be performed immediately, early or late. Immediate excision is only recommended for burns of under 20% TBSA where the patient is otherwise healthy and there are no complicating fac-tors. The burn response is attenuated or terminated and the patient can be treated as having trauma with blood loss (Frame, et al 1990). The major problem with operating at this time is increased wound vascularity and consequent large blood losses.

The early excision and grafting of the burn wound has been one of the major advances in burn care over the last 20 years. It has resulted in de-creased hospital stay, decreased infection rates, and earlier restoration of function when compared to conservative treatment with topical antimicro-bial therapy and skin grafting after separation of the eschar (Herndon et al 1989).

Early excision is performed after a successful resuscitation has been completed, usually about 72 h post burn (but can be as early as 36 h). The aim is to remove the dead and dying tissue and achieve skin cover at the earliest time. Excision is limited to approximately 20% TBSA per opera-tion session. This will reduce the trauma response, limit the blood loss and heat loss, decrease the possibility of a consumptive coagulopathy, and al-low the rotation of graft donor sites. Infection rates will decrease and the metabolic load will be attenuated. In large burns, important functional areas such as the hands, face, eyelids, neck and joints are given priority to re-ceive grafts. As venous access secured through unburned skin decreases mortality, it may be wise to discuss with the surgeon at this time graft access sites such as the neck, clavicles and groin to ensure clean venous access for the future.

If the burn is deep or in highly vascular areas, the excision may be per-formed down to deep fascia. This is usually avoided as it will be aestheti-cally mutilating. The method of choice is termed tangential excision (Janzekovic 1975). Here the damaged tissue is progressively shaved off in layers until a viable bed for the graft is reached. This method is slower and results in a greater blood loss but is cosmetically more acceptable. Subcu-taneous infiltration under both the wound and donor sites with a solution of 15 mg phenylephrine BP in 1 litre of Hartmann's solution BP or saline 0.9% BP will decrease the blood loss dramatically. Swabs soaked in the same solution may also be applied topically.

Small burns will be covered with sheet autograft, punctured to allow blood to be expressed. Sheet autograft will also be used on the functional areas. Where the wound is more extensive, meshed autograft will be used in varying mesh ratios ranging from 1 : 1.5 to 1 : 9 if donor skin is sparse. The greater the mesh the less satisfactory is the cosmetic result. Temporary coverage may be obtained using the skin of close relatives, cadaver skin, porcine skin or proprietary biological dressings. Cyclosporin may be administered in an attempt to prevent skin rejection where autograft has not been used. The adverse side-effects of this drug that may be encountered are hepatic and renal impairment, hyperkalaemia and hypertension. This technique has so far proved of limited success. Cultured epithelial cells from victims   of massive burns have been applied as graft but have a poor cosmetic outcome, poor mechanical strength, is expensive and remains experimental.

The limit of 20% TBSA excision per visit to the operating room may mean that a patient with a large burn may return every 2–3 days. It may be wise to sedate and mechanically ventilate these patients in the meantime, to ensure adequate analgesia and to instigate invasive cardiovascular monitoring to ensure satisfactory blood and plasma volume replacement.

Dressing and debridement procedures

Dressing changes are carried out at regular intervals of 2 days. These can be performed without anaesthesia but it is a painful and degrading procedure. A variety of techniques have been used for this procedure including ketamine BP, self-administered Entonox (with or without an inhalation agent) and opiates; all with or without an anaesthetist present. With the advent of agents such as propofol and alfentanil, short anaesthetics can be administered safely with the minimum of distraction to the patient's ongoing care and nutrition. Under an anaesthetic these procedures can be performed more swiftly and with less nursing staff, making it not only more acceptable to the patient but more cost effective in the long run.

If the patient is being nursed in an intensive care or high dependency environment, short procedures may be performed in the patient's own room provided there is adequate assistance, monitoring and facilities for resuscitation (Rylah 1989).

Reconstructive operations

Reconstruction of form and function is needed after the initial debridement and grafting operations have been completed and full skin coverage has been obtained. However, this is an arbitrary classification as the grafting procedures should have been performed with the need for further operations in mind. Great efforts are taken by the burn team members to prevent contractures, limit scarring and preserve function by the use of physiotherapy, pressure garments and splints. However, in a major burn, contractures are likely to occur and anaesthesia for their release will be necessary. The various types of operation needed by these patients may go on for many years, thus it is important to plan well ahead.

Planning the operative sequence in conjunction with the surgeon is important both in terms of priority and fitness for surgery. The functional areas are covered first, i.e. the hands, feet, face and perineum; then the arms, legs, chest and back.

Contracture release on the neck may require special skills from the anaesthetist as the airway may be particularly difficult to intubate. Other problems that will be encountered are difficult venous access, maintenance of anaesthesia, monitoring, positioning, fluid replacement, hypotensive techniques, analgesia and postoperative care, all of which are discussed below.

The airway

Tracheal intubation may prove difficult in the immediate management due to tissue oedema either related to the burn injury or precipitated by the fluids used in the resuscitation. Suspected airway involvement will necessitate aggressive treatment and the airway must be secured immediately. As mentioned earlier, tracheostomy is not recommended, being associated with a higher mortality. Most injuries needing airway management will have burns around the face and neck which are likely to become infected. If a tracheostomy is performed, this may then lead to septicaemia, mediastinitis or chest infection, ultimately causing the demise of the patient.

Scarring and contractures may limit head and neck movements, making intubation difficult or impossible. The burned skin is greasy and slippery; therefore, retaining a rubber face mask on a patient with facial burns may prove very difficult and exhausting.

Airway management for shorter procedures may be facilitated by the use of the laryngeal mask. For longer operations, those on the head and neck and those requiring special positioning or moving of the patient, tracheal intubation is advisable both to guarantee the airway and allow mechanical ventilation.

Intubation may be facilitated with a competitive muscle relaxant if difficulty is not anticipated. Suxamethonium is contraindicated after the first 48 h post burn (see below). If difficulty is anticipated many other methods of intubation can be considered (Goudsouzian & Szyfelbein 1985). These include inhalation induction followed by direct laryngoscopy or with blind nasal intubation, awake fibre-optic intubation, cricothyroidotomy with jet ventilation, cricothyroid puncture and retrograde cannulation or percutaneous tracheostomy. If the difficulty is due to contractures around the neck, it may be possible to release these under local anaesthesia, facilitating the intubation. The laryngeal mask has proved its worth and is an acceptable alternative method to try (Russell & Judkins 1990).

Intravenous access and fluid balance

Preoperative fasting must be kept to a minimum and any calorie deficit should be replaced postoperatively. Hypovolaemia and anaemia must be recognized prior to operation and rectified if time permits. If the operation must go ahead, it is wise to begin transfusion before blood loss occurs. Red cell loss may be minimized by haemodilution with a plasma substitute prior to the commencement of surgery or by replacing the volume but not the red cells until the required haemoglobin concentration is attained.

A 20% TBSA excision can present the anaesthetist with a massive blood loss. It is therefore essential that adequate, secure venous access is guaranteed. Cannulation sites are at a premium post burn and there may not be many to choose from. Peripheral sites are chosen first, then groin, followed by internal jugular and subclavian veins. The central route may be all that is available in the early stages and therefore must be used. Central lines must be removed after their need has subsided as infection of these portals will lead to a septic crisis.

In children and some adults, inhalation induction may be necessary before cannulation can be attempted. This must be considered a necessity, not a nicety, as these patients will undergo many more operations and must be given as much support as they need. Aseptic technique must be adhered to and cannulae placed through non-burned tissue if possible. If a large excision is contemplated, it is advisable to insert two large-bore cannulae (14 G in an adult). Due to the complexity of the anaesthesia and fluid management, two anaesthetists should be present at all operations. One should look after the anaesthetic management and the second should solely look after the fluid replacement and documentation. Both must communicate with each other and with the surgeon at all times.

Both invasive and non-invasive techniques are used to assess the required fluid replacement. Tachycardia is common in burned patients but in those with adequate analgesia a rate above 120 may be the earliest sign of hypovolaemia. This will be followed by reduced capillary refill and then hypotension. Finally, the urinary output will fall and the patient will become anuric.

Blood loss during the primary excision can be estimated by weighing swabs, colorimetric techniques and other methods but is difficult to assess accurately and is usually estimated on clinical grounds. On average, an excision will lose between 100 and 200 ml of blood per cent TBSA excised (Howie 1987, Dye 1993). Blood loss can be very rapid, especially in areas with little or no deep fascia, such as the shoulders, face, neck and buttock.

Positioning and handling

Both active and passive movements may be limited by pain, scarring or contractures. Thus positioning and handling of these patients becomes very important. It is recommended that the patient should be anaesthetized on the ward bed and then transferred to the operating table. Similarly, the patient should be placed on the ward bed before the termination of the anaesthetic.

The surgeon may require the patient to be placed in any position. The airway and the intravenous access sites must be guarded and carefully watched throughout the procedure. Previous graft sites may be vulnerable to damage; bony prominences may be left unprotected, being only covered by burned tissue; the eyes may not close and may need to be protected with ointment and covers. Care must also be taken when repositioning the patient during and after the operation.

ANAESTHESIA

Whilst there is no single technique that may be regarded as ideal, a number of general principles apply. Skin grafting or free-tissue transfers must not be jeopardized by poor perfusion during or after anaesthesia. The use of hypotensive techniques, smooth balanced anaesthesia and excellent analgesia with good fluid replacement will contribute to a successful outcome and will avoid anaesthesia being blamed for poor surgical technique (Rylah & Underwood 1992).

Induction of anaesthesia

Non-invasive monitoring should be placed in situ prior to induction of anaesthesia. The hypermetabolic patient will become desaturated very quickly and should receive preoxygenation. If the trachea is assessed as being easy to intubate, fentanyl at 3–5 µg/kg body weight may be given by slow intravenous injection. This may be followed with an induction dose of propofol (1–2 mg/kg). This technique will allow for rapid recovery and minimize postoperative cognitive disturbances. Lignocaine 1% (1–1.5 mg/kg) may be given prior to induction to depress the cardiac response to intubation and enhance the potency of fentanyl. Droperidol may also be administered as an antiemetic (10–20 µg/kg).

The laryngeal mask may be used for shorter procedures but intubation can be facilitated with a competitive muscle relaxant. Suxamethonium is contraindicated. The area of proposed surgery will dictate the positioning of the tracheal tube. Securing the tube may prove difficult especially with facial burns. Suturing the tube to the teeth may be the only safe alternative available (Jensen & Kealey 1992).

Inhalational induction of anaesthesia may be necessary if venous access proves impossible with an awake adult or child. The possibility of a difficult airway has been discussed (see above).

Maintenance

Controlled ventilation, facilitated with muscle relaxation, is the method of choice for all but the shortest procedures, i.e. dressing changes. This technique reduces oxygen consumption and makes it possible to increase the minute volume to ensure that normal carbon dioxide levels are maintained in these highly catabolic patients. The anaesthetist will have to cope with poor gaseous exchange and a low compliance during the early phases and may require positive end-expiratory pressure (PEEP) and other ventilatory adjuncts to maintain oxygenation. The effects of positive pressure ventilation, PEEP and hypovolaemia may summate to have a deleterious effect on the cardiac output and renal function and must be avoided by ensuring adequate intravascular volume.

The burned patient has a relative resistance to competitive muscle relaxants (Martyn et al 1983). Accumulation of tubocurarine and pancuronium may make reversal difficult as large doses may need to be given. The newer generation of relaxants (atracurium, vecuronium and mivacurium) easily overcome this problem. Theoretically, larger doses of vecuronium may accumulate but in practice this does not seem to occur.

Inhalation agents may be used to provide balanced anaesthesia, enflurane and isoflurane being quickly excreted. Recovery after desflurane anaesthesia would be expected to be quicker, though this has yet to be shown in this group of patients. Halothane may prolong the recovery period enough to interfere with nutrition. Despite reports of halothane having no adverse effects when used for repeated anaesthesia in this group of patients (Gronert et al 1968), it is wise to avoid its use now that there are better agents available. The prolonged or repeated use of nitrous oxide may decrease erythropoesis by inhibition of vitamin B_{12} but this can be overcome by hydroxycobalamin injection if thought to be a problem. Nitrous oxide and oxygen may be substituted by an air and oxygen mix if this is available. The current revival in circle systems with a carbon dioxide absorber will reduce theatre pollution, warm and humidify the inspired gases and decrease the amount of inhalation agent used.

Reversal of the muscle relaxant is usually not necessary but all the common techniques may be used. It is humane to complete the dressings and place the patient on the ward bed before terminating anaesthesia.

Monitoring

Conventional monitoring techniques may be difficult or impossible to use on patients with major burns. The level of monitoring should match the severity of the injury but sometimes decisions may rest with clinical acumen alone.

Electrocardiography may require steel sutures or staples to be placed through burned tissue as adhesive electrodes will not adhere to the wound or skin. Oesophageal electrodes are an expensive alternative. The positioning of the pulse oximetry probe may be difficult and sites such as the tongue, the nares, the penis and the labia have all been used.

As surgery may involve all limbs, rotation of the non-invasive blood pressure cuff may be necessary. The Finapres (Ohmeda) may be used where a digit is available, giving both blood pressure and beat-to-beat variation. Invasive arterial monitoring is essential in large burns or when using hypotensive techniques as it will give beat-to-beat information and allow sampling of arterial blood gases (including haemoglobin estimation) during the operative procedure.

Central venous cannulation will give limited data. It would be better to place a pulmonary artery catheter enabling cardiac output and pulmonary occlusion pressures to be obtained. Either must be removed when no longer of vital use as catheter-related sepsis is common. Large-bore central catheters will be of great assistance when faced with massive fluid and blood loss perioperatively.

All patients with major burns will have a urinary catheter. Adequate fluid replacement will ensure a good urine output but a decreased output is a late sign of inadequate replacement. Temperature control is a major problem and heat loss can be enormous. Both core and peripheral temperatures must be monitored. Heat loss is minimized by warming all fluid, especially those used to prepare the skin for surgery. The thermoneutral temperature for these patients is between 31°C and 33°C (Wilmore et al 1982). This would be extremely uncomfortable for the working staff. A compromise of between 27°C and 30°C is usually made. All areas not being operated upon must be covered; overhead heaters and heating blankets should be used, especially on children; and simply covering the head will make a noticeable difference. A falling peripheral temperature may be due to an inadequate plasma volume if the core temperature is remaining static.

POSTOPERATIVE CARE

Excellent analgesia during the operation is imperative and a relative overdose must not be reversed with antagonists. It is better to support ventilation for a few hours than to reverse analgesia and subject the patient to the subsequent pain or discomfort that will ensue. If the patient awakes complaining of pain, an opioid should be titrated intravenously to obtain the required effect.

The anaesthetic management will have ensured that the patient returns from theatre in the best possible state. However, it is likely that there has been a large blood loss, that the patient's temperature has fallen and that nutrition has been interrupted. Normal postoperative monitoring must be instituted with the addition of the invasive techniques used during the operation. Blood is given to replace that lost and that which will continue to be lost from the wounds as erythropoesis is inhibited and this loss will not be regenerated by the normal means. Clotting studies will indicate whether fresh frozen plasma or platelet concentrate needs to be administered but this is not a substitute for good surgical haemostasis. Fluid replacement is given to ensure a urine output of 0.5 ml/kg per hour usually in the form of dextrose 4% with saline 0.18%. Volume can be replaced with 4.5% human albumin solution BP or 6% hetastarch solution BP.

Rewarming the patient is another priority in the recovery phase. This will decrease shivering and thus oxygen consumption; it will also reverse the anticoagulant effect of hypothermia. Nutrition should be started as soon as possible, usually via a fine-bore nasogastric tube.

It is imperative that experienced staff look after these patients. Occult bleeding is common and a distinction has to be made early as to whether this is surgical or haematological in origin. Despite the immensity of the operation, with good anaesthetic management the patient may be eating within an hour or two of awakening.

Hypotensive techniques

Hypotensive anaesthesia will facilitate reconstructive surgery by improving the operative field; in so doing it will decrease operative time, limit blood loss and enable better use from the limited resources of the blood bank. The physiological effects of induced hypotension are well documented and the risks involved must be calculated individually against the perceived benefits. In skilled hands these techniques are remarkably safe.

The cornerstone to a successful hypotensive anaesthetic is good analgesia, an unimpeded airway and reliable monitoring. There are many techniques available and the reader is referred to a specialist review (Enderby 1985). However, the use of moderate doses of fentanyl (5–10 µg/kg) and droperidol (50–75 µg/kg) given prior to induction will produce a moderate fall in blood pressure without the effect extending into the postoperative period, as will controlled ventilation using tubocurare as the muscle relaxant of choice. Other techniques may involve the use of ganglion-blocking drugs such as pentolinium and trimetaphan, while in some instances sodium nitroprusside and hydrallazine may be necessary. Hypotension may also be produced by the use of drugs with combined α- and β-adrenergic blocking properties.

Invasive arterial monitoring is mandatory when mean arterial pressures of 50 mmHg are attempted. ST segment analysis would be advantageous, if available. The non-invasive Finapres (Ohmeda) gives beat-to-beat waveforms and pressures and may be an alternative to an invasive technique.

Local and regional analgesia

Infiltration of donor sites with local anaesthetic agents with a vasoconstrictor will reduce both the blood loss and the pain produced by these wounds. If the donor site is small, topical application of EMLA cream (Astra) is highly effective if anaesthesia is not indicated.

The burn wound is classified as an infected area. Thus peripheral nerve blocks and regional techniques are relatively contraindicated as the risk of introducing infection is high. If the burn is small and the area limited such as a hand burn, a brachial block may be contemplated (Randalls 1990).

During the reconstructive phase, when these patients are no longer considered as potentially infected cases, local and regional techniques may be used. The sympathetic blockade produced will increase blood flow to grafts and dilate vessels, facilitating free tissue transfers. The limits for these techniques is the same as in other branches of surgery, namely patient acceptability, length of operation, site of operation, allowing time for the block to be effective and recognizing the potential for toxicity or overdose of local analgesic agent.

ANALGESIA

Thermal injury can produce severe and protracted pain and discomfort. There is a wide variation in the perception of pain between patients and in a single patient over the course of treatment. It is vital to understand the different components of pain which are produced by the burn injury so that rational and effective therapy can be provided during the different phases of treatment (Choiniere 1989, Kinsella & Booth 1991).

Whilst full-thickness injury destroys the pain nerve endings and may therefore be pain free, partial-thickness wounds may be agonizingly painful. Most injuries have a mixed depth and therefore are painful. Pain has been shown to increase with the %TBSA full-thickness injury (Atchison et al 1991), the pain being constant in nature and exacerbated by movement. Donor sites produce a similar pain to a superficial or partial-thickness burn and have been reported as being more painful than the site of injury.

Therapeutic procedures such as dressing changes, debridement and physiotherapy may be excruciatingly painful and may be necessary for months after the injury has occurred. The intensity of the pain seems not to decrease with time, sometimes increasing due to a lowering of the pain threshold or other psychological factors including depression.

The healing process itself can result in areas of hyperaesthesia, para-aesthesia and severe itching. These can lead to marked discomfort and have been known to lead to severe responses by the patient, including suicide. Itching can be countered by the use of a partial agonist such as buprenorphine or nalbuphine. If analgesia is not required, naloxone can be used.

The psychological effect of the injury must not be forgotten. The pain, fear, helplessness and dependency, coupled with the possibility of deformities, scarring and even death, will result in depression, distress, lethargy and other psychological manifestations. These manifestations will be exacerbated by pain. It is therefore essential to ensure that excellent analgesia and psychological support are given from the outset to prevent any loss of confidence by the patient in the burn team.

Pain severity is measured objectively to obtain information about efficacy of technique. There are many methods available, such as the visual analogue scales. Treatment is based upon the results. Preconceived ideas relating to addiction, tolerance, and the nature and history of the pain often result in these patients not being given adequate doses or strong enough drugs to cope with the intensity of their problem. Opioid requirements may increase with time due to tolerance occurring and some physical dependence may be evident, but it is rare for a psychological dependence to occur in this group of patients.

Debridement, escharotomy and the taking of the donor skin are painful (usually increasing the area and the sites of pain). The recurrent painful, distressing, and sometimes degrading procedures of debriding, grafting and dressing changes necessitate the use of the best postoperative pain relief techniques available. Strong analgesics are needed and intravenous opiate or opioids should be used. With the fluid shifts that these patients encounter, intramuscular or subcutaneous injection is unreliable. Slow-release oral preparations are extremely useful in the longer-term management of pain. In the shorter term, patient-controlled analgesia is the method of choice if not limited by age, understanding or disability. These machines can usually have their trigger mechanisms adapted to allow most patients to benefit. This will return a degree of autonomy to the patient which is important for his self-image. If the patient cannot operate such a machine, a continual background infusion would be preferable to intermittent intramuscular injections as these will have a variable effect due to the cardiovascular instability experienced after surgery.

A technique for anaesthesia for burn dressing has already been mentioned (see above). However, relative analgesia has been used with the injection of fentanyl, alfentanil or other opioids and self-administration of Entonox with or without enflurane. Alternative therapies such as hypnosis and acupuncture have been tried with varying success but can be very time consuming and labour intensive.

The pharmacokinetics of the opioids is altered in burns. The high metabolic rate, increased cardiac output and liver blood flow lead to higher doses being required than in the general surgical population. However, this is a complicated picture and these are not the only component factors. Fentanyl and alfentanil are excellent analgesics for use in burns. Morphine can also be used, but the accumulation of its metabolites may cause long-standing disorientation and renal impairment, especially if used for sedation in the intensive care unit.

Once the patient can tolerate oral medication, slow-release oral morphine preparations are excellent for the relief of background pain. Finally, non-steroidal anti-inflammatory drugs may be used for short terms but their toxicity must be kept in mind when using them for more than a few days.

PHARMACOKINETICS AND PHARMACODYNAMICS

A burn of over 20% TBSA results in an altered pharmacological profile for the majority of drugs. As previously mentioned there are many reasons, mostly unknown. The inter- and intra-patient variation makes studies of this group very difficult (Martyn 1990).

The loss of vascular integrity results in a redistribution of both fluid and protein throughout the body. There is a two- to three-fold increase in α_1-acid glycoprotein and albumin levels may be decreased by half. This will result in a changed free fraction of the drug, which will either increase or decrease the effect. The result of the albumin loss is the relative reduction of protein binding of any acidic or neutral drugs that are administered and therefore an increase in their volume of distribution. Thus albumin-bound drugs such as diazepam, phenytoin and salicylic acid will increase their potency while α_1-acid glycoprotein-bound drugs will have a relative de-creased effect (i.e. lignocaine, propranolol and pethidine). The pathologi-cal process and the aggressive fluid resuscitation together with some hypoperfusion, oedema formation, hypoxaemia and the production of tox-ins from the burn wound will affect cardiovascular function, the central nervous system, the liver, the kidneys, and the gastrointestinal tract. These will all contribute to the altered efficacy and pharmacological profile of any administered drugs.

Phase I hepatic metabolism is depressed and the drugs metabolized by the liver will have a prolonged half-life (lignocaine and pethidine). In con-trast, phase II reactions, exemplified by lorazepam and morphine, are unimpaired and will therefore be unaltered by the burn injury (Bonate 1990). Thus the complicated assessment of drug efficacy in a burned pa-tient is shown above in the effects the injury has on pethidine and lignocaine. The surest way to administer drugs is by intravenous injection and to monitor the effect or level of the drug.

During the hypermetabolic phase the increased cardiac output results in a supernormal organ perfusion, resulting in a more rapid uptake and clearance. The volume of distribution will be altered by the formation of oedema and the loss of fluid from the wound. Enzyme induction may occur through the ad-ministration of one drug altering the efficacy of other prescribed agents.

Opioids

Clinically, the requirements of opioids by burned patients is very high and has been shown to increase with the severity of the injury. Studies have shown that clearance is similar to controls but because of the wide variations in these patients it has been impossible to show any other trends that can be used practically. The amount of the chosen analgesic is that which is enough to give the required effect in that patient and at that time.

Induction agents

The increased metabolic rate and cardiac output result in a fast onset of anaesthesia as arm/brain circulation time is greatly decreased. These patients must be considered to be hypovolaemic and, as with all critically ill patients, induction must be carried out with extra care. The rapid recovery from propofol makes it the obvious choice but it must be used carefully by skilled operators. The extreme bradycardia that may occur with propofol combined with fentanyl is uncommon as these patients have a high resting pulse rate due to their increased metabolic rate, thus the relative fall in pulse rate is less significant but can be reversed with atropine if necessary.

Volatile agents

Increased liver blood flow may be the reason behind the safe use of halothane in this group. However, the use of agents with little or no postoperative side-effects are preferred in patients needing to feed soon after their operation.

Muscle relaxants

Suxamethonium, a depolarizing relaxant, is contraindicated in burns in all but the first 48 h. Administration after this time may produce an acute hyperkalaemia resulting in cardiac arrest and death (Gronert & Theye 1975). This sensitivity lasts until skin coverage is complete and healed. However, it has been shown to be present over 2 years post burn and should be avoided in all patients who have sustained a large burn (Martyn et al 1982). The effect of suxamethonium may also be enhanced by the decreased levels of plasma cholinesterase as a result of decreased production.

Conversely, there is a resistance to the competitive muscle relaxants, resulting in a two- to five-fold requirement increase. This increase reaches a maximum 2 weeks post burn and gradually falls as the burn wound heals. Many theories are put forward for this effect, including changed drug binding, increased acetylcholine receptors, burn toxins, inhibitory substances present in the plasma and all the common effects previously mentioned.

PAEDIATRIC BURNS

Thermal injury in the child is a common occurrence, accounting for up to 40% of burn admissions. Most of these are minor scalds but even these can be life threatening if sepsis develops. Children are not just small adults, especially when burned. There are many differences to be considered.

Throughout childhood, the body surface area-to-weight ratio is increased, tending towards the adult ratio the older the child gets. This results in a more severe physiological response to the burn injury. The rise in temperature may cause febrile convulsions and it may be necessary to actively cool the child. The resuscitation formulae must be adjusted to the needs of the child. Drug dosage, fluid requirements and nutritional needs are more accurately assessed if based on the surface area rather than the weight.

The inability to communicate well in the younger child will present the anaesthetist with a frightened, often crying, child at the preoperative visit. It is important to attempt to gain the child's confidence at this time.

As intravenous access may be difficult, an inhalation induction can be performed and a cannula placed into a vein after the child is asleep. The use of EMLA cream (Astra) will help allay further fears associated with blood sampling and intravenous cannulation. Heat loss is greater in the child because of the greater surface area-to-weight ratio, thin skin and higher cardiac output. Every effort must be made to maintain normal temperatures during surgery. Smaller children can be operated upon under infrared heaters. Intraoperative monitoring may prove difficult, as previously mentioned, but the size of the patient will add to these difficulties. Fluid replacement, blood loss and drugs will need special care as these will be affected by the basal temperature, the cardiac output, the size of the burn, the size of the child and the nutritional status. The nutritional requirements are high and preoperative starvation should be kept to an absolute minimum. Hypoglycaemia is common in very small children and must be guarded against by constant monitoring and an adequate dextrose infusion.

Ketamine has been used in children as the occurrence of postoperative problems associated with hallucinations is reported to be low. This may be due to inadequacy of communication skills in the child. Other techniques are preferred that will ensure minimal starvation, swift recovery and early feeding.

Blood loss, when over 10% of the estimated blood volume, should be replaced, as erythropoesis is impaired and there is an increased need of good oxygen transport so that healing will be satisfactory.

Pain relief should be measured objectively. Smiling faces instead of the visual analogue scale may prove successful. A child can be taught to use a patient controlled analgesic device if of school age (Gaukroger et al 1991). Oral analgesics should be instituted as early as possible. Many novel ways of administering analgesia have been tried, all with some success. These include fentanyl lollipops, fentanyl skin patches and intranasal fentanyl. Some of these are now commercially available.

SUMMARY

The burn patient can present the anaesthetist with a formidable challenge. Airway management may be extremely difficult. Blood and heat loss, if not attended to with care, may cause the anaesthetist to stop the procedure. Intravenous access may test the skill and patience, whilst monitoring difficulties may mean improvisation and the need for clinical acumen. In all, the anaesthetist can play a very significant part in the treatment and healing of the burned patient by being thoughtful, careful and skillful.

REFERENCES

Atchison N E, Osgood P F, Carr D B, Szylfelbein S K 1991. Pain during burn dressing change in children: relationship to burn area, depth and analgesic regimens. Pain 47: 41–45

Bonate P L 1990 Pathophysiology and pharmacokinetics following burn injury. Clin Pharmacokinet 18: 391–395

Choiniere M 1989 The pain of burns. In: Wall P D, Melzack R (eds) Textbook of pain, (2nd edn). Churchill Livingstone, Edinburgh.

Deitch E A 1990 The management of burns. N Engl J Med 323: 1249–1253

Dye D J 1993 Requirement for crossed matched blood in burns surgery. Burns 19: 524–528

Eckhauser F E, Billote J, Burke J F, Quinby W C 1974 Tracheostomy complicating massive burn injury: a plea for conservation. Am J Surg 126: 418–423

Enderby G E H 1985. Hypotensive anaesthesia. Churchill Livingstone, Edinburgh.

Frame J D, Taweepoke P, Moieman N, Rylah L 1990 Immediate fascial flap reconstruction of joints and use of Biobrane in the burned limb. Burns 16: 381–384

Gaukroger P B, Chapman M J, Davey R B 1991 Pain control in paediatric burns: the use of patient controlled analgesia. Burns 17: 396–399

Goudsouzian N, Szyfelbein S K 1985. Management of the upper airway following burns. In Martyn J A J (ed) Acute management of the burned patient. Saunders, Philadelphia, pp 46–65

Gronert G A, Schauer P I, Gunter R C 1968 Multiple anaesthesia in burned patients. JAMA 205: 878

Gronert G A, Theye R A 1975 Pathophysiology of hyperkalaemia induced by succinylcholine. Anaesthesiology 43: 89–99

Herndon D N, Barrow R E, Rutan R L et al 1989 A comparison versus early excision therapies in severely burned patients. Ann Surg 209: 547–553

Howie C C M 1987. Anaesthesia for grafting procedures. In: Judkins K C (ed) Baillière's clinical anesthesiology, Baillière Tindall, London, Vol. 1, pp 619–633

Hu Y P, Ho S T, Wang J J et al 1993 Evaluation of gastric emptying in severe burn injured patients. Crit Care Med 21: 527–531

Hunt J L, Monafo W W, Purdue G F, Rylah L T A 1992 Resuscitation S F major burns. In: Rylah L T A (ed) Critical care of the burned patient. Cambridge University Press, Cambridge, pp 44–58

Janzekovic Z 1975 A new concept in early excision and immediate grafting of burns. J Trauma 15: 42–62

Jensen N F, Kealey G P 1992 Securing an endotracheal tube in the presence of facial burns or instability. (Letter.) Anaesth Analg 75: 641–642

Kinsella J, Booth M G 1991 Pain relief in burns. James Laing memorial essay 1990. Burns 17: 391–395

Martyn J A J, Matteo R S, Szyfelbein S K, Kaplan R F 1982 Unprecedented resistance to neuromuscular blocking effects of metocurine with persistence after complete recovery in a burned patient. Anesth Analg 61: 614–617

Martyn J A J, Goldhill D R, Goudsouzian N G 1983. Clinical pharmacology of neuromuscular relaxants in patients with burns. J Clin Pharmacol 26: 680–685

Martyn J A J 1990 Clinical pharmacology and therapeutics in burns. In: Martyn J A J (ed) Acute management of the burned patient. Saunders, Philadelphia, pp 180–200

Milner S M, Bennet J, Rylah L T A 1995 The advanced burn wheel. Burns (in press)

Muller M J, Herndon D N 1994. The Challenge of Burns. Lancet i: 216–220

Randalls B 1990 Continual brachial plexus blockade: a case report. Anaesthesia 45: 143–144

Russell R, Judkins K C 1990 The laryngeal mask airway and facial burns. (Letter.) Anaesthesia 45: 894

Rylah L T A 1989. 'Diprivan' in a regional burns unit. Diprivan Casebook, Vol 2, No 1. ICI.

Rylah L T A, Underwood S M 1992 In: Rylah L T A (ed) Critical care of the burned patient. Cambridge University Press, Cambridge, pp 137–149

Wilmore D W, Mason A D, Johnson D W, Pruitt B A 1982 Effect of ambient temperature on heat loss in burned patients. J Appl Physiol 38: 593–597

14

Update

L. Kaufman

ABDOMINAL ANAESTHESIA

Smith et al (1993) found that in a study of nearly 800 cases of upper gastrointestinal endoscopy many endoscopists were using unnecessarily large doses of intravenous sedation. Satisfactory conditions were provided with a mean dose of 4.65 mg of midazolam given as a bolus intravenously in sedating patients under 70 years of age, but in patients over 70 the mean dose was as little as 1.89 mg. Topical pharyngeal analgesia was not required.

There have been many studies suggesting that requirements of drugs depend on the underlying medical disorder such as chronic inflammatory bowel disease. Gesink-van der Veer et al (1993) found increased requirements of alfentanil during abdominal surgery in patients with Crohn's disease and suggested this was due to a change in pharmacodynamics, but Crohn's disease has little effect on pharmacokinetics. This was based on a small series of cases, but in the author's experience in over 100 cases of Crohn's disease alfentanil requirements were similar in patients undergoing major abdominal surgery either for Crohn's disease, ulcerative colitis or carcinoma.

In the management of patients prior to abdominal surgery the bowel is prepared either by purging or even by the use of antibiotics. It is interesting to note that respiratory tract infection is very common in patients requiring ventilation in intensive care units and that selective decontamination of the alimentary tract reduces the incidence of infection in the lungs by 63% (Selective Decontamination of the Digestive Tract Trialists' Collaborative Group 1993).

Reservations have been expressed about the use of nitrous oxide in colonic surgery, in that nitrous oxide might distend the bowel during operation and may even prolong postoperative convalescence. But in a controlled trial Krogh et al (1994) were unable to confirm the deleterious effects of nitrous oxide on the outcome of colonic surgery.

Rodriguez & Jick (1994) are aware that non-steroidal anti-inflammatory drugs (NSAIDs) increase the risk of upper gastric intestinal bleeding and perforation; risk factors include advanced age, smoking, history of peptic ulcer and the use of oral steroids or anticoagulants. Langman et al (1994) only advocate the use of NSAIDs when other analgesics have failed and the least toxic NSAID should be used in the lowest possible dosage. Apparently ibuprofen is the least toxic of the NSAIDs, whereas piroxicam and azapropazone are much more hazardous (Bateman 1994).

REFERENCES

Bateman D N 1994 NSAIDs: time to re-evaluate gut toxicity. Lancet 343: 1051–1052
Gesink-van der Veer B J, Burm A G L, Vletter A A, Bovill J G 1993 Influence of Crohn's disease on the pharmacokinetics and pharmacodynamics of alfentanil. Br J Anaesth 71: 827–834
Krogh B, Jern Jensen P, Henneberg S W et al 1994 Nitrous oxide does not influence operating conditions or postoperative course in colonic surgery. Br J Anaesth 72: 55–57
Langman M J S, Weil J, Wainwright P et al 1994 Risks of bleeding peptic ulcer associated with individual non-steroidal anti-inflammatory drugs. Lancet 343: 1075–1078
Rodriguez L A G, Jick H 1994 Risk of upper gastrointestinal bleeding and perforation associated with individual non-steroidal anti-inflammatory drugs. Lancet 343: 769–772
Selective Decontamination of the Digestive Tract Trialists' Collaborative Group 1993 Meta-analysis of randomised controlled trials of selective decontamination of the digestive tract. Br Med J 307: 525–532
Smith M R, Bell G D, Quine M A et al 1993 Small bolus injections of intravenous midazolam for upper gastrointestinal endoscopy: a study of 788 consecutive cases. Br J Clin Pharmacol 36: 573–578

MUSCLE RELAXANTS

Rocuronium

The proceedings of a workshop on rocuronium bromide held in 1993 have been published in a supplement of the *European Journal of Anaesthesiology* (Denissen et al 1994). Rocuronium is a non-depolarizing muscle relaxant whose onset appears to be as rapid as suxamethonium but without many of its side effects. Intubation conditions are described as being satisfactory and it is said there are no major side effects. The cardiovascular system is said to be stable, although some investigators have reported tachycardia. Histamine is not released and elimination is primarily by the biliary system and does not depend on the kidney for excretion. Duration of action is 20–35 min and it is effectively antagonized by both edrophonium and neostigmine. It appears to be of value in the rapid induction of anaesthesia and may replace suxamethonium, especially when that drug is contraindicated. It lowers intraocular pressure and therefore it may be suitable for perforated eye injury, and as it has little effect on intracranial pressure it may have a place in neurosurgery.

Harper et al (1994) studied the effect of neostigmine on reversing atracurium. They found that 20 µg/kg was the optimum dose for antagonizing light blockade (40–50% recovery) and 40 µg/kg for profound blockade (5–10% recovery). No benefit was achieved by increasing the dose to 80 µg/kg.

REFERENCES

Denissen P A F, Wierda J M K H, Vickers M D (eds) 1994 Rocuronium bromide
investigators' workshop. Eur J Anaesth 11 (Suppl 9): 1–140
Harper N J N, Wallace M, Hall I A 1994 Optimum dose of neostigmine at two levels of
atracurium-induced neuromuscular block. Br J Anaesth 72: 82–85

PHAEOCHROMOCYTOMA

Neumann et al (1993) have drawn attention to the fact that phaeochromocytoma is present in two autosomal disorders: (1) multiple endocrine
malignancy (medullary thyroid carcinoma, hyperparathyroidism); and
(2) von Hippel-Lindau disease (angioma of the retina, central nervous
haemangioblastoma, renal cell carcinoma, pancreatic cysts and cysto-
adenoma of the epididymus).

It is inevitable that the virtues of new agents should be exploited in the
management of phaeochromocytoma. Lippmann et al (1994) described the
use of desflurane, which seems a surprising choice in that it stimulates
sympathetic activity. During induction, when 3% desflurane was administered the blood pressure decreased to 70/40 mmHg, while during removal
of the tumour the blood pressure reached 190/120 mmHg despite an increase in the concentration of desflurane to 8%.

REFERENCES

Lippmann M, Ford M, Lee C et al 1994 Use of desflurane during resection of
phaeochromocytoma. Br J Anaesth 72: 707–709
Neumann H P H, Berger D P, Sigmund G, Blum U et al 1993 Pheochromocytomas,
multiple endocrine neoplasia type 2, and von Hippel–Lindau disease. N Engl J Med
329: 1531–1538

INTRAVENOUS THERAPY

Hyponatraemia not infrequently results from the postoperative use of
hypotonic fluids (Arieff et al 1992, Sterns 1987). Other causes include the
use of hypotonic fluids during transurethral prostatectomy and endometrial
ablation. Morbidity is high in children and in menstruant women. Morbidity increases when there are signs of hyponatraemic encephalopathy,
which results in oedema of the brain, respiratory insufficiency and
hypoxaemia. Treatment includes the use of hypertonic sodium chloride
(514 mmol) together with a loop diuretic such as frusemide. The serum
sodium should not be increased by more than 25 mmol in the initial 24–
48 h of treatment (Arieff 1993).

REFERENCES

Arieff A I, Ayus J C, Fraser C L 1992 Hyponatraemia and death or permanent brain
damage in healthy children. Br Med J 304: 1218–1222

Arieff A I 1993 Management of hyponatraemia. Br Med J 307: 305–308
Sterens R H 1987 Severe symptomatic hyponatremia: treatment and outcome: a study of
   64 cases. Ann Intern Med 107: 656–664

BLOOD TRANSFUSION

Royston (1993) has discussed means of reducing perioperative bleeding.
The choice is between lysine analogues such as tranexamic acid and ε-
aminocaproic acid and the serine protease inhibitors such as aprotinin,
nefamostat and gabexate. Both groups of drugs appear equally effective
although the cost of the former is less.

Errors in blood transfusion in Britain have been highlighted by McClelland
& Phillips (1994), most being due to errors in labelling samples for testing or
failure to identify the patient with his own blood group. Most of the deaths are
due to ABO incompatibility and in one study 1 in 3330 patients received
ABO-incompatible blood (Contreras & de Silva 1994).

There have been many studies suggesting that blood transfusion has
influenced the outcome of patients undergoing surgery for colorectal
cancer. Houbiers et al (1994), however, have shown conclusively that the
recurrence rate of carcinoma was not influenced by blood transfusion, but
the 3-year survival rate of patients who had blood was lower than non-
transfused patients. The reduced survival rate was attributed to infection,
especially in patients who received more than 3 units of blood.

REFERENCES

Contreras M, de Silva M 1994 Preventing incompatible tranfusions. Br Med J 308:
   1180–1181
Houbiers J G A, Brand A, van de Watering L M G et al 1994 Randomized controlled
   trial comparing transfusion of leucocyte-depleted or buffy-coat-depleted blood in
   surgery for colorectal cancer. Lancet 344: 573–578
McClelland D B L, Phillips P 1994 Errors in blood transfusion in Britain: survey of
   hospital haematology departments. Br Med J 308: 1205–1206
Royston D 1993 Perioperative bleeding: drugs for surgical blood loss. Lancet 341: 1629

SPINAL AND EXTRADURAL

Standl & Beck (1993) have studied radiologically the position of 28 gauge
spinal catheters inserted intrathecally and suggest that the catheter should
be inserted with the patient in the sitting position and the depth of insertion should not exceed 4 cm.

REFERENCE

Standl T, Beck H 1993 Radiological examination of the intrathecal position of micro-
   catheters in continuous spinal anaesthesia. Br J Anaesth 71: 803–806

EXTRAVASATION INJURIES

Gault (1993) has outlined in detail the management of extravasation injuries and this has been reiterated by Martin et al (1994), who agreed that when extravasation of drugs occurs in subcutaneous tissues active management is indicated. The manufacturer's data sheets, especially of cytotoxic drugs, should be followed closely: these agents should be given as a bolus injection into a fast-running intravenous drip, preferably into a large vein and not one on the dorsum of the hand. Results of soft tissue injury are usually more than observed initially and treatment should not be delayed. This involves washing out the tissues with saline and liposuction. Stanley & Root (1992) also suggest the use of intravenous hydrocortisone and injecting hydrocortisone subcutaneously around the margins of the extravasation. Hyaluronidase should be avoided with vesicant drugs to avoid encouraging their spread through tissues.

REFERENCES

Gault D T 1993 Extravasation injuries. Br J Plast Surg 46: 91–96
Martin P H, Carver H, Petros A J 1994 Use of liposuction and saline washout for the treatment of extensive subcutaneous extravasation of corrosive drugs. Br J Anaesth 72: 702–704
Stanley A, Root T 1992 Extravasation In: Allwood M, Wright P (eds) Cytotoxics handbook (2nd edn). Radcliffe Medical Press, Oxford, pp 77–89

PAEDIATRICS

Indomethacin has been used as a tocolytic agent and appears to have little effect on the neonate of 32 weeks' gestation. However, there is a high fetal morbidity in those born prior to 32 weeks and these include necrotizing enterocolitis, intracranial haemorrhage and patent ductus arteriosus (Norton et al 1993).

Fetal thoracic surgery is now more widely practised and the indications for surgical intervention are outlined by Adzick & Harrison (1994). Fetal movements may make the procedures more difficult, but this can be minimized by the use of muscle relaxants. Fan et al (1994) favoured the use of pipecuronium as pancuronium could lead to fetal tachycardia and absence of beat-to-beat variability.

Sudden infant death syndrome (SIDS)

The prone sleeping position has been advocated for many years, but it has recently been found to lead to an increase in SIDS, especially when the child's mattress contains natural fibre, there is a history of recent illness, there is heating in the bedroom and the child is wrapped in a sheet or light blanket (Ponsonby et al 1993, Poets & Southall 1993).

Neonatal anaemia

Anaemia is frequently present in premature infants who require repeated blood transfusions. Maier et al (1994) found that erythropoietin, given in the first 6 weeks of life, reduced the need for blood transfusion (see Strauss 1994).

Fetal monitoring

Bucher et al (1994) have drawn attention to errors in the interpretation of arterial oxygen saturation in neonates; when there is venous congestion (30–40 mmHg pressure) the veins may become pulsatile and give false readings of pSO_2 (oxygen saturation).

REFERENCES

Adzick N S, Harrison M R 1994 Fetal surgical therapy. Lancet 343: 897–902
Bucher H U, Keel M, Woolf M et al 1994 Artifactual pulse-oximetry estimation in neonates. Lancet 343: 1135–1136
Fan S Z, Susetio L, Tsai M C 1994 Neuromuscular blockade of the fetus with pancuronium or pipecuronium for intra-uterine procedures. Anaesthesia 49: 284–286
Maier R F, Obladen M, Scigalla P et al 1994 The effect of epoetin beta (recombinant human erythropoietin) on the need for transfusion in very-low-birth-weight infants. N Engl J Med 330: 1173–1178
Norton M E, Merrill J, Cooper B A B et al 1993 Neonatal complications after the administration of indomethacin for preterm labor. N Engl J Med 329: 1602–1607
Poets C F, Southall D P 1993 Prone sleeping position and sudden infant death. N Engl J Med 329: 425–426
Ponsonby A-L, Dwyer T, Gibbons L E et al 1993 Factors potentiating the risk of sudden infant death syndrome associated with the prone position. N Engl J Med 329: 377–382
Strauss R G 1994 Erythropoietin and neonatal anemia. N Engl J Med 330: 1227–1228

OBSTETRICS

Rodgers & Morgan (1994) have reiterated the possible dangers of anaesthetizing patients on tocolytic drugs, as exemplified by the β_2 agonists such as ritodrine, salbutamol and isoxuprine. Although they inhibit uterine contractions they have major cardiac effects, including tachycardia and hypokalaemia. In addition, to promote fetal maturity steroids are also given during late pregnancy, but they also cause salt and water retention. Ergometrine can cause arterial and venoconstriction. Oxytocin can cause salt and water retention and all these factors are likely to lead to pulmonary oedema.

Pulmonary oedema following the use of ritrodrine has also recently been reported by Clesham (1994), and this was previously discussed by Robertson (1982), whos reported a case of pulmonary oedema during induction of anaesthesia in a patient who was on ritodrine and high-dose steroids; she also reviewed the drug interactions and cardiovascular problems in patients on tocolytic agents.

Eisenmenger's syndrome

Patients with this syndrome are at a high degree of risk during pregnancy. Kahn (1993) has warned of the dangers of heparin to prevent pulmonary thromboemboli. He reported a case given heparin in the postpartum period who developed vaginal bleeding resulting in tachycardia and a decrease in systemic blood pressure, the patient dying presumably because the pulmonary artery pressure exceeded the systemic blood pressure. In a personal series of five cases of Eisenmenger's syndrome (four for obstetrics) all survived operative deliveries, although one patient died 1 week later following immersion in a hot bath, presumably from vasodilatation and hypotension. At postmortem there was a large ventriculoseptal defect.

Epilepsy

Antiepileptic drugs such as phenytoin, carbamazepine, phenobarbitone and primidone are enzyme inducers and may cause reduction in vitamin K-dependent clotting factors and therefore vitamin K_1 should be given at least a week prior to delivery (O'Brien & Gilmour-White 1993). There is an increase in fetal abnormalities in patients on antiepileptic drugs, especially hare lip and cleft palate and even congenital heart defects. Phenytoin appears to be implicated and carbamazepine appears to be the safest drug. Folic acid supplements may be necessary. For patients on oral contraceptives the dose should be increased.

REFERENCES

Clesham G J 1994 β-Adrenergic agonists and pulmonary oedema in preterm labour. Br Med J 308: 260–262
Kahn M L 1993 Eisenmenger's syndrome in pregnancy. N Engl J Med 329: 887–888
O'Brien M D, Gilmour-White S 1993 Epilepsy and pregnancy. Br Med J 307: 492–495
Robertson M J S 1982 Pulmonary oedema: recent developments. In Kaufman L (ed) Anaesthesia review 2. Churchill Livingstone, Edinburgh pp 55–64
Rodgers S J, Morgan M 1994 Tocolysis, $β_2$ agonists and anaesthesia. Anaesthesia 49: 185–187

PAIN

Control of pain relief following third molar surgery is still problematical, especially for day stay patients. Rectal NSAIDs are of great value. Moore et al (1994) considered the use of a morphine gel inserted into the tooth socket, but found it to be of no value. Hannington-Kiff & Dunne (1993) found that the topical application of 1% guanethidine to exposed dentine relieved the pain. They suggested that there was an anti-noradrenergic blockade.

For many years it was believed that opioids only acted centrally and it is of interest that Alexander Wood, who introduced the syringe in 1854, injected a painful spot with morphine. It is believed that opioid receptors are located on peripheral sensory nerve terminals and upregulated in the presence of inflammation. It has also been shown that endogenous opioid peptides are present in inflamed synovial tissue (Stein et al 1993). Tennant et al (1993) in fact found that topical morphine applied as a cream relieved localized pain when applied over painful areas on the back. Many agents, apart from analgesics, have been used in the management of chronic back pain and Filos et al (1993) have now reported on the use of a calcium antagonist, nimodipine, in the treatment of pain due to carcinoma.

Bromley & Woolf (1993) found that intravenous administration of morphine prior to surgical stimulation reduced the requirements for postoperative analgesia. This effect is not apparent with the use of local analgesia. Turner & Chalkiadis (1994) infiltrated the line of the incision with 1.5% lignocaine prior to appendicectomy and found that this had little effect on postoperative analgesic requirement. It is possible that the local anaesthetic solution had little effect on the pain due to peritoneal irritation.

REFERENCES

Bromley L M, Woolf C J 1993 Preoperative morphine pre-empts postoperative pain. Lancet 342: 73–75
Filos K S, Goudas L C, Patroni, Tassoudis V 1993 Analgesia with epidural nimodipine. Lancet 342: 1047
Hannington-Kiff J G, Dunne S M 1993 Topical guanethidine relieves dentinal hypersensitivity and pain. J R Soc Med 86: 514–515
Moore U J, Seymour R A, Gilroy J, Rawlins M D 1994 The efficacy of locally applied morphine in postoperative pain after bilateral third molar surgery. Br J Clin Pharmacol 37: 227–230
Stein C, Hassan A H S, Lehrberger K et al 1993 Local analgesic effect of endogenous opioid peptides. Lancet 343: 321–324
Tennant F, Moll D and DePaulo V 1993 Topical morphine for peripheral pain. Lancet 342: 1047–1048
Turner G A, Chalkiadis G 1994 Comparison of preoperative with postoperative lignocaine infiltration on postoperative analgesia requirements. Br J Anaesth 72: 541–543

ANALGESIC AGENTS

Morphine

Morphine can also be given transdermally; 10 mg of morphine given transdermally results in a constant plasma concentration over 11 h, although there was a considerable delay until the metabolites were detectable in the plasma (morphine-6-glucuronide and morphine-3-glucuronide). The non-analgesic effects of morphine were less pronounced than when the drug was given intravenously (Westerling et al 1994).

Fentanyl

Transdermal fentanyl is now available as 'duragesic', but there have been reports of deaths due to hypoventilation following its use for analgesia for relatively minor operations such as tonsillectomy and extraction of wisdom teeth. It is now recommended that the drug is not used transdermally in the management of acute or postoperative pain for outpatient surgery or for children under 12. Its use should be limited to severe chronic pain that cannot be controlled by less potent agents (McCarthy 1994).

Bell et al (1994) studied the effect of propofol and fentanyl anaesthesia in patients with low cardiac output undergoing cardiac surgery and found that arterial pressure fell by 20% although myocardial contractility was not adversely affected. However, the heart rate was slower in patients given propofol and low-dose fentanyl compared with midazolam and high-dose fentanyl. The affect on heart rate may be compounded if the patients are also given suxamethonium. In the presence of fentanyl vecuronium may cause profound bradycardia (Inoue & Reichelt 1987).

Alfentanil

Increased muscle rigidity has also been reported with alfentanil. Strong & Matson (1989) have reported a case of apparent seizure following the use of alfentanil. This was not confirmed by EEG.

Naloxone

Naloxone in high doses is known to have cardiovascular effects (class III), including antiarrhythmic activity in animals following coronary artery occlusion. However, the racemic mixture of naloxone had no clinical effect in man although studies of isomers suggest they may be of value (Oldroyd et al 1994).

REFERENCES

Bell J, Sartain J, Wilkinson G A L, Sherry K M 1994 Propofol and fentanyl anaesthesia for patients with low cardiac output state undergoing cardiac surgery: comparison with high-dose fentanyl anaesthesia. Br J Anaesth 73: 162–166
Inoue K, Reichelt W 1987 Combination of fentanyl, etomidate and vecuronium may cause severe vagotonic state. Br J Anaesth 59: 1475–1479
McCarthy M 1994 Fentanyl patch misuse. Lancet 343: 351
Oldroyd K G, Rankin A C, Gray C E et al 1994 Failure to reproduce the in vitro cardiac electrophysiological effects of naloxone in humans. Br J Clin Pharmacol 37: 289–294
Strong W E, Matson M 1989 Probable seizure after alfentanil. Anaesth Analg 68: 692–693
Westerling D, Hoglund P, Lundin S, Svedman P 1994 Transdermal administration of morphine to healthy subjects. Br J Clin Pharmacol 37: 571–576

ENDOCRINE

The mechanism for release of hormones in response to surgical stimulation is still unclear. Moore et al (1994) were unable to incriminate interleukin 6 (IL-6) during extradural anaesthesia. Crozier et al (1994) confirmed that IL-6 does not initiate the release of cortisol in response to surgical trauma under general anaesthesia. They were able to suppress the release of IL-6 with the administration of fentanyl, but unable to prevent the release of cortisol.

Guillou (1993) has discussed the biological variation in the development of sepsis following surgery or trauma. Within hours of major surgery there are increased levels of IL-1β and IL-6 and in uncomplicated cases the cytokine levels decline within 24 h. Monocytes release cytokines and prostaglandin E$_2$. There is a relationship between the development of postoperative sepsis and the 'monocyte expression of MHC class II antigens'. In patients who recover from severe trauma the HLA-DR expression returned to normal within 1 week, but in those who developed infection it took 3 weeks for it to return to normal levels, and in those who subsequently died it did not return to normal. The importance of the monocyte in the immune response to surgery is that it is mediated by the release of cytokines, especially IL-1, IL-6 interleukin-6 and tumour necrosis factor α, which appear to act on the hypothalamus, stimulating the synthesis and release of the corticotrophin-releasing hormone (CRF) (Reichlin 1993).

REFERENCES

Crozier T A, Muller J E, Quittkat D et al 1994 Effect of anaesthesia on the cytokine responses to abdominal surgery. Br J Anaesth 72: 280–285
Guillou P J 1993 Biological variation in the development of sepsis after surgery or trauma. Lancet 342: 217–220
Moore C M, Desborough J P, Powell H et al 1994 Effects of extradural anaesthesia on interleukin-6 and acute phase response to surgery. Br J Anaesth 72: 272–279
Reichlin S 1993 Neuroendocrine–immune interactions. N Engl J Med 329: 1246–1253

ANTIHISTAMINE AGENTS

Lorenz et al (1994) advocate the routine use of antihistamine agents such as dimetindene H$_1$ and cimetidine H$_2$ receptor blockers at operation. They found a high incidence of histamines release in patients who were anaesthetized with alcuronium, fentanyl, thiopentone and suxamethonium. The incidence of histamine-related problems was increased if patients also received haemaccel. In a commentary on this paper Dahl (1994) debated whether anaesthetists would in fact advocate the routine use of antihistamine agents or elect to administer drugs which are less likely to provoke histamine release. Preparations of haemaccel in the past were known to have a high incidence of allergic responses. Alcuronium is less used in the UK and fentanyl is known also to produce bradycardia. The incidence of complications seen by Lorenz et al (1994) is undoubtedly high and it would seem preferable to avoid the technique they advocate.

REFERENCES

Dahl J B 1994 Antihistamine prophylaxis and general anaesthesia. Lancet 343: 929–930
Lorenz W, Duda D, Wolfgang D et al 1994 Incidence and clinical importance of
  perioperative histamine release: randomised study of volume loading and antihista-
  mines after induction of anaesthesia. Lancet 343: 933–940

ANTIEMETICS

The mechanism of the emetic response has been outlined by Grunberg & Hesketh (1993). This involves the vomiting centre and the chemoreceptor trigger zone, which is outside the blood–brain barrier and which cannot initiate vomiting, but can only do so by stimulating the vomiting centre. Other afferent stimuli include the vestibular system, the pharynx and gastrointestinal tract and the higher brain stem and cortex. Histamine and acetylcholine may be involved in nausea and vomiting, while the nausea and vomiting resulting from morphine may be due to stimulation of delta or kappa receptors, although mu receptors have an antiemetic effect. D2 (dopamine) receptors do not appear to be involved in producing vomiting. $5-HT_3$ receptors are present not only in the gastrointestinal tract but also in the area postrema and in the nucleus of the tractus solitarius. $5-HT_3$ antagonists are effective antiemetic agents, not only in controlling chemotherapy-induced emesis but also in the management of postoperative nausea and vomiting. Although D2 receptors do not appear to be involved in initiating vomiting the D2 antagonist metopimazine was effective when given with the $5-HT_3$ antagonist ondansetron, and this combination is more effective than ondansetron alone (Herrstedt et al 1993). The anti-vomiting mechanism of steroids is still unknown and, again, when dexamethasone is given in combination with ondansetron it is more effective than ondansetron alone (Levitt et al 1993). Ondansetron clearance is mostly by hepatic phase I metabolism and it appears that cytochrome P-450 2D6 is not exclusively involved. In addition the fate of the drug is unaffected whether patients are poor or rapid metabolizers (Ashforth et al 1994).

Another antagonist recently marketed is granisetron (Kytril). The only side effects which have been reported are that of headache and a decrease in intestinal activity, which may simulate subacute intestinal obstruction.

REFERENCES

Ashforth I E L, Palmer J L, Bye A, Bedding A 1994 The pharmacokinetics of
  ondansetron after intravenous injection in healthy volunteers phenotyped as poor or
  extensive metabolisers of debrisoquine. Br J Clin Pharmacol 37: 389–391
Grunberg S M, Hesketh P J 1993 Control of chemotheraphy-induced emesis. N Engl J
  Med 329: 1790–1796
Herrstedt J, Sigsgaard T, Boesgaard M et al 1993 Ondansetron plus metopimazine
  compared with ondansetron alone in patients receiving moderately emetogenic
  chemotherapy. N Engl J Med 328: 1076–1080
Levitt M, Warr D, Yelle L et al 1993 Ondansetron compared with dexamethasone and
  metoclopramide as antiemetics in the chemotherapy of breast cancer with
  cyclophosphamide, methotrexate and fluorouracil. N Eng J Med 328: 1081–1084

APPARATUS

Spinal needles

Patel et al (1994) have compared the flow characteristics of spinal needles, 120 mm in length, and found that resistance to fluid flow of the 26-gauge Braun needle was twice that of the 27-gauge Becton-Dickinson needle. The result of this was that it took three times as long, when using the finer needle, for CSF to appear at the hub of the needle.

MC mask

Ooi et al (1992) have investigated the use of the MC mask for administration of nitrous oxide and oxygen to supplement analgesia in regional techniques. They found that the inspired concentration of nitrous oxide and oxygen were determined by the total fresh gas flow, the concentrations and the peak inspiratory flow rate. A mixture of equal portions of nitrous oxide and oxygen with a flow rate of 4–6 litres/min was recommended to achieve adequate oxygenation and nitrous oxide in a concentration of 20–30%.

REFERENCES

Ooi R, Joshi P, Soni N 1992 Nitrous oxide–oxygen analgesia: the performance of the MC mask delivery system. J R Soc Med 85: 534–536
Patel M, Samsoon G, Swami A, Morgan B M 1994 Flow characteristics of long spinal needles. Anaesthesia 49: 223–225

GENERAL ANAESTHETIC AGENTS

The celluar and molecular aspects of anaesthesia are discussed in great detail in a symposium in the postgraduate educational number of the *British Journal of Anaesthesia* 1993 (Halsey et al 1993).

Another intravenous agent, eltanolene (pregnanolone), may soon be available and this is three times more potent than propofol and six times more potent than thiopentone (Hemelrijck et al 1994).

Halothane

Smith et al (1993) have identified a carboxylesterase isozyme in human livers and found there were antibodies present in the sera of patients with halothane hepatitis. This antibody response is seen in patients with halothane hepatitis, but not in those exposed to halothane who do not develop hepatitis. The use of this isozyme may identify patients likely to develop halothane hepatitis.

Although halothane is often blamed for hepatitis in relation to operation there are many other causes such as viral hepatitis, vascular causes resulting in hepatic ischaemia, as well as many other toxins. Other idiosyncratic reactions may be due not only to halothane but also to sulphonamides and phenytoin, and even amiodarone (Tharakan et al 1993, see also O'Grady et al 1993). Hepatic failure results in encephalopathy and cerebral oedema, coagulopathy, hypotension, hypovolaemia and renal failure. There are also metabolic changes with hypoglycaemia, hypokalaemia and hyponatraemia. Oxygen extraction is decreased.

REFERENCES

Halsey M J, Prys Roberts C, Strunin L 1993 Receptors and transmembrane signalling: cellular and molecular aspects of anaesthesia. Br J Anaesth 71: 1
Hemelrijck J V, Muller P Van Aken H et al 1994 Relative potency of eltanolene, propofol and thiopentone for induction of anaesthesia. Anesthesiology 80: 36–41
O'Grady J G, Schalm S W, Williams R 1993 Acute liver failure: redefining the syndromes. Lancet 342: 273–275
Smith G C M, Kenna J G, Harrison D J et al 1993 Autoantibodies to hepatic microsomal carboxylesterase in halothane hepatitis. Lancet 342: 963–964
Tharakan J, Bannerjee D B, Smith D A, Carroll S 1993 Amiodarone-induced hepatic failure. Hosp Update (March) 180–182

BENZODIAZEPINE

The calcium channel blockers diltiazem and verapamil affect the metabolism of oral midazolam, resulting in prolonged and profound sedation. The action of midazolam is also prolonged in patients taking erythromycin and the mechanism of this is probably due to enzyme inhibition. Midazolam is metabolized in the liver by cytochrome P-450 IIIA. Diltiazem and verapamil inhibit hepatic cytochrome P-450 and also increase hepatic blood flow, which would reduce first-pass metabolism (Olkkola et al 1994).

Fever may lead to convulsions, especially in children, and oral diazepam given when the fever is present reduces the risk of recurrent febrile seizures (Rosman et al 1993).

REFERENCES

Olkkola K T, Aranko K, Himberg J J, Neuvonen P J 1994 Dose of midazolam should be reduced during diltiazem and verapamil treatments. Br J Clin Pharmacol 37: 221–225
Rosman N P, Colton T, Labazzo J et al 1993 A controlled trial of diazepam administered drug febrile illnesses to prevent recurrence of febrile seizures. N Eng J Med 329: 79–84

ANAESTHETIC TECHNIQUE

Atelectasis commonly occurs following general anaesthesia. Atelectasis was not reduced by inflating the lungs with a tidal volume or even double the tidal volume (sigh), but only by inflating to vital capacity (airway pressure of 40 cm H_2O) (Rothen et al 1993).

Nolan (1994) has reviewed the cardiovascular and respiratory implications of patients undergoing total hip replacement. There have been numerous reports of hypotensive episodes during insertion of cemented prostheses and it has been shown that methylmethacrylate could produce hypotension and hypoxaemia in animals, but not in humans. Micro-pulmonary emboli may result from reaming the bone, especially as insertion of a cemented femoral prothesis may give rise to a high intramedullary pressure. Nolan (1994), however, showed that a cemented prosthesis resulted in a marked decrease in mean arterial oxygen tension and an increase in mean arterial blood pressure.

Laparoscopy

During laparoscopy the end-tidal carbon dioxide is likely to rise and Baraka et al (1994) found that it reached a peak after about 40 min. However, normocapnia could be obtained by increasing the ventilation by 25%.

Prolonged insufflatation of carbon dioxide into the abdominal cavity may lead to hyperkalaemia, with its attendant cardiovascular problems (Pearson & Sander 1994).

REFERENCES

Baraka A, Jabbour S, Hammond R et al 1994 End-tidal carbon dioxide tension during laparoscopic cholecystectomy: correlation with the baseline value prior to carbon dioxide insufflation. Anaesthesia 49: 304–306
Nolan J P 1994 Arterial oxygenation and mean arterial blood pressure in patients undergoing total hip replacement: cemented versus uncemented components. Anaesthesia 49: 293–299
Pearson M R B, Sander M L 1994 Hyperkalaemia associated with prolonged insufflation of carbon dioxide into the peritoneal cavity. Br J Anaesth 72: 602–604
Rothen H U, Sporre B, Engberg G, Wegenius G, Hedenstierna 1993 Re-expansion of atelectasis during general anaesthesia: a computed tomography study. Br J Anaesth 71: 788–795

DRUG METABOLISM

The importance of plasma protein binding displacement as a cause of drug interactions appears to have been overrated (Rolan 1994). Protein binding is only of importance when there is low clearance of a drug, a low therapeutic index and a small volume of distribution. There may be a temporary increase in plasma levels and this effect would only apply to drugs such as warfarin, phenytoin and tolbutamide.

The dose of drugs administered to critically ill patients should be reduced on first principles, but the mechanism for reduced metabolism is unknown. Park et al (1994) have produced a model and found there was a substance in the plasma which affected the ability of hepatocytes to glucuronidate progesterone.

Kupffer cells exposed to hypoxia lost only 25% of their number but following reoxygenation all the Kupffer cells became non-viable. The release following reoxygenation may in fact produce oxygen radicals and hydrolytic enzymes which destroy all cell activity (Rymsa et al 1990).

The main metabolites of morphine are morphine-3-glucuronide and morphine-6-glucuronide, especially 3-glucuronide. Clinical trials are in progress to determine the efficacy of these metabolites in management of pain, since they are able to cross the blood–brain barrier directly, which morphine is unable to do. Although the liver is said to be the main site of metabolism, Sear (1991) concluded that there is significant renal involvement as well (also see Sloan et al 1991).

Although there is a decrease in plasma albumin associated with age and renal failure, Viani et al (1992) demonstrated that there was a negative correlation between albumin concentration and age in healthy patients, but no correlation in those with poor renal function.

There is a circadian rhythm affecting estimated hepatic blood flow which is greatest at 8 am (Lemmer & Nold 1991). Conjugation pathways are depressed in liver disease, but enzyme activity is substrate dependent (Pacifici et al 1990). Sulphotransferase, acetyltransferase, glutathione transferase and thiomethyltransferase are affected but not glucuronyltransferase. In patients with cirrhosis, the half-lives of morphine and oxazepam, which are essentially destroyed by glucuronidation, are less affected than that suffered by paracetamol and chloramphenicol, which undergo more complicated metabolic destruction. Hepatic clearance of midazolam may be altered by erythromycin inhibiting hepatic metabolism (Hiller et al (1990).

Idiosyncratic drug reactions are discussed by Park et al (1992). Adverse drug reactions can be classified as follows:

Type A: these are predictable, e.g. hypoglycaemia.
Type B: idiosyncratic. There is no correlation between the dose and toxicity.
Type C: reactions associated with long-term drug therapy, e.g. renal damage from analgesics. These reactions can be anticipated.
Type D: delayed effects such as carcinogenic activity.

Current aspects of diagnosis and prevention of anaphylaxis during anaesthesia are discussed by Fisher & Baldo (1994). Anaphylaxis was associated with drugs such as althesin and propanidid which contain cremophor, and when these drugs were withdrawn it became apparent that neuromuscular blocking agents were often the cause of life-threatening reactions and these were mediated by IgE.

REFERENCES

Hiller A, Olkkola K T, Isohanni P, Saarnivaara L 1990 Unconsciousness associated with midazolam and erythromycin. Br J Anaesth 65: 826–828
Fisher M, Baldo B A 1994 Anaphylaxis during anaesthesia: current aspects of diagnosis and prevention. Eur J Anaesthesiol 11: 263–284
Lemmer B, Nold G 1991 Circadian changes in estimated hepatic blood flow in healthy subjects. Br J Clin Pharmacol 32: 627–629
Pacifici G M, Viani A, Franchi M, Santerini S et al 1990 Conjugation pathways in liver disease. Br J Clin Pharmacol 30: 427–435
Park B K, Pirohamed M, Kitteringham N R 1992 Idiosyncratic drug reactions: a mechanistic evaluation of risk factors. Br J Clin Pharmacol 34: 377–395

Park G R, Pichard L, Tinel M et al 1994 What changes drug metabolism in critically ill patients? Two preliminary studies in isolated human hepatocytes. Anaesthesia 49: 188–191

Rolan P E 1994 Plasma protein binding displacement interactions: why are they still regarded as clinically important? Br J Clin Pharmacol 37: 125–128

Rymsa B, Becker H D, Lauchart W, de Groot H 1990 Hypoxia/reoxygenation injury in liver: Kupffer cells are much more vulnerable to reoxygenation than to hypoxia. Res Commun Chem Pathol Pharmacol 68: 283–286

Sear J W 1991 Drug biotransformation by the kidney: how important is it, and how much do we really know? Br J Anaesth 67: 369–370

Sloan P A, Mather L E, McLean C F, Rutten A J et al 1991 Physiological disposition of iv morphine in sheep. Br J Anaesth 67: 378–386

Viani A, Rizzo G, Carrai M, Pacifici G M 1992 The effect of ageing on plasma albumin and plasma protein binding of diazepam, salicylic acid and digitoxin in healthy subjects and patients with renal impairment. Br J Clin Pharmacol 33: 229–304

Index